Coronary Care
for the
House Officer

Coronary Care
for the
House Officer

Edited by:

Michael W. Rich, M.D., F.A.C.C.

Director, Coronary Care Unit
Director, Geriatric Cardiology
Jewish Hospital at Washington University Medical Center
St. Louis, Missouri

WILLIAMS & WILKINS
Baltimore • Hong Kong • London • Sydney

Editor: Michael Fisher
Associate Editor: Carol Eckhart
Copy Editor: Judith F. Minkove
Design: Dan Pfisterer
Illustration Planning: Lorraine Wrzosek
Production: Raymond E. Reter
Cover Design: Dan Pfisterer

Copyright © 1989
Williams & Wilkins
428 East Preston Street
Baltimore, MD 21202, USA

Accurate indications, adverse reactions, and dosage schedules for drugs are provided in this book, but it is possible that they may change. The reader is urged to review the package information data of the manufacturers of the medications mentioned.

Printed in the United States of America

Library of Congress Cataloging in Publication Data

Rich, Michael W.
    Coronary care for the house officer/Michael W. Rich.
        p. cm.
    Includes bibliographies and index.
    ISBN 0-683-07254-4
    1. Heart—Diseases—Handbooks, manuals, etc. 2. Medical emergencies—Handbooks, manuals, etc. 3. Coronary care units—Handbooks, manuals, etc. I. Title.
    [DNLM: 1. Coronary Care Units—handbooks. 2. Coronary Disease—handbooks. WG 39 R499c]
RC682.R53   1989
616.1'2—dc19
DNLM/DLC
for Library of Congress   89-5358
                                                                                     CIP

                                                                   89   90   91   92
                                              1   2   3   4   5   6   7   8   9   10

For my wife, Vicki,
and for my children,
Sarah, Daniel, Beth, and Madeline

Preface

When a house officer or medical student enters the coronary care unit for the first time, he or she is often confronted with an intimidating and seemingly hostile array of technology which does little to relieve the preconceived anxiety that there is a potential "emergency" lurking in every room. In reality, there is little to fear since the CCU presents one of the more controlled environments in the hospital, the support staff is usually capable of dealing with common problems, and although it may be appropriate to maintain an "anything can happen" attitude, it is important to recognize that most things won't happen (or at least not all at once). It is also worth noting that the types of problems that arise commonly in the CCU are relatively limited, and that for each problem, the number of treatment options is generally small. Similarly, the practical aspects of CCU technology are readily comprehensible in a short period of time.

Despite these considerations, it is my experience that house officers (as well as medical students, cardiology fellows, and nurses) find it useful to have an easy to use reference guide which spells out the specifics of how to recognize and treat typical problems that occur in the CCU. The present manual grew out of such a need in the house staff training program at our institution. The manual was first written and distributed to our house staff in 1984, and had extensive revisions in 1985 and 1986. It received favorable reviews from our normally very critical house officers, several of whom suggested that it be submitted for formal publication. The manuscript was therefore sent to Williams & Wilkins and, following its preliminary acceptance, much of the last year was spent revising, editing, and updating the text.

As is readily apparent, my intent in writing this manual is not to provide a comprehensive review of cardiology or critical care, but to give the house officer an information source that can be read in its entirety in just a few hours and which deals with the very practical aspects of direct patient care. Specific recommendations in the manual are based on standard practices, current literature, and clinical experience. Areas of controversy or treatment protocols based on local preference are noted as such, and a list of references is provided at the end of most chapters.

At the beginning of this project, I did not conceive of the tremendous amount of work required in producing even such a small volume as this. I would therefore like to express my appreciation to the following individuals who have contributed substantially towards making this book possible. First, I wish to thank all of the contributing authors for their excellent work, and give special thanks to Dr. Robert E. Kleiger for his editorial review of the manuscript. I would also like to thank the entire office staff of the Jewish Hospital Cardiology Division, but most importantly Shelly Rifken, Marge Leaders, Barbara Woodson, Sharon Anglim, and James Havranek for their outstanding work in preparing the manuscript. The book would also not have been possible without the support and suggestions of the many medical house officers who have used prior incarnations of the manual as they rotated through the Coronary Care Unit. Finally, I am indebted to Nancy Collins, Carol Eckhart, and the rest of the staff at Williams & Wilkins, without whose guidance this book could not have become a reality.

M.W.R.

Contributors

Jean T. Barbey, M.D., F.A.C.C.
Director, Telemetry Unit
Jewish Hospital at Washington University
Chapter 38

Stanley I. Biel, M.D., F.A.C.C.
Chapter 37

Robert M. Carney, Ph.D.
Associate Professor of Psychology
Director, Behavioral Medicine
Jewish Hospital at Washington University
Chapter 31

Patricia L. Cole, M.D.
Staff Cardiologist
Jewish Hospital at Washington University
Chapters 29, 34, 35, and 36

Stephen S. Lefrak, M.D., F.A.C.C.P.
Professor of Medicine
Director, Medical Intensive Care Unit
Jewish Hospital at Washington University
Chapters 8 and 9

Stephen Liggett, M.D.
Fellow, Respiratory and Critical Care Division
Washington University School of Medicine
Chapters 8 and 9

Edward C. Miller, M.D., F.A.C.C.
Co-Director, Cardiac Graphics
Jewish Hospital at Washington University
Chapters 16, 18, and 30

Allen D. Soffer, M.D.
Staff Cardiologist
Jewish Hospital at Washington University
Chapters 24 and 26

Contents

Preface   vii

Contributors   ix

Section I.   Introduction

1. Introduction to the Coronary Care Unit   1
2. Routine Admission Orders   4
3. Approach to the Patient with Chest Pain   6
4. Management of Chest Pain   10
5. Approach to Arrhythmias   15
6. Management of Specific Arrhythmias   24
7. Cardiac Arrest   34
8. Interpretation of Arterial Blood Gases   47
9. Mechanical Ventilation in the Coronary Care Unit   54

Section II.   Acute Myocardial Infarction

10. Diagnosis and Early Management   64
11. Limitation of Myocardial Infarct Size   70
12. Thrombolytic Therapy   78
13. Intravenous Beta Blockade   88
14. Acute Angioplasty and Bypass Surgery   92
15. Arrhythmias and Conduction Disturbances   95
16. Temporary Pacemakers   102
17. Hypoperfusion, Congestive Heart Failure, and Shock   109
18. Invasive Hemodynamic Monitoring   117
19. Right Ventricular Infarction   130
20. Mechanical Complications   135
21. Other Complications: Thromboembolism, Recurrent Ischemia, and Pericarditis   142
22. Prognosis in Myocardial Infarction   147
23. Secondary Prevention of Recurrent Cardiac Events   154
24. Cardiac Rehabilitation after Myocardial Infarction   160

Section III.   Other Problems in the CCU

25. Unstable Angina and Variant Angina   165
26. Pericardial Disease   172
27. Congestive Heart Failure and Pulmonary Edema   179
28. Hypertensive Emergencies and Urgencies   186
29. Percutaneous Transluminal Coronary Angioplasty   190
30. Dissection of the Aorta   193
31. Psychosocial Aspects of Coronary Care   198
32. The Geriatric Patient in the Coronary Care Unit   202

Section IV.   Procedures

33. Cardioversion   209
34. Central Venous and Pulmonary Artery Catheterization   212
35. Temporary Pacemaker Insertion   220
36. Arterial Lines   225
37. Intra-Aortic Balloon Pumps   228

Section V.   Medications

38. Cardiovascular Drug Pharmacology   233

Appendix

A. Abbreviations Used in the Text   251
B. Formulas   253
C. Normal Hemodynamic Values   255
D. Dosages of Dopamine and Dobutamine   256
E. Body Surface Area   258

Index   259

Chapter 1

Introduction to the Coronary Care Unit

The coronary care unit (CCU) is an intensive care nursing facility designed for optimal management of acute or threatened myocardial infarction (MI), unstable coronary ischemic syndromes, refractory congestive heart failure, and other potentially life-threatening cardiovascular disorders. The CCU is staffed by highly trained nurses and technicians skilled in the recognition and initial management of cardiac arrhythmias and conduction disturbances, and in the use of an array of invasive and non-invasive monitoring devices. Routine telemetric monitoring, often with computerized arrhythmia detection and rate-triggered alarm systems, and the ability to monitor arterial and intracardiac pressures via indwelling catheters are now standard equipment in most CCUs. Additional capabilities that may be available include respiratory monitoring, fluoroscopy to facilitate placement of specialized catheters and pacemakers, intra-aortic balloon counterpulsation, ventricular assist devices, and internal electrode systems for the detection and treatment of tachyarrhythmias.

Coronary care units first became popularized in the 1960s, and have been credited with reducing in-hospital mortality rate in acute MI patients from 25-30% to 10-15%, largely through the prompt recognition and treatment of life-threatening arrhythmias occurring within the first 24-48 hours of admission (1-2). This beneficial effect gave rise to the development of Mobile Intensive Care Units, which have contributed to a reduction in the pre-hospital arrhythmic death rate (3-4). Despite these successes and the development of sophisticated techniques for hemodynamic monitoring, as well as the availability of more potent and/or less toxic inotropic agents, until recently CCUs have had little demonstrable effect on hospital mortality resulting from pump failure following acute MI. Strategies designed to limit infarct size and decrease the incidence of pump failure have therefore undergone extensive testing, and two of these strategies—thrombolytic therapy and intravenous beta blockade—have now been proven to be efficacious (see Chapters 11-13).

In recent years, there has been a gradual shift in the demographics and presentation of CCU patients. As a result of the general aging of the population and the increasing incidence of coronary heart disease with advancing age, especially in females, more elderly patients and women are now being admitted to the CCU (Chapter

32). In addition, as a result of improved public awareness of the symptoms and signs of acute myocardial ischemia, more patients are presenting early in the course of infarction or with unstable or pre-infarctional angina. Finally, with the advent and widespread use of technological advances, more admissions to the CCU are procedure-related (e.g., for pulmonary artery catheterization or following coronary angioplasty). In this author's opinion, all of these changes represent an appropriate evolution in the utilization of the CCU. In particular, the increased admission of patients with unstable angina allows the CCU physician to intervene before an infarct occurs, thus optimizing myocardial salvage and functional outcome.

What is the future of CCUs? Although the incidence of ischemic heart disease is on the decline, current projections do not indicate that there will be a substantial reduction in the number of patients in the population with coronary heart disease within the next two decades. The development of more effective means for managing patients with acute ischemic syndromes and other acute cardiovascular problems will also continue to support the need for CCUs. On the other hand, growing concerns about cost containment may mandate closer scrutiny of CCU utilization and its effect on total cost of care (5). Algorithms for admission and transfer of patients to and from the CCU have been developed (6-8) but are not in general use; this may change as hospitals try to meet the demands of the prospective payment system. Finally, difficult questions regarding to-treat-or-not-to-treat issues in patients with little hope of significant functional recovery may need to be addressed, as they already have been in other countries.

With this brief background, we now proceed to the more practical aspects of current coronary care.

REFERENCES

1. Lown B, Fakhro AM, Hood WB, Thorn GW. The coronary care unit. New perspectives and directions. JAMA 1967;199:188-198.

2. Goldman L. Coronary care units. A perspective on their epidemiologic impact. Int J Cardiol 1982;2:284-287.

3. Pantridge JF, Adgey AAJ. Pre-hospital coronary care. The mobile coronary care unit. Am J Cardiol 1969;24:666-673.

4. Crampton RS, Aldrich RF, Gascho JA, Miles JR, Stillerman R. Reduction of pre-hospital, ambulance, and community coronary death rates by the community-wide emergency cardiac care system. Am J Med 1975;58:151-165.

5. Thibault GE. Making the coronary care unit cost effective. Am J Cardiol 1985;56:35C-39C.

6. Mulley AG, Thibault GE, Hughes RA, Barnett GO, Reder VA, Sherman EL. The course of patients with suspected myocardial infarction. The identification of low-risk patients for early transfer from intensive care. N Engl J Med 1980;302:943-948.

7. Pozen MW, D'Agostino RB, Selker HP, Sytkowski PA, Hood WB. A predictive instrument to improve coronary care unit admission practices in acute ischemic heart disease. N Engl J Med 1984;310:1273-1278.

8. Fineberg HV, Scadden D, Goldman L. Care of patients with a low probability of acute myocardial infarction. Cost effectiveness of alternatives to coronary care unit admission. N Engl J Med 1984; 310:1301-1307.

Chapter 2

Routine Admission Orders

The majority of CCU admissions will be for acute myocardial infarction, unstable angina, or "rule-out MI." As the initial management is similar in most of these patients, a standard set of routine admission orders is useful. These orders also help ensure consistency in the approach to patient care. Such orders vary according to local practices; the following are currently in use at our hospital.

1. Admitting diagnosis:
2. Major secondary diagnoses:
3. Condition:
4. Medication allergies:
5. Continuous ECG monitoring. Low rate alarm: _____ min
                                 High rate alarm: _____ min
6. Routine vital signs on admission, then:
       _____ Stable patient: q 1 hr x 4, then q 4 hrs
       _____ Unstable patient: q 15 min x 4, progress as indicated
7. Diet: Full liquid, no added salt x 24 hrs
           No very hot or cold items for 24 hrs
           Progress to regular diet as tolerated
8. Activity: Bedrest with bedside commode x 24 hrs
               Then may be up in chair if stable
9. Input and output q shift
10. Daily weights
11. Nasal O_2: _____ L/min x 48 hrs
12. Heparin lock. Flush q 6 hrs with 1 cc 1:10 heparin/saline
13. Intravenous fluids (if indicated):
14. ECG on admission, then q AM x 3 days (mark precordial leads)
15. Cardiac enzymes:
        CK with MB q 6 hrs x 4, then CK only q 8 hrs x 3
        LDH with isoenzymes on admission, then q AM x 2
16. Heparin 5000 U subcutaneously q 12 hrs unless contraindicated
17. Enteric coated aspirin 325 mg on admission, then q AM
18. Stool softener: Docusate sodium 100 mg p.o. qhs
19. Sedative:
20. Sleeping pill: Triazolam 0.25 mg p.o. qhs (Use 0.125 mg if
        patient is 70 years or older)

21. Other medications:
        Nitrates:
        Beta blocker:
        Calcium channel blocker:
        Other:
22. Other laboratory:
23. Physician signature:

These orders are applicable to most patients admitted to the CCU, but should be construed as general guidelines only. Appropriate additions and deletions should be made as indicated. Note that prophylactic lidocaine is not included in the standard admission orders. We recommend lidocaine prophylaxis in selected patients with documented acute myocardial infarction or life-threatening ventricular arrhythmias (see Chapter 15). A separate order sheet with the following lidocaine protocol is used for these patients.

1. Patients < 70 years without CHF or liver disease:
        1 mg/kg bolus x 2 at 15 minute intervals, then 0.4% infusion (1 g/250 cc) at 2 or 3 mg/min (Circle one)
2. Patients ≥ 70 years or with CHF or liver disease:
        1 mg/kg bolus followed by 0.5 mg/kg bolus in 15 minutes, then 0.4% infusion (1 g/250 cc) at 1 or 2 mg/min (Circle one)
3. Lidocaine levels are obtained:
        a. 4 hours after initiating therapy
        b. Daily for the duration of therapy
        c. Anytime there is a suspicion of toxicity
        d. 4 hours after any dosage change
4. In the absence of ongoing ischemia or serious arrhythmias, discontinue prophylactic lidocaine after 48 hours (sooner if clinically indicated).
5. Physician signature:

Chapter 3

Approach to the Patient with Chest Pain

Chest pain or discomfort is one of the most common symptoms leading the patient to seek medical attention. This in part reflects the fact that patients recognize chest pain as a cardinal manifestation of heart disease and there is considerable anxiety associated with the thought that one may be having a "heart attack." Because it is often difficult to exclude an acute coronary ischemic event with certainty at the time of initial presentation, patients with a variety of chest pain syndromes may be admitted to the CCU to rule-out MI. It is therefore important for the CCU physician to have an understanding of the broad differential diagnosis of chest pain, and to approach each patient with an open mind regarding possible causes of that patient's symptoms.

Table 3.1 is a partial listing of common causes of cardiac and non-cardiac chest pain which may lead to admission to the CCU, and Table 3.2 summarizes typical findings in selected conditions. These should be viewed as general guidelines and may not apply to individual patients.

In approaching the patient with chest pain, the physician should make a prompt assessment of the apparent severity of illness, as this will affect the timing of the remainder of the evaluation and initiation of treatment. Following this, the single most valuable piece of information is the patient's history. (Note that 6 of 10 features in Table 3.2 relate to historical items.) It is therefore of great importance to obtain an accurate history of the patient's symptoms and relevant past medical problems as expeditiously as possible. In acutely ill patients, this should take no more than 5-10 minutes so as to avoid unnecessary delays in starting therapy. A brief physical examination should then be performed, focusing on the cardiovascular system, lungs, abdomen, and chest wall. An electrocardiogram is often obtained prior to the patient's transfer to the CCU but may need to be repeated if the patient's symptoms have progressed and the initial ECG was non-diagnostic. A chest x-ray and arterial blood gas determination are often helpful, both in narrowing the differential diagnosis and in assessing clinical status.

Table 3.1
Common Causes of Chest Pain

  I. Cardiovascular
     A. Typical angina pectoris
     B. Variant angina (Prinzmetal's or vasospastic angina)
     C. Unstable angina
     D. Acute myocardial infarction
     E. Pericarditis
     F. Aortic aneurysm or dissection
     G. Myocarditis or cardiomyopathy
     H. Aortic valve disease
     I. Severe hypertension
     J. Hypertrophic cardiomyopathy with or without obstruction
     K. Mitral valve prolapse
     L. Syndrome X (ischemic chest pain with normal coronaries)
     M. Arrhythmias

 II. Gastrointestinal
     A. Esophageal reflux, spasm, or rupture
     B. Esophageal tumor, web, diverticulum, or foreign body
     C. Gastritis
     D. Peptic ulcer disease
     E. Pancreatic disease
     F. Gall bladder disease
     G. Hepatic disease

III. Pulmonary
     A. Pulmonary embolism or infarction
     B. Pleurisy or pleurodynia
     C. Pneumothorax
     D. Pneumonia
     E. Pulmonary hypertension

 IV. Musculoskeletal
     A. Chest wall twinge syndrome
     B. Costochondritis
     C. Radiculopathy
     D. Disorders of the shoulder joint
     E. Rib fracture or tumor involvement
     F. Muscle strain
     G. Trauma

  V. Psychogenic
     A. Hyperventilation syndrome
     B. Depression or anxiety
     C. Malingering

Table 3.2
Features of Selected Causes of Chest Pain

	Quality	Duration	Associated Symptoms	Intensity	Exacerbation	Relief	Exam	ECG	CXR	ABG
Angina	Pressure, heaviness	5-15 min	Dyspnea, diaphoresis, weakness	Mild to moderate	Exertion, emotional stress	Rest, nitroglycerin	Transient S_4 or murmur (uncommon)	ST-T changes	Normal	Usually normal
Acute MI	Squeezing, smothering	30 min	Dyspnea, N/V, diaphoresis, weakness, palpitations	Mild-severe		Nitroglycerin, morphine	Often normal	ST-T changes, Q-waves	Normal or CHF	↑pH, ↓pO_2, ↓pCO_2
Pericarditis	Sharp, pleuritic	Hours	Fever, dyspnea	Mild-severe	Deep breath, supine position	Sitting up, anti-inflam agents	Friction rub	↑HR, diffuse ST elev.	Normal	Usually normal
Dissection of the aorta	Tearing, radiation to back	Minutes-hours	Neurological symptoms, limb ischemia	Severe		Analgesics, lowering the BP	↑BP, pulse deficit, AI murmur	LVH common	Wide mediastinum	Often normal
Pulmonary embolus	Aching, pleuritic	Minutes-hours	Dyspnea	Mild-severe	Deep breath	Analgesics, anti-inflam agents	Tachypnea, ↑HR, ↑P2, crackles	↑HR, RAD, RV strain	Normal or atelectasis	↑pH, ↓pO_2, ↓pCO_2
Musculo-skeletal	Sharp, aching, superficial	Seconds-days	Occasional dyspnea	Mild-moderate	Deep breath, positional changes	Analgesics, anti-inflam agents	Tenderness	Normal	Normal or skeletal abnormality	Usually normal
Gastro-intestinal	Visceral, waxing-waning	Minutes-hours	Nausea, vomiting, change in bowel habits	Mild-severe	Eating	Antacids, vomiting, belching, bowel movement	Abdominal tenderness	Non-specific ST-T changes	Normal	Normal
Hyperventilation	Pressure, heaviness	Minutes	Anxiety, dyspnea, paresthesias	Mild	Emotional stress	Sedation, breathing CO_2	Anxious	Normal	Normal	↑pH, ↑pO_2, ↓pCO_2
Mitral valve prolapse	Pressure, sharp, aching	Seconds-hours	Dyspnea, palpitations	Mild-moderate	Emotional stress	Beta blocker	Click, murmur	Non-specific	Normal	Normal

In an acutely ill patient, the evaluation outlined in the above paragraph should be completed within 15-20 minutes so that therapy can be initiated promptly. In many severely ill patients, therapy should begin <u>during</u> the initial assessment; critically ill patients may require treatment prior to obtaining even basic information. In all cases, the physician should go back and perform a more comprehensive history and physicial, once the patient has stabilized, again keeping in mind the broad differential diagnosis of chest pain and endeavoring to further clarify the nature of the patient's problem.

FURTHER READING

1. Braunwald E. Chest discomfort and palpitation. In: Harrison's principles of internal medicine, 11th ed. McGraw-Hill Book Co, New York, 1987:17-23.

2. DeGowin RL. Pain in the chest. In: DeGowin and DeGowin's bedside diagnostic examination, 5th ed. MacMillan Publishing Co, New York, 1987:227-251.

3. Walsh RA, O'Rourke RA. Chest pain. In: Stein JH, editor-in-chief. Internal medicine. Little, Brown & Co, Boston, 1983:471-474.

Chapter 4

Management of Chest Pain

As discussed in Chapter 3, the possible causes of chest pain are numerous. To further complicate matters, the symptomatology of cardiac ischemia is highly variable. It is therefore not possible to set forth specific criteria as to which symptoms are likely to be anginal and which are not. Careful attention to the clinical setting, including age, sex, presence of coronary risk factors, prior cardiac history, and the precise nature of the presenting symptoms is required to make a reasonable assessment of the likelihood of cardiac ischemia. Cardiac auscultation should be performed during chest pain when possible, since the presence of transient murmurs, gallops, or rales is highly suggestive of ischemic pain. Examination of the pulse may reveal arrhythmias or pulsus alternans. An ECG obtained before or shortly after chest pain is helpful if ischemic ST-segment or T-wave changes are present. However, a normal ECG should never be used as the sole criterion for excluding ischemic pain. If after a careful review of the clinical findings and differential diagnosis, cardiac ischemia still cannot be excluded with reasonable certainty, it is generally safer to treat the patient for presumptive ischemia until proven otherwise. The management of chest pain in specific situations is outlined below.

Acute Transmural Myocardial Infarction

The term "transmural" MI has fallen into disfavor but is retained for this discussion to include those MIs likely to be associated with total occlusion of a major coronary artery or branch (1), as indicated by the presence of a subepicardial injury pattern on the initial ECG and the subsequent development of pathologic Q-waves, tall R-waves in V1 and V2 (posterior MI), or significant loss of R-wave voltage.

Patients with documented transmural infarction may experience chest pain for up to 24 hours after initial onset. This pain, termed peri-infarctional, may be due to continued stimulation of pain fibers within the necrosing muscle rather than to ongoing ischemia per se. In either case, the drug of first choice in this situation is intravenous morphine sulfate (not nitrates). An initial dose of 4 mg followed by repeat 2-4 mg doses at 5-minute intervals as needed up to a total dose of 10-40 mg is usually effective and well-tolerated in this setting. Heart rate, blood pressure, respiratory rate, and level of consciousness should be carefully monitored, and therapy discontinued if significant bradycardia, hypotension, respiratory depression, or obtundation occurs. Elderly patients and those with severe lung disease may be more susceptable to the adverse effects of morphine, and dosage should be adjusted accordingly. Patients intolerant of morphine may be treated with equivalent doses of hydromorphone (Dilaudid) or meperidine (Demerol). Bradycardia induced by these agents usually responds to atropine. If other severe adverse reactions occur, naloxone (Narcan) 0.4 mg should be administered. It is important to recognize that the peak respiratory depressant effect of narcotics may lag behind the analgesic effect, so that patients receiving these drugs should be monitored closely for delayed development of respiratory compromise.

If narcotic analgesics are not tolerated, fail to provide adequate pain relief in sufficient doses, or if recurrent prolonged pain occurs, institution of nitroglycerin either topically or by intravenous infusion is warranted. Sublingual nitroglycerin may also be used but is more likely to produce hypotension leading to worsening ischemia. Patients with intravascular volume contraction or inferior infarction, particularly when associated with right ventricular infarction, are most prone to develop hypotension from nitroglycerin.

Intravenous metoprolol, 5 mg every 2 minutes up to a total of 15 mg, propranolol, 0.1 mg/kg up to 10 mg, or verapamil, 2.5–10 mg may be useful in the management of refractory ischemic pain, especially if hypertension and/or tachycardia are present. Moderate or severe left ventricular dysfunction and overt congestive heart failure are contraindications to using these agents. Combination therapy with an intravenous beta blocker and verapamil should be avoided, since profound depression of left ventricular contractility may ensue.

If chest pain persists despite the above measures, particularly when associated with increasing evidence of ischemic injury on ECG, urgent cardiac catheterization should be considered. Selected patients may benefit from thrombolytic therapy, placement of an intra-aortic balloon pump, or emergency angioplasty or bypass surgery.

Peri-infarctional pain will usually subside within 24 hours after the onset of infarction. Pain occurring more than 24 hours after the acute event usually indicates recurrent ischemia, infarct extension pericarditis, impending myocardial rupture, or, less frequently, non-cardiac disorder.

Non-Q Myocardial Infarction

Non-Q MI (also called non-transmural or subendocardial MI) i usually associated with incomplete occlusion of the infarct-relate vessel (2). Infarcts tend to be smaller, and the in-hospita prognosis is better than for transmural MI (3). However, patient with initial non-Q MI have a higher incidence of early and lat reinfarction, and the long-term prognosis is not substantial. different than for patients with transmural MI (4-8). This is mos likely due to the fact that patients with non-Q MI continue to have significant myocardium at risk in the region of the infarct artery (9).

For these reasons, recurrent chest pain following non-Q MI has important prognostic implications and should be managed aggressively. Pericarditis and cardiac rupture are infrequent complications of non-Q MI, so that chest pain should be presumed ischemic until proven otherwise. At present, only the calcium antagonist diltiazem in doses of 240-360 mg/day has been shown to reduce the short-term incidence of reinfarction in patients with non-Q MI (10); treatment with diltiazem is therefore recommended as soon as the diagnosis is confirmed. Concomitant use of nitrates and/or a beta blocker may also be beneficial (10).

In patients with non-Q MI, reinfarction due to acute thrombotic reocclusion has been reported in up to 43% of patients an average of 10 days after the initial event (4). Reinfarction is associated with a substantial increase in early mortality and decline in ventricular function (4). In order to further decrease the likelihood of these events, aspirin 160-325 mg/day is warranted (11,12). Full heparinization may be used in patients who cannot tolerate aspirin, or for whom there is a high likelihood of early cardiac surgery, since aspirin is associated with increased of peri-operative bleeding.

Chest pain following non-Q MI should be managed with nitrates and/or morphine. Prolonged pain lasting 30 minutes or longer is likely to be associated with enzymatic evidence for infarct extension. An ECG should be obtained and if there is evidence of acute injury intravenous beta blockade, thrombolytic therapy, and/or urgent cardiac catheterization should be considered (Chapters 11-14).

Ischemic Pain Without Definite Evidence of MI

Ischemic pain of short duration (< 30 minutes) should be treated with sublingual nitroglycerin, repeated at 5-minute intervals as needed until the pain resolves. Intravenous morphine sulfate 2-4 mg should be used if nitroglycerin fails to provide adequate relief. Additional therapeutic options include intravenous beta blockade or verapamil and sublingual nifedipine, but these measures are not usually required.

For more prolonged pain (> 30 minutes), acute MI should be suspected. If there are definite ECG changes, the pain should be managed as previously described, and intravenous beta blockade and/or thrombolytic therapy for limitation of infarct size should be considered (Chapters 11-13). If there are no ECG changes, a trial of sublingual nitroglycerin is appropriate if the patient is hemodynamically stable. If this is ineffective, morphine should be administered, but if pain persists intravenous nitroglycerin and urgent cardiac catheterization may be necessary.

Following treatment of the acute episode, institution of standard anti-anginal therapy with nitrates, a beta blocker, and/or a calcium antagonist is usually indicated.

Ischemic Pain Occurring More than 24 Hours After Acute MI

Whether the patient has had a transmural or non-Q MI, recurrent pain more than 24 hours after the initial event is a poor prognostic sign, indicating additional jeopardized myocardium. In transmural MI, this is often in an area remote from the initial event and therefore implies multivessel disease. The acute episode of pain should be managed as described above, followed by aggressive therapy with standard anti-anginal agents and either aspirin or heparin. In addition, early cardiac catheterization is usually warranted.

REFERENCES

1. DeWood MA, Spores J, Notske R, et al. Prevalence of total coronary occlusion during the early hours of transmural myocardial infarction. N Engl J Med 1980;303:897-902.

2. DeWood MA, Stifter WF, Simpson CS, et al. Coronary arteriographic findings soon after non-Q-wave myocardial infarction. N Engl J Med 1986;315:417-423.

3. Thanavaro S, Krone RJ, Kleiger RE, et al. In-hospital prognosis of patients with first nontransmural and transmural infarctions. Circulation 1980;61:29-33.

4. Marmor A, Sobel BE, Roberts R. Factors presaging early recurrent myocardial infarction ("extension"). Am J Cardiol 1981;48:603-610.

5. Marmor A, Geltman EM, Schechtman K, Sobel BE, Roberts R. Recurrent myocardial infarction: Clinical predictors and prognostic implications. Circulation 1982;66:415-421.

6. Krone RJ, Friedman E, Thanavaro S, Miller JP, Kleiger RE, Oliver GC. Long-term prognosis after first Q-wave (transmural) or non-Q-wave (nontransmural) myocardial infarction: Analysis of 593 patients. Am J Cardiol 1983;52:234-239.

7. Hutter AM, DeSanctis RW, Flynn T, Yeatman LA. Nontransmural myocardial infarction: A comparison of hospital and late clinical course of patients with that of matched patients with transmural anterior and transmural inferior myocardial infarction. Am J Cardiol 1981;48:595-602.

8. Maisel AS, Ahnve S, Gilpin E, et al. Prognosis after extension of myocardial infarct: The role of Q-wave or non-Q-wave infarction. Circulation 1985;71:211-217.

9. Gibson RS, Beller GA, Gheorghiade M, et al. The prevalence and clinical significance of residual myocardial ischemia two weeks after uncomplicated non-Q-wave infarction: A prospective natural history study. Circulation 1986;73:1186-1188.

10. Gibson RS, Boden WE, Theroux P, et al. Diltiazem and reinfarction in patients with non-Q-wave myocardial infarction: Results of a double-blind, randomized, multicenter trial. N Engl J Med 1986;315:423-429.

11. Lewis HD, Davis JW, Archibald DG, et al. Protective effects of aspirin against acute myocardial infarction and death in men with unstable angina. N Engl J Med 1983;309:396-403.

12. Cairns JA, Gent M, Singer J, et al. Aspirin, sulfinpyrazone, or both in unstable angina: Results of a Canadian multicenter trial. N Engl J Med 1985;313:1369-1375.

Chapter 5

Approach to Arrhythmias

Questions concerning the identification and management of arrhythmias arise frequently. Although each case requires individual analysis, the guidelines summarized below and in Tables 5.1–5.5 should prove useful in diagnosing common rhythm disturbances.

Tachycardias

Table 5.1 reviews the differential diagnosis of tachyarrhythmias, broken down by whether the QRS complex is narrow (< 0.12 sec) or wide (≥ 0.12 sec), and by whether the rhythm is regular or irregular. Note that a single or even dual channel rhythm strip will not reliably distinguish narrow from wide QRS tachycardias in all cases. Therefore, when confronted with an undiagnosed tachyarrhythmia, a standard 12-lead ECG is mandatory if the patient's condition permits.

Consistently narrow QRS tachycardias are invariably supraventricular or junctional in origin, and the precise nature of the arrhythmia can usually be delineated from the clinical setting and an analysis of the atrial activity (Table 5.2). Regular tachycardias in which atrial activity is not readily discernible may cause difficulty, particularly if the ventricular rate is near 150/min, since sinus tachycardia, paroxysmal supraventricular tachycardia, junctional tachycardia, and atrial flutter with 2:1 block may all appear similar. If the patient is hemodynamically stable, vagal stimulation (by carotid sinus massage or the Valsalva maneuver) or intravenous verapamil 2.5–20 mg may slow the rate and allow the underlying atrial rhythm to become manifest. Alternatively, placement of an esophageal or intra-atrial lead may be helpful in identifying atrial activity.

Wide QRS tachycardias pose a greater diagnostic dilemma. The importance of performing a careful search for atrial activity on the 12-lead ECG cannot be overemphasized (1). If the arrhythmia is sustained and grossly irregular, atrial fibrillation with aberrant ventricular conduction is the most likely diagnosis. If A-V dissociation is present, as evidenced by cannon A-waves on physical examination or by independent atrial and ventricular activity on the ECG, ventricular tachycardia should be presumed. By contrast, 1:1 association between P-waves and QRS complexes does not always imply a supraventricular origin, since ventricular tachycardia with retrograde conduction to the atria will also display this pattern (although the P-waves will usually be inverted). Other clues to the diagnosis of wide QRS tachycardia are listed in Table 5.3. If atrial activity cannot be identified, an esophageal lead may aid in determining whether A-V dissociation is present. Rarely, a patient with recurrent wide QRS tachycardia of undetermined origin will require an electrophysiologic study to establish the diagnosis and guide therapy.

Table 5.1
Differential Diagnosis of Tachycardia

Narrow QRS (< 0.12 sec)
    Regular
        Sinus tachycardia
        Paroxysmal supraventricular tachycardia
        Atrial tachycardia
        Atrial flutter with fixed A-V conduction
        Junctional tachycardia
    Irregular
        Atrial fibrillation
        Multifocal atrial tachycardia
        Atrial flutter with variable A-V conduction

Wide QRS (≥ 0.12 sec)
    Regular
        Ventricular tachycardia
        Supraventricular tachycardia with aberrancy
        Supraventricular tachycardia with antegrade conduction
            over an accessory pathway
    Irregular
        Ventricular tachycardia
        Atrial fibrillation with aberrancy
        Atrial flutter with variable A-V conduction and aberrancy
        Multifocal atrial tachycardia with aberrancy
        Atrial fibrillation with accessory pathway conduction

Treatment of specific arrhythmias is discussed in detail in the next chapter, but some general comments are warranted at this point. First, in a clinically unstable patient with evidence of tissue hypoperfusion (significant hypotension, altered mental status, clammy skin, oliguria), immediate electrical cardioversion (see Chapter 33) is indicated, regardless of whether the arrhythmia is supraventricular or ventricular in origin (exceptions: sinus tachycardia and multifocal atrial tachycardia do not respond to cardioversion). In cases where the nature of the arrhythmia is not immediately apparent, 50 joules is an appropriate energy level with which to initiate cardioversion. Although it is useful to have a 12-lead ECG prior to therapy so that prophylaxis against recurrences can be initiated, excess time should not be wasted obtaining an ECG in a critically ill patient.

Table 5.2
Distinguishing Features of Supraventricular Tachycardia

	Ventricular Rate	Atrial Activity
Sinus tachycardia	100–180	Normal P-waves, normal PR interval
PSVT	120–240	P-waves inapparent or inverted close to QRS
Atrial tachycardia	120–240	P-waves normal or inverted
Junctional tachycardia	70–200	Usually inapparent; P-wave inverted and close to QRS if seen
Atrial flutter	75–150	Atrial rate 250–350 with 2:1, 4:1, or variable A-V block; regular flutter waves, often best seen in V1; saw-tooth pattern in inferior leads
Atrial fibrillation	50–240, irregular	Fine or coarse fibrillatory waves without regularity
MAT	120–220, irregular	Multiple P-wave morphologies with no consistent pattern

PSVT: Paroxysmal supraventricular tachycardia
MAT: Multifocal atrial tachycardia

In a hemodynamically stable patient, there is no immediate urgency to treat the arrhythmia. Rather, an aggressive attempt should be made to identify the nature of the rhythm disturbance. A common error is to treat a stable arrhythmia incorrectly because proper steps were not taken to first identify the problem.

Table 5.3
Differential Diagnosis of Wide-QRS Tachycardia

	Supraventricular	Ventricular
Physical Findings		
Cannon A waves	Uncommon	Common*
Response to vagal maneuvers	May slow	Unchanged
ECG findings		
QRS morphology	RBBB more common	LBBB more common
QRS duration	< 0.14 sec	> 0.14 sec
A-V dissociation	Rare	Common*
Fusion beats	Rare	Occasional*
Marked left axis deviation	Uncommon	Occasional
Mode of initiation	APC	VPC
Response to therapy		
Verapamil	Slows or breaks	May worsen
Lidocaine	No change	May break

*Presence of these findings strongly suggests ventricular tachycardia.

RBBB: right bundle branch block, LBBB: left bundle branch block, APC: atrial premature contraction, VPC: ventricular premature contraction

Finally, a word of caution about "empiric" treatment of wide QRS tachycardia. There is a common misconception that if a patient is hemodynamically stable, ventricular tachycardia is unlikely (2,3). Treatment of such patients with verapamil for presumed supraventricular tachycardia is often associated with hemodynamic deterioration (3,4). Therefore, in patients with wide QRS tachycardia in whom a ventricular origin cannot be excluded, verapamil should be avoided, and procainamide is preferable as a first choice agent (5).

Bradyarrhythmias

By definition, bradycardia is present when the average ventricular rate is less than 60/minute. Common etiologies of bradycardia include sinus bradycardia, atrial fibrillation or atrial flutter with a slow ventricular response, second degree A-V block (types I and II), complete heart block, and junctional and ventricular escape rhythms. Sinus pauses are also a form of bradyarrhythmia, although the average heart rate may not be less than 60/minute in this situation.

From the diagnostic standpoint, differentiation of Mobitz I from Mobitz II 2° A-V block and the evaluation of A-V dissociation pose the greatest difficulties. Table 5.4 summarizes features which help distinguish A-V nodal block (Mobitz I) from infranodal block (Mobitz II). This distinction is important because Mobitz I A-V block often has a benign course and can be managed conservatively, whereas Mobitz II block may be associated with sudden progression to complete heart block with an inadequate escape mechanism, resulting in marked hemodynamic compromise or death. Mobitz II block therefore usually mandates pacemaker implantation (see Chapters 6, 15, and 16).

Table 5.4
Differential Features of Second Degree A-V Block

	Proximal 2° A-V Block	Distal 2° A-V Block
Nomenclature	Mobitz I	Mobitz II
Location of block	A-V node	Infranodal
PR interval	Lengthens prior to non-conducted beat	Constant
Ventricular rate	Accelerates prior to non-conducted beat	Constant
QRS morphology	Usually narrow	Wide
Escape focus	Junctional	Ventricular
Clinical setting	Inferior MI	Anterior MI
Carotid massage	↑Block	No change or ↓block
Atropine	↓Block	No change or ↑block

It is important to recognize that when 2:1 second degree A-V block occurs (i.e., every other P-wave is conducted), it may not be immediately apparent whether A-V nodal or infranodal block is present. A common error is to assume that since the PR interval remains constant, the block must be Mobitz II. However, if the QRS is narrow or block occurs in the setting of an inferior MI, Mobitz I is much more likely. If the QRS is wide (≥ 0.12 sec), or block occurs in the setting of an anterior MI, it is reasonable to assume that the block is infranodal.

Note that in Table 5.4 and in the above discussion, the term "Wenckebach" has been avoided. Classical Wenckebach conduction describes a characteristic electrocardiographic pattern in which there is progressive lengthening of the PR interval prior to the occurrence of a non-conducted P-wave. Although over 90% of classical Wenckebach occurs at the level of the A-V node, the Wenckebach pattern can in fact arise from anywhere in the conduction system, including the sinoatrial node (S-A Wenckebach) and the infranodal tissues. In addition, as discussed above, A-V nodal block can occur without Wenckebach when there is 2:1 A-V conduction. Therefore, Wenckebach should not be considered synonomous with Mobitz I block.

A-V Dissociation

As the term implies, A-V dissociation (6) indicates a condition in which the atria and ventricles are beating independently. The criteria for diagnosing complete A-V dissociation are:

1. Regular P-waves (exceptions: atrial fibrillation, multifocal atrial tachycardia, marked sinus arrhythmia, frequent atrial premature contractions);

2. Regular QRS complexes;

3. No identifiable association between atrial activity and the QRS complexes. If the atrial rate is regular, variable "PR" intervals will usually be seen.

The importance of criterion #2 cannot be overemphasized. Since escape rhythms of junctional or ventricular origin are very regular, the absence of QRS regularity virtually excludes complete A-V dissociation and suggests that a different mechanism for the observed findings should be sought. The most common disorders masquerading as complete A-V dissociation are Mobitz I 2° A-V block with junctional escape beats and incomplete A-V dissociation with intermittent normally conducted beats. By contrast, isorhythmic A-V dissociation (7), where the atrial and ventricular rates are nearly identical, may superficially resemble a normal rhythm (Fig. 5.1A). Also, A-V dissociation may go unrecognized in the presence of atrial fibrillation with a superimposed junctional rhythm (Fig. 5.1B). This arrhythmia is particularly important to identify because it frequently indicates digitalis intoxication.

Once A-V dissociation has been diagnosed, its mechanism should be determined. The three major mechanisms (8) of A-V dissociation are:

1. Default, in which the sinus node slows to a level that permits subsidiary pacemakers in the A-V junction or ventricle to assume control of the pacemaking function. In order for complete A-V dissociation to occur by this mechanism, there must also be retrograde block preventing the impulse from the subsidiary pacemaker from depolarizing the atria. This mechanism for A-V dissociation is most commonly seen as a normal variant in healthy young patients, in the setting of sick sinus syndrome or inferior myocardial infarction, or as a result of medication (Table 5.5).

2. Interference or usurpation, in which an accelerated junctional or ventricular rhythm produces concealed conduction into the A-V node, thus preventing the normal transmission of supraventricular impulses to the ventricles. This is the usual mechanism whereby ventricular tachycardia produces A-V dissociation.

3. Heart block, whereby there is delayed or absent electrical communication between the atria and ventricles. Heart block can be either incomplete (1° or 2°) or complete (3°). Note that although complete heart block is one mechanism for A-V dissociation, the two terms refer to different phenomena, and should not be used interchangeably.

A.

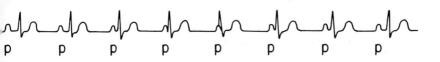

A. Isorhythmic A-V dissociation giving appearance of normal sinus
    rhythm but note that P-waves "march through" the QRSs.

B.

B. Atrial fibrillation with A-V dissociation and accelerated
    junctional rhythm due to digitalis toxicity.

Figure 5.1. Isorhythmic A-V dissociation (A), and atrial fibrillation
with accelerated junctional rhythm (B).

The importance of differentiating these three mechanisms is that
in mechanisms 1 and 3, a pacemaker may be required if there is
infranodal complete heart block or if severe hemodynamically
significant bradycardia does not respond to conservative therapy.   In
mechanism 2, treatment is usually directed at the interfering rhythm
rather than at the A-V dissociation itself.

Occasionally A-V dissociation will be due to more than one
mechanism. For example, in inferior myocardial infarction complete
A-V dissociation may arise as a result of 2° heart block (Mobitz I)
combined with interference from a junctional escape rhythm.   In this
situation, some P-waves are blocked, others are nonconducted due to
interference.   Failure to recognize this combination may lead to
unnecessary pacemaker insertion.

Thus, the presence of A-V dissociation should prompt an
investigation of the underlying etiology and mechanism, which will
then dictate proper therapy.   In many circumstances, no treatment
other than close observation will be required.   Table 5.5 lists common
causes of A-V dissociation.   For a more detailed discussion of this
problem, see references 6-8.

Table 5.5
Causes of A-V Dissociation

Mechanism: Default
    Normal variant in healthy young people
    Inferior myocardial infarction
    Sick sinus syndrome
    Drugs
        Beta blockers
        Verapamil, diltiazem
        Digitalis
        Anti-arrhythmic agents
        Miscellaneous

Mechanism: Interference
    Accelerated junctional rhythm
    Junctional tachycardia
    Accelerated idioventricular rhythm
    Ventricular tachycardia

Mechanism: Heart block
    Congenital complete heart block
    Acquired conduction system disease
        Acute myocardial infarction
        Chronic ischemic heart disease
        Cardiomyopathies
        Valvular heart disease
            Aortic stenosis
            Calcified mitral valve anulus
    Primary conduction system disease
    Drugs (see above)

REFERENCES

1. Wellens HJJ, Bar F, Lie KI. The value of the electrocardiogram in the differential diagnosis of a tachycardia with a widened QRS complex. Am J Med 1978;64:27-33.

2. Morady F, Baerman JM, DiCarlo LA, DeBuitleir M, Kool RB, Wahr DW. A prevalent misconception regarding wide-complex tachycardias. JAMA 1985;254:2790-2792.

3. Dancy M, Camm AJ, Ward D. Misdiagnosis of chronic recurrent ventricular tachycardia. Lancet 1985;II:320-323.

4. Stewart RB, Bardy GH, Greene HL. Wide complex tachycardia: Misdiagnosis and outcome after emergent therapy. Ann Intern Med 1986;104:766-771.

5. Wellens HJJ. The wide QRS tachycardia. Ann Intern Med 1986;104:879.

6. Jacobs DR, Donoso E, Friedberg CK. A-V dissociation: A relatively frequent arrhythmia. Medicine 1961;40:101-118.

7. Levy MN, Edelstein J. The mechanism of synchronization in isorhythmic A-V dissociation. Circulation 1970;42:689-699.

8. Pick A. A-V dissociation. A proposal for a comprehensive classification and consistent terminology. Am Heart J 1963;66:147-150.

FURTHER READING

1. Chou TC. Electrocardiography in clinical practice, 2nd ed. Grune & Stratton, Inc., Orlando, FL, 1986.

2. Friedman HH. Diagnostic electrocardiography and vector-cardiography, 3rd ed. McGraw-Hill Book Company, New York, 1985.

3. Pick A, Langendorf R. Interpretation of complex arrhythmias. Lea & Febiger, Philadelphia, 1979.

Chapter 6

Management of Specific Arrhythmias

Detailed discussion of the management of all arrhythmias is beyond the scope of this manual and can be found in standard references. Selected features of arrhythmias commonly seen in the CCU will be reviewed.

Supraventricular Arrhythmias

Etiology

In treating arrhythmias, possible causative mechanisms should be kept in mind and remedied when possible. Digitalis increases atrial, junctional, and ventricular automaticity while decreasing A-V nodal conduction. Digitalis excess may therefore be associated with a wide range of arrhythmias and conduction abnormalities. Paroxysmal supraventricular tachycardia with block and non-paroxysmal junctional tachycardia (rate 70-120/min) are particularly suggestive of digitalis intoxication. Theophylline derivatives, sympathomimetic agents and amrinone are other commonly used agents which may induce arrhythmias. Other common causes of supraventricular arrhythmias in the CCU are listed in Table 6.1.

Sinus Tachycardia

In addition to the etiologies in Table 6.1, sinus tachycardia may result from fever, anemia, infections, heightened adrenergic tone and/or diminished parasympathetic tone, or as a compensatory response to decreased cardiac output. Although low cardiac output is often due to severe left ventricular dysfunction, remediable causes, such as intravascular volume contraction, acute mitral regurgitation or ventricular septal rupture, and ventricular aneurysm should not be overlooked. A careful search for treatable causes of sinus tachycardia is important, since tachycardia increases myocardial oxygen demand and may therefore exacerbate ischemia. If low cardiac output is suspected, pulmonary artery catheterization may be indicated to exclude hypovolemia and other treatable disorders. If the pulmonary artery occlusive pressure is ≤15 mm Hg, cautious administration of fluids is warranted while assessing the effect of this intervention on overall hemodynamics (see Chapter 18).

Table 6.1
Causes of Supraventricular Arrhythmias in the CCU

Drugs
   Theophylline derivatives
   Digitalis
   Sympathomimetic agents
   Amrinone
   Alcohol
Heart failure of any etiology
Uncontrolled hypertension
Valvular heart disease
   Mitral regurgitation
   Mitral stenosis
   Mitral valve prolapse
   Mitral valve anulus calcification
   Aortic stenosis
Pericarditis
Chronic ischemic heart disease
Atrial ischemia or infarction
Hyperthyroidism
Primary conduction system disease
   Sick sinus syndrome
   Re-entrant tachycardias
   Accessory pathway
   Idiopathic
Left atrial enlargement of any etiology
Pulmonary disease
   Pulmonary embolus
   Chronic lung disease
Hypokalemia

In general, treatment of sinus tachycardia should be directed at the underlying cause since in most cases the tachycardia represents an appropriate response to some pathologic stimulus. Occasionally, a patient will exhibit an inappropriate sinus tachycardia due to increased sympathetic tone, and a cautious trial of beta blockade is appropriate therapy in such cases. Patients with persistent sinus tachycardia following acute myocardial infarction have a poor prognosis; careful evaluation and follow-up are therefore required.

Atrial Premature Contractions (APCs)

Frequent APCs may indicate the presence of one or more of the processes shown in Table 6.1, and may be the harbinger of more sustained supraventricular arrhythmias. However, APCs per se generally require no specific treatment unless they are highly symptomatic or precipitate sustained tachycardia. Type IA and IC anti-arrhythmic agents (quinidine, procainamide, disopyramide, encainide, and flecainide) are usually effective in suppressing APCs (see Chapter 38). Beta blockers are also useful in selected patients.

Atrial Fibrillation and Atrial Flutter

In hemodynamically unstable patients, immediate cardioversion is indicated (Chapter 33). We recommend initial energy levels of 50-100 joules for atrial fibrillation and 20-30 joules for atrial flutter.

In stable patients, the ventricular response should be controlled with digitalis, a beta blocker, verapamil, or diltiazem. This therapy alone or in conjunction with treatment of the underlying etiology may result in reversion to sinus rhythm, although a recent study suggests that conversion occurs no more frequently in patients treated with digitalis than in untreated controls (1). In patients who remain in atrial fibrillation or flutter, quinidine or other type IA or IC anti-arrhythmic agents will often produce conversion to sinus rhythm. If atrial fibrillation persists for more than a few days, conversion to sinus rhythm may result in systemic embolization; anti-coagulation prior to cardioversion is therefore recommended (2-4). Finally, refractory or poorly tolerated atrial fibrillation or flutter of recent onset should be electrically cardioverted using the energy levels suggested above (see also Chapter 33).

Paroxysmal Supraventricular Tachycardia (PSVT)

The mechanism of PSVT is A-V nodal re-entry in 60% of cases, an accessory pathway in 30-40%, and sinus nodal or atrial re-entry in less than 10%. Intravenous verapamil 2.5-20 mg given slowly will terminate the arrhythmia in over 80% of cases (5,6). Other effective agents include digitalis and beta blockers.

PSVT with 2:1 or variable A-V conduction is caused by digitalis intoxication in about 50% of cases and severe organic heart disease in the remainder. Withhold digitalis and maintain serum potassium at 4.0-5.0 meq/L. If significant ventricular arrhythmias develop, phenytoin or lidocaine in full anti-arrhythmic doses should be administered.

Junctional Tachycardia

Junctional tachycardias are of two types: non-paroxysmal (rate 70-120/min) and paroxysmal (rate 120-200/min). Non-paroxysmal junctional tachycardia is probably caused by increased automaticity of an ectopic pacemaker, and is often drug-induced. Common offenders include digitalis, theophylline derivatives, and sympathomimetic agents. Digitalis should be withheld and serum potassium normalized. If the patient is receiving a theophylline preparation, a serum level should be obtained and the dose reduced as indicated. Similarly, the dosage of sympathomimetic agents may require adjustment.

Paroxysmal junctional tachycardia is usually due to re-entry; its significance and therapy are similar to PSVT.

Multifocal Atrial Tachycardia (MAT)

MAT is usually seen in the setting of severe pulmonary or cardiac decompensation. Primary treatment is directed at improving cardiopulmonary function. Recently, intravenous verapamil has been shown to decrease both the atrial and ventricular rates in patients with MAT (7,8). However, this agent should not be given to patients with severe left ventricular dysfunction. Other anti-arrhythmic agents are ineffective, and MAT may be exacerbated by digitalis or theophylline. In addition, MAT does not respond to cardioversion. Occasionally, MAT will convert to atrial fibrillation, which should be managed in the usual manner.

Ventricular Arrhythmias

Etiology

Table 6.2 lists common causes of ventricular arrhythmias in the CCU. Although a precise cause cannot always be identified, it is important to search for treatable factors in all cases, and to correct underlying abnormalities whenever possible.

Table 6.2
Causes of Ventricular Arrhythmias in the CCU

Drugs
    Anti-arrhythmic agents
    Digitalis
    Sympathomimetic agents
    Theophylline derivatives
    Tricyclic antidepressants
    Major tranquilizers
    Alcohol
Metabolic factors
    Acidosis
    Hyperkalemia and hypokalemia
    Hypomagnesemia
Acute MI or ischemia
Chronic ischemic heart disease
Congestive heart failure
Valvular heart disease (including mitral valve prolapse)
Cardiomyopathies
Hypertensive heart disease, esp. with LVH
Low cardiac output state
Chronic lung disease
Hypoxemia of any etiology
Anxiety or depression
Catheter-induced (e.g., pacemaker or pulmonary artery catheter)

Ventricular Premature Contractions (VPCs)

VPCs are exceedingly common in patients with and without organic cardiovascular disease (9,10). Although frequent VPCs are associated with an increased risk of sudden cardiac death in patients with chronic ischemic heart disease and left ventricular dysfunction (11), and possibly in other circumstances as well, at present there is no convincing evidence that empiric anti-arrhythmic therapy improves prognosis. In addition, all available anti-arrhythmic agents have the potential for exacerbating arrhythimas (pro-arrhythmic effect), and may be associated with other side effects as well. Therefore, treatment of VPCs is generally directed at correction of any precipitating or exacerbating factors, and at relieving symptoms. Some experts also recommend treating frequent, multifocal VPCs in patients with severe left ventricular dysfunction, especially if ventricular couplets or triplets are also present.

The choice of anti-arrhythmic therapy in the treatment of chronic VPCs is variable. Type I agents are effective in suppressing VPCs, but side effects are common. Beta blockers are less effective, but in patients with ischemic heart disease, they are anti-ischemic and have been shown to decrease sudden death after myocardial infarction. In addition, they have no known pro-arrhythmic effect other than bradycardia, which is rarely life-threatening. Type III agents are also effective but are rarely indicated as first line therapy (Chapter 38). Treatment of ventricular ectopy in the setting of acute MI and the use of prophylactic lidocaine are discussed in Chapter 15.

Accelerated Idioventricular Rhythm (AIVR)

AIVR is defined as 3 or more consecutive VPCs at a regular rate of less than 120/min. This rhythm is commonly seen in acute MI, particularly anterior MI, and as a reperfusion arrhythmia following thrombolytic therapy. AIVR may persist or recur for a period of several hours, but is generally self-limited and does not usually result in hemodynamic compromise. In such cases, no specific treatment is necessary. If the patient develops hemodynamic compromise attributable to the arrhythmia, or if AIVR degenerates into a more malignant ventricular arrhythmia, initiation of lidocaine is indicated (see Chapter 38 for dosing). Warning: Occasionally, AIVR may be confused with accelerated ventricular escape rhythm. Be sure A-V conduction is intact prior to administering lidocaine, since suppression of a ventricular escape rhythm in the presence of A-V block may result in severe bradycardia or asystole.

Non-Sustained Ventricular Tachycardia

Non-sustained ventricular tachycardia may be defined as 3 beats to 30 seconds of self-terminating, non-hemodynamically compromising ventricular tachycardia (VT) at a rate greater than 120/min. In the setting of acute MI or other ischemic event, suppression of non-sustained VT with lidocaine or other anti-arrhythmic therapy is warranted. In the chronic setting, it has not been shown that treatment of this arrhythmia prolongs survival. Nonetheless, many experts recommend anti-arrhythmic therapy if the rate is fast (over 150/min), if runs are frequent and relatively long (more than 5 or 6 beats), or if there is significant left ventricular dysfunction (ejection fraction < 40%).

Sustained Ventricular Tachycardia (VT)

Sustained VT refers to a run of ventricular ectopic activity at a rate greater than 120/min lasting at least 30 seconds or associated with hemodynamic decompensation. This is a potentially lethal arrhythmia which usually requires aggressive therapy. If there is prolonged hemodynamic compromise, immediate cardioversion is indicated (recommended initial energy: 50 joules; see Chapter 33). If the patient is stable and VT persists, lidocaine is the agent of first choice. If adequate doses of this drug are ineffective, intravenous procainamide (loading dose: 10-15 mg/kg given at a rate of 25 mg/min; maintenance dose: 1-4 mg/min) or bretylium (loading dose: 5 mg/kg over 5 minutes; maintenance dose: 1-4 mg/min) should be tried. If none of these agents is effective, electrical cardioversion is appropriate. Long-term management of this arrhythmia can be guided by empiric trial if the rhythm occurs frequently, but electrophysiologic study should be considered if it occurs infrequently and is associated with significant hemodynamic impairment.

Torsade de Pointes (14)

This is a highly malignant form of VT characterized by shifting of the QRS axis in a cyclic pattern (Figure 6.1). It is usually seen in the setting of a prolonged QT interval. Table 6.3 lists common etiologic factors. Among anti-arrhythmic agents, quinidine has been associated with the highest incidence of torsade de pointes VT.

Treatment of torsade de pointes starts with removal of the inciting agent. Atrial or ventricular pacing at rates of 100-120/min is usually effective in preventing recurrence. Intravenous isoproterenol, propranolol, phenytoin, and lidocaine at usual dosages have all been used in treating this arrhythmia. Occasionally, patients may respond to magnesium sulfate 1 gram intravenously, repeated as necessary (15). If the arrhythmia degenerates to ventricular fibrillation, prompt defibrillation is mandatory.

Ventricular Fibrillation (VF)

Ventricular fibrillation (VF) is seen in the CCU in three different contexts. Primary VF occurs during the early hours of acute myocardial infarction and is due to transient electrical instability within the ischemic zone. The incidence of primary VF is greatest in the first hour of acute MI and accounts for the majority of out-of-hospital deaths following acute coronary occlusion. In the absence of prophylactic lidocaine, primary VF occurs in 3-7% of

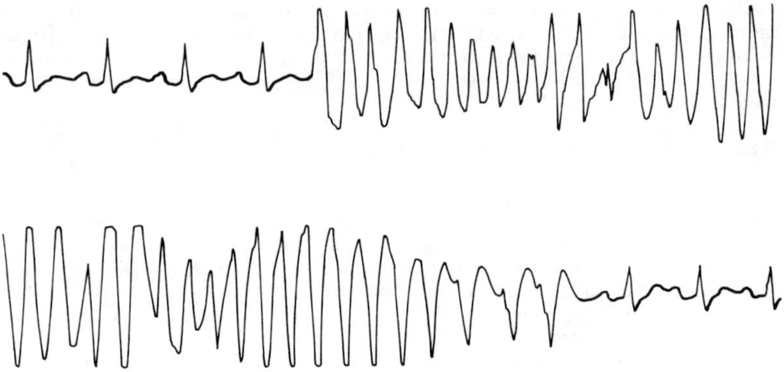

Figure 6.1. Torsade de pointes ventricular tachycardia. Note cyclic shifting of QRS axis giving rise to changing QRS morphology. (Courtesy of A. Quattromani, M.D.)

Table 6.3
Causes of Torsade de Pointes Ventricular Tachycardia

    Drugs
        Anti-arrhythmic agents, esp. Type IA
        Tri-cyclic antidepressants
        Major tranquilizers
        Miscellaneous

    Electrolyte Disturbances
        Hypokalemia
        Hypomagnesemia

    Repolarization abnormalities associated with
        myocardial ischemia or neurologic disease

    Hereditary prolonged QT syndrome

    Severe bradycardia of any etiology

patients admitted with acute MI and tends to respond readily to prompt defibrillation. This form of VF, when treated successfully, is associated with a relatively benign long-term prognosis, although a recent series found that hospital mortality was twofold higher in patients suffering primary VF (16). In this study, thrombolytic therapy failed to protect against primary VF, but patients over 65 years of age had a lower incidence of this arrhythmia than younger patients.

Secondary VF usually occurs in the setting of severe left ventricular dysfunction with low cardiac output and congestive heart failure. This arrhythmia is often a pre-terminal or terminal event, and although it may initially respond to anti-arrhythmic therapy or defibrillation, the prognosis is poor due to the severity of the underlying disease. Occasionally, secondary VF may be drug-induced or result from a metabolic abnormality. Correction of the etiologic disturbance may be curative, and the prognosis is more favorable.

Late VF after MI is a leading cause of sudden cardiac death. It may be due to recurrent ischemia or electrical instability in the peri-infarctional myocardium. If diagnosed promptly, late VF often responds to defibrillation, but it may recur without warning. Anti-arrhythmic therapy guided by electrophysiologic testing is indicated. The prognosis is intermediate between primary and secondary VF. Spontaneous ventricular fibrillation occurring in the absence of MI is usually associated with severe ischemic heart disease or cardiomyopathy; management and prognosis are similar to late VF.

The acute management of VF includes prompt cardiopulmonary resuscitation and immediate defibrillation. Subsequent management in refractory cases should follow the American Heart Association guidelines for advanced cardiac life support outlined in the next chapter (17). Following successful resuscitation, any treatable precipitating factors should be corrected, and anti-arrhythmic therapy, usually with intravenous lidocaine, procainamide, or bretylium should be instituted. In survivors of late VF or secondary VF, an electrophysiologic study may be needed to guide further therapy.

Bradyarrhythmias

The proper management of bradyarrhythmias is dependent on the clinical setting in which they occur as well as the specific nature of the arrhythmia. The treatment of bradycardia and conduction disturbances in acute MI is discussed in Chapter 15, and management in cardiac arrest is outlined in Chapter 7.

Patients with chronic Mobitz II second degree A-V block (Chapter 5) or complete heart block with a ventricular escape mechanism are at risk for developing asystole; permanent pacemaker insertion is usually indicated. Most other bradyarrhythmias are not life-threatening, and treatment is based on the presence of symptoms (e.g., dizziness, syncope) or evidence of hemodynamic compromise. Any medications contributing to the bradycardia should be discontinued. If acute treatment is indicated, atropine 0.5-1.0 mg should be given subcutaneously or intravenously. This can be repeated in 5-10 minutes if necessary. If significant bradycardia persists, a temporary or permanent pacemaker is usually warranted. If the patient is severely compromised, isoproterenol may be given while awaiting pacemaker insertion. Alternatively, transcutaneous pacing may be used (18).

Patients with uncomplicated bradycardia can be managed conservatively. Discontinue all offending drugs. A trial of atropine may be considered if bradycardia is profound (ventricular rate <35-40/min). In most cases, these arrhythmias will require no additional therapy, but continued close observation for evidence of hemodynamic compromise is warranted.

REFERENCES

1. Falk RH, Knowlton AA, Bernard SA, Gotlieb NE, Battinelli NJ. Digoxin for converting recent onset atrial fibrillation to sinus rhythm. Ann Intern Med 1987;106:503-506.

2. Mancini GBJ, Goldberger AL. Cardioversion of atrial fibrillation: Consideration of embolization, anticoagulation, prophylactic pacemaker and long-term success. Am Heart J 1982;104:617-621.

3. Dunn M, Alexander J, deSilva R, Hildner F. Antithrombotic therapy in atrial fibrillation. Chest 1986;89(Suppl):68S-74S.

4. Olshansky B, Waldo AL. Atrial fibrillation: Update on mechanism, diagnosis, and management. Mod Conc Cardiovasc Dis 1987;56:23-27.

5. Rinkenberger RL, Prystowsky EN, Heger JJ, Troup PJ, Jackman WM, Zipes DP. Effects on intravenous and chronic oral verapamil administration in patients with supraventricular tachyarrhythmias. Circulation 1980;62:996-1010.

6. Sung RJ, Elser B, McAllister RG. Intravenous verapamil for termination of re-entrant supraventricular tachycardias. Ann Intern Med 1980;93:682-689.

7. Levine JH, Michael JR, Guarnieri T. Treatment of multifocal atrial tachycardia with verapamil. N Engl J Med 1985;312:21-25.

8. Salerno DM, Anderson B, Sharkey PJ, Iber C. Intravenous verapamil for treatment of multifocal atrial tachycardia with and without calcium pretreatment. Ann Intern Med 1987;107:623-628.

9. Vlay SC, Reid PR. Ventricular ectopy: Etiology, evaluation, and therapy. Am J Med 1982;73:899-913.

10. Kennedy HL, Whitlock JA, Sprague MK, Kennedy LJ, Buckingham TA, Goldberg RJ. Long-term follow-up of asymptomatic healthy subjects with frequent and complex ventricular ectopy. N Engl J Med 1985;312:193-197.

11. Bigger JT. Definition of benign versus malignant ventricular arrhythmias: Targets for treatment. Am J Cardiol 1983;52:47C-54C.

12. Kleiger RE, Miller JP, Thanavaro S, Province MA, Martin TF, Oliver GC. Relationship between clinical features of acute myocardial infarction and ventricular runs two weeks to one year after infarction. Circulation 1981;63:64-70.

13. Follansbee WP, Michelson EL, Morganroth J. Nonsustained ventricular tachycardia in ambulatory patients: Characteristics and association with sudden cardiac death. Ann Intern Med 1980;92:741-747.

14. Smith WM, Gallagher JJ. "Les Torsades de Pointes": An unusual ventricular arrhythmia. Ann Intern Med 1980;93:578-584.

15. Tzivoni D, Keren A, Cohen AM, et al. Magnesium therapy for torsades de pointes. Am J Cardiol 1984;53:528-530.

16. Volpi A, Maggioni A, Franzosi MG, Pampallona S, Mauri F, Tognoni G. In-hospital prognosis of patients with acute myocardial infarction complicated by primary ventricular fibrillation. N Engl J Med 1987;317:257-261.

17. Standards for cardiopulmonary resuscitation and emergency cardiac care. Part III: Adult advanced cardiac life support. JAMA 1986;255:2933-2954.

18. Zoll PM, Zoll RH, Falk RH, Clinton JE, Eitel DR, Antman EM. External noninvasive temporary cardiac pacing: Clinical trials. Circulation 1985;71:937-944.

FURTHER READING

1. Zipes DP. Specific arrhythmias: Diagnosis and treatment. In: Braunwald E, ed. Heart disease: A textbook of cardiovascular medicine, 3rd ed. W. B. Saunders Co, Philadelphia, 1988:658-716.

Chapter 7

Cardiac Arrest

General Considerations

Several factors simplify the management of cardiac arrest in the CCU. These include: immediate recognition of the onset of arrest (i.e. all arrests are "witnessed"), rapid identification of the primary rhythm disorder, pre-existing intravenous access to facilitate drug administration, and the availability of necessary equipment and skilled staff. Detailed guidelines of the management of cardiac arrest are beyond the scope of this manual and have been published elsewhere (1,2). Selected features relevant to cardiac arrest in the CCU will be summarized in this chapter.

To maximize outcome of patients experiencing cardiac arrest, all team members participating in the arrest must respond rapidly and function efficiently according to pre-defined roles. One person, often a medical resident, should "run" the arrest, assigning specific tasks to other participants and supervising administration of medications and other procedures. To do this, the house officer must be well versed in the techniques of basic life support (CPR), current standards in advanced life support (1), and in local policies regarding adjuncts to advanced life support and the termination of resuscitative efforts.

If the patient is unconscious or pulseless, basic CPR should be initiated by the first qualified person entering the room. A rapid assessment of the cardiac rhythm should be made and treatment instituted according to the algorithms set forth by the American Heart Association (1) and reproduced in Figures 7.1-7.4. Adequate intravenous access should be secured, an arterial blood gas obtained to permit optimal management of acid-base balance and, if the patient does not respond promptly to resuscitation, endotracheal intubation should be performed to control ventilation. Accomplishment of these tasks, however, should not take precedence over performing basic CPR and prompt defibrillation, since time to initiation of CPR and defibrillation correlate closely with eventual outcome (3-5).

Once the above procedures have been initiated, consideration should be given to the mechanism of the arrest and treatment of specific factors which may be reversible (see also Chapter 6). Ventricular tachycardia and ventricular fibrillation account for over

34

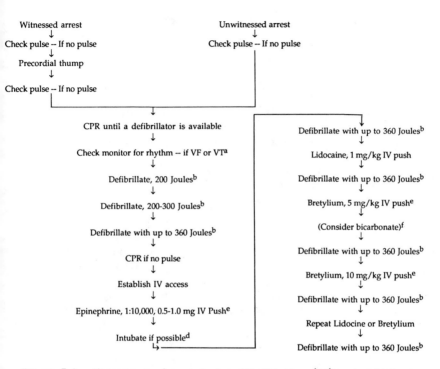

Figure 7.1. Management of ventricular fibrillation (VF) and pulseless ventricular tachycardia (VT).

  [a] Pulseless VT should be treated identically to VF.
  [b] Check pulse and rhythm after each shock.
  [c] Repeat epinephrine every 5 minutes.
  [d] Defibrillation and epinephrine are more important initially than intubation if the patient can be effectively ventilated without intubation.
  [e] Repeat boluses of lidocaine, up to a total dose of 3 mg/kg, are an acceptable alternative.
  [f] Sodium bicarbonate is not recommended routinely in cardiac arrest. Consideration of its use in a dose of 1 meq/kg is appropriate at this point.

From: Standards and guidelines for cardiopulmonary resuscitation and emergency cardiac care. JAMA 1986;255:2946. Copyright 1986, American Heart Association; used with permission.

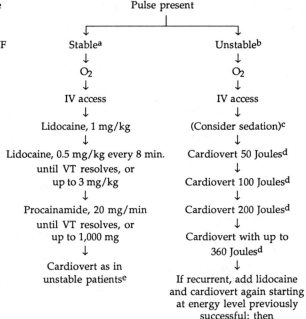

No pulse   Pulse present

↓   │

Treat as VF   Stable[a]   Unstable[b]

Stable[a]	Unstable[b]
↓	↓
O_2	O_2
↓	↓
IV access	IV access
↓	↓
Lidocaine, 1 mg/kg	(Consider sedation)[c]
↓	↓
Lidocaine, 0.5 mg/kg every 8 min. until VT resolves, or up to 3 mg/kg	Cardiovert 50 Joules[d]
↓	↓
Procainamide, 20 mg/min until VT resolves, or up to 1,000 mg	Cardiovert 100 Joules[d]
↓	↓
Cardiovert as in unstable patients[e]	Cardiovert 200 Joules[d]
	↓
	Cardiovert with up to 360 Joules[d]
	↓
	If recurrent, add lidocaine and cardiovert again starting at energy level previously successful; then procainamide or bretylium[f]

Figure 7.2.   Management of ventricular tachycardia (VT).
 [a] If patient becomes unstable (note b), move to unstable arm.
 [b] Presence of chest pain, dyspnea, hypotension (systolic blood
    pressure < 90 mm Hg), congestive heart failure, ischemia, or
    infarction.
 [c] Sedation should be considered except in the presence of severe
    instability.
 [d] To avoid delay in markedly unstable patients, use unsynchronized
    cardioversion, otherwise cardioversion should be synchronized.
 [e] In severely unstable patients, a precordial thump may be used
    prior to cardioversion.
 [f] Once VT has resolved, begin intravenous anti-arrhythmic therapy.
From: Standards and guidelines for cardiopulmonary resuscitation and
emergency cardiac care.   JAMA 1986;255:2947.   Copyright 1986, American
Heart Association; used with permission.

If rhythm is unclear and possibly ventricular fibrillation
defibrillate as for VF. If asystole is present[a]

↓

Continue CPR

↓

Establish IV access

↓

Epinephrine, 1:10,000, 0.5 - 1.0 mg IV push[b]

↓

Intubate when possible[c]

↓

Atropine, 1.0 mg IV push (repeated in 5 min.)

↓

(Consider bicarbonate)[d]

↓

Consider pacing

Figure 7.3. Management of asystole (cardiac standstill).
[a] Asystole should be confirmed in at least 2 leads.
[b] Repeat epinephrine every 5 minutes.
[c] CPR and epinephrine are more important initially than intubation
if the patient can be effectively ventilated without intubation.
[d] Sodium bicarbonate is not recommended routinely in cardiac
arrest. Consideration of its use in a dose of 1 meq/kg is
appropriate at this point.
From: Standards and guidelines for cardiopulmonary resuscitation and
emergency cardiac care. JAMA 1986;255:2947. Copyright 1986, American
Heart Association; used with permission.

70% of cardiac arrests in the CCU. Precipitating factors include
acute MI or other ischemic episode, congestive heart failure, drugs
(digitalis, anti-arrhythmics, sympathomimetics), electrolyte disturbances (hypokalemia, hyperkalemia, hypomagnesemia), and pulmonary
disorders.

Bradycardias and electromechanical dissociation (i.e. failure of
a synchronous electrical impulse to produce myocardial contraction)
are less frequent causes of cardiac arrest, but are generally
associated with a poorer prognosis. Common etiologies of bradycardia
include ischemia, severe hypoxemia of any cause, acidosis
hyperkalemia, and drugs (digitalis, beta blockers, verapamil
diltiazem, anti-arrhythmics). Electromechanical dissociation usuall
connotes profound left ventricular dysfunction or hypoxemia
pericardial tamponade, tension pneumothorax, pulmonary embolism, or
severe electrolyte or acid-base disturbance.

Continue CPR
↓
Establish IV access
↓
Epinephrine, 1:10,000, 0.5 - 1.0 mg IV push[a]
↓
Intubate when possible[b]
↓
(Consider bicarbonate)[c]
↓
Consider hypovolemia,
cardiac tamponade,
tension pneumothorax,
hypoxemia,
acidosis,
pulmonary embolism

Figure 7.4.   Management of electromechanical dissociation.
[a] Repeat epinephrine every 5 minutes.
[b] Epinephrine is more important initially than intubation if the patient can be effectively ventilated without intubation.
[c] Sodium bicarbonate is not recommended routinely in cardiac arrest. Consideration of its use in a dose of 1 meq/kg is appropriate at this point.
From: Standards and guidelines for cardiopulmonary resuscitation and emergency cardiac care. JAMA 1986;255:2947. Copyright 1986, American Heart Association; used with permission.

Use of the arrhythmia treatment algorithms (Figs. 7.1-7.4) is self-explanatory, but it is worth emphasizing that the algorithms are intended only as general guidelines, and not as a substitute for a careful clinical assessment in each individual situation. Details of the algorithms will not be reviewed, but some recent changes bear further comment. First, the recommended initial energy level for defibrillation is now 200 joules as a result of recent studies indicating high efficacy and a potential for fewer complications with lower energies (6,7).

Second, calcium is no longer recommended routinely in the management of asystole or electromechanical dissociation because recent studies have failed to demonstrate benefit from this agent (8-10). Furthermore, calcium has been implicated as a cause of post-anoxic tissue damage in both the heart and brain, and administration of calcium may result in dangerously high serum levels (11). Thus, calcium is now recommended for use only in the moribund patient with severe hyperkalemia, hypocalcemia, or calcium antagonist intoxication.

Routine administration of sodium bicarbonate is also unproven in the management of cardiac arrest (12,13). In addition, its use may be associated with a variety of adverse effects, including a shift to the left in the oxyhemoglobin saturation curve, paradoxical central nervous system acidosis, depression of myocardial contractility, inactiviation of catecholamines, congestive heart failure, arrhythmias, and hypernatremia (13). Use of sodium bicarbonate is not recommended within the first 10 minutes of cardiac arrest, and hyperventilation should be the primary treatment for acidosis. Refractory metabolic acidosis not responsive to hyperventilation, particularly when associated with severe hyperkalemia, may be treated with bicarbonate. It should also be noted that use of the arterial pH for monitoring acid-base status in cardiac arrest has been questioned; assessing central venous pH and pCO_2 may be more appropriate (13,14).

Special Considerations

Digitalis Intoxication

As discussed in Chapter 6, digitalis can produce both tachy- and bradyarrhythmias, either of which may result in cardiac arrest. Calcium and sympathomimetic agents may exacerbate digitalis-induced arrhythmias and should be avoided. Quinidine, verapamil and amiodarone increase serum digoxin concentrations and are also contraindicated.

In addition to standard treatment for ventricular tachycardia or fibrillation, serum potassium should be maintained in the range of 4.0-5.0 meq/L, and phenytoin 250 mg slow IV push (not more than 50 mg/min) or lidocaine (1 mg/kg, repeated after 10 min) should be given. Intravenous propranolol may also be of benefit.

For life-threatening digitalis-induced bradycardias, atropine, phenytoin, and temporary pacing are appropriate therapy. Potassium may exacerbate heart block even in hypokalemic patients and should be used cautiously unless a pacemaker is in place. Lidocaine and other anti-arrhythmic drugs may suppress ventricular escape mechanisms and should not be used in bradycardic patients.

Recently, Fab fragments of specific antibodies to digoxin (also effective against digitoxin) have been released for clinical use, representing a major advance in the treatment of life-threatening digitalis intoxication (15,16). This modality is quite expensive, and the efficacy of repetitive administration remains uncertain; use of this treatment should be reserved for patients with imminently life-threatening arrhythmias in the presence of documented or strongly suspected digitalis intoxication. A suggested protocol for using this agent is given in Table 7.1.

Digoxin-specific Fab fragments should be used only when conventional methods of treatment fail. A serum digoxin (or digitoxin) level should be obtained prior to initiating therapy

Table 7.1
Use of Digoxin-Specific Fab Fragments (Digibind)

I. Indications

    A. Life-threatening arrhythmias due to digitalis intoxication
        1. Ventricular tachycardia or fibrillation
        2. Progressive bradyarrhythmias
    B. Digitalis intoxication with rising [K+], esp. > 5 meq/L

II. Dosage

    A. 1 vial (40 mg) will neutralize 0.6 mg digoxin
    B. # vials needed = .0093 x dig level x wt (kg) = .0042 x dig
        level x wt (1b)
    C. Usual dose for unintentional digitalis intoxication: 200-400
        mg (5-10 vials)

III. Administration

    A. Infuse over 15-30 minutes in isotonic saline solution
    B. May be given IV "push" in emergencies

IV. Monitor

    A. Frequent serum potassium levels in first few hours
    B. Observe for worsening CHF or acceleration of ventricular rate
        in atrial fibrillation
    C. Serum digoxin levels not helpful after drug given
    D. If there is no response to an adequate dose, digitalis
        intoxication is unlikely

whenever feasible. A typical dose for an accidental overdose is
200-400 mg, or 5-10 vials. The drug produces a rapid fall in the
serum level of free digoxin, with favorable changes in rhythm
typically occurring after 15-30 minutes. The peak drug effect is at
about 60-80 minutes. The elimination half-life is 15-20 hours in
patients with normal renal function; longer if renal function is
impaired. Serum digoxin levels following drug administration are of
little value for several days, since most of the glycoside is bound to
the Fab fragments and is therefore inactive.

Rapid removal of digitalis from the tissues will permit
intracellular potassium influx, resulting in a fall in serum potassium
concentration. Potassium levels should, therefore, be monitored
closely for the first few hours after the drug is given. Removal of
digoxin may also produce exacerbation of congestive heart failure or
an increase in the ventricular rate in patients with atrial
fibrillation or flutter. CHF should be treated with diuretics and
vasodilators. Sympathomimetic agents are best avoided since they may
exacerbate digitalis-induced arrhythmias. Digitalis should not be

resumed until after the Fab fragments have been cleared, typically several days to more than a week. Finally, failure of the patient to respond to an adequate dose of Fab fragments should prompt investigation into other possible etiologies for the arrhythmia.

Hyperkalemia

Hyperkalemia is associated with a series of progressive electrocardiographic changes as the serum potassium level rises. These include:

(1) Tall, narrow, peaked (or tented) T-waves
(2) Widening of the QRS with intraventricular conduction delay
(3) Progressive loss of P-wave amplitude until P-waves become absent
(4) ST segment shifts mimicking ischemia (current of injury)
(5) Bradyarrhythmias, tachyarrhythmias, A-V conduction defects

Since hyperkalemia produces a broad array of ECG changes and arrhythmias, a high index of suspicion must be maintained. Any markedly widened, bizarre QRS, particularly in association with diminished atrial activity, should be considered a possible manifestation of severe hyperkalemia. Note that tall, peaked T-waves, often thought to be the sine qua non of hyperkalemia, may be subtle and frequently disappear as hyperkalemia progresses.

Treatment of severe hyperkalemia includes:

(1) Calcium gluconate 10-30 cc of 10% solution intravenously (direct antagonist to cardiac and neuromuscular toxicity of potassium)
(2) Sodium bicarbonate 22-88 meq (1/2-2 ampules), especially if acidosis is present
(3) 50% glucose, 1-2 ampules (D50W, 50-100 cc)
(4) Regular insulin 10 units IV or subcutaneously (optional)

The combination of bicarbonate, glucose, and insulin effectively drives the potassium intracellularly, an effect which persists for several hours. Following acute management, adminitration of an exchange resin (e.g. Kayexelate) or diuretic may be needed to deplete potassium stores. Dialysis may be required in severe cases and in renal patients. (Note: Severe Type I anti-arrhythmic excess may also give rise to marked QRS widening and atrial suppression, and this possibility should be considered in patients taking these agents. Not infrequently, hyperkalemia and anti-arrhythmic drug toxicity may coexist.)

Pericardial Tamponade

Pericardial tamponade may produce ventricular fibrillation, asystole, or electromechanical dissociation. The diagnosis should be suspected if the patient develops rapid hemodynamic deterioration without other evident cause, particularly following acute myocardial infarction (suggesting myocardial rupture, Chapter 20) or an invasive cardiac procedure (suggesting perforation).

If cardiac arrest develops, immediate pericardiocentesis is mandatory, since all other therapy, including CPR, will be ineffective. Using the protocol suggested in Table 7.2, emergency pericardiocentesis is a simple and relatively safe procedure to perform, even for the novice. Typically, removal of 50-100 cc of pericardial fluid will be sufficient to stabilize the patient. Hemorrhagic pericardial fluid may sometimes be differentiated from intracardiac blood by the absence of pulsatile flow or by a failure to clot when left standing for 10 minutes. Following effective pericardiocentesis, more definitive treatment with a pericardial catheter or surgical procedure is often required.

Table 7.2
Emergency Pericardiocentesis: Subxiphoid Approach

1. Rapidly clean subxiphoid area with betadine or other sterile cleansing fluid.*

2. Make a quick stab wound with a scalpel immediately to the left of the xiphoid process and 1-2 cm inferior to the costal margin.

3. Insert a long, sterile pericardial or intracardiac needle attached to a 20-50 cc syringe.

4. Angle the needle directly at the RIGHT shoulder.

5. Aspirate the syringe while slowly advancing the needle until fluid is recovered.

6. Continue aspirating 50-100 cc of fluid.

*Excessive delay in accomplishing this step in a moribund patient is contraindicated.

Pulmonary Embolus and Tension Pneumothorax

Massive pulmonary embolus or tension pneumothorax will occasionally be the etiology of cardiac arrest, usually presenting as profound hypotension with bradycardia or electromechanical dissociation. In massive pulmonary embolus, thrombolytic therapy or emergency embolectomy may life-saving. Tension pneumothorax most commonly occurs in intubated patients, particularly when positive end-expiratory pressure (PEEP) is in use, or following procedures such as central line placement or thoracentesis, but it may occur spontaneously as well. Needle aspiration on the side of the chest with absent breath sounds may be a life-saving maneuver; insertion of a chest tube constitutes definitive therapy.

Complications of Cardiac Arrest and Post-Arrest Management

Neurological Sequelae

It is well known that irreversible brain damage begins within 4-6 minutes of complete cessation of cerebral blood flow, and in most cases is virtually complete within 8-12 minutes. Because successful cardiopulmonary resuscitation with unsuccessful cerebral resuscitation is undesirable, increased attention has been given to methods of protecting the brain during and after cardiac arrest. Comprehensive reviews of this topic have been published elsewhere (17,18); current recommendations are summarized in Table 7.3. The role of other interventions, including barbiturate loading (19), paralysis with pancuronium bromide, corticosteroids, free-radical scavengers, calcium antagonists, and hypothermia remains investigational (18).

Persistent Hemodynamic Instability

Hypotension persisting for more than 30 minutes following successful cardiopulmonary resuscitation warrants a search for an underlying cause, e.g. sepsis, bleeding, ongoing myocardial ischemia, pericardial tamponade, etc. Optimal management may require insertion of a pulmonary artery catheter, particularly if congestive heart failure is also present.

Persistent hypertension and bradycardia may indicate the presence of increased intracranial pressure. A careful neurologic examination, including evaluation of the eye grounds, should be performed; a computed tomographic scan may also be indicated. If hypertension fails to respond to conventional agents, intravenous nitroprusside should be instituted, titrating the mean arterial pressure to 90-100 mm Hg using an intra-arterial pressure line. Pulmonary artery catheterization may also be required.

Oliguria and Acute Renal Failure

Oliguria and acute renal failure occur commonly following prolonged cardiac arrest. Try to maintain urine output at 30 cc/hour or greater with furosemide in boluses up to 500 mg or by an intra-venous infusion of 20% mannitol solution at 60-120 cc/hour. The latter agent should be avoided in the presence of congestive heart failure and discontinued promptly if no response is seen. Dopamine in doses up to 4 mcg/kg/min may also be helpful in increasing renal blood flow and maintaining urine output.

Hypoxemia

Hypoxemia may be due to congestive heart failure, non-cardiac pulmonary edema (adult respiratory distress syndrome), ventilation/

Table 7.3
Current Recommendations for Reducing Post-Anoxic Cerebral Injury*

1. Induce brief, mild hypertension (mean arterial pressure 120-140 mm Hg) for 1-5 minutes following restoration of spontaneous circulation

2. Maintain normotension subsequently (mean pressure 90 mm Hg, systolic pressure 120-130 mm Hg); mild hypertension is preferable to hypotension

3. Elevate head approximately 30°

4. Maintain normothermia

5. Maintain pCO_2 at 25-35 mm Hg

6. Maintain arterial pH at 7.3-7.6

7. Maintain blood glucose at 100-300 mg/dl

8. Control seizures, restlessness, and straining with phenobarbital, phenytoin, or diazepam as needed

9. Avoid vigorous tracheal suctioning, as it increases intracranial pressure

*Adapted from Safar P. Cerebral resuscitation after cardiac arrest: A review. Circulation 1986;74(Suppl. IV):IV-143. Used by permission of the American Heart Association, Inc.

perfusion mismatching, pleural effusion, pneumothorax, intubation of the right mainstem bronchus, or a variety of other causes. Careful auscultation of the chest should be performed, noting the presence of wheezing, rales, or unilaterally diminished breath sounds. A chest x-ray should be obtained and the position of the endotracheal tube (proper position is 2-3 cm above the carina) as well as other catheters and tubes should be noted. Evidence of pulmonary congestion, pleural or pericardial effusion, or pneumothroax should be sought. Treatment should be directed at the underlying cause, using arterial blood gases to assess response.

Prevention of Recurrence

After the patient has been stabilized, a more thorough diagnostic evaluation of potential factors contributing to the arrest should be undertaken. Although the primary cause may be evident (e.g., acute MI), other factors, such as electrolyte disturbances or drugs, should not be overlooked. Short-term prophylaxis against recurrence usually consists of lidocaine for ventricular tachyarrhythmias or a temporary pacemaker for persistent bradycardia (see also Chapters 5 and 16). In surviving patients for whom no apparent cause for the arrest can be identified, further evaluation with an electrophysiologic study may be justified.

REFERENCES

1.   Standards and guidelines for cardiopulmonary resuscitation (CPR) and emergency cardiac care (ECC). JAMA 1986;255:2905-2989.

2.   Proceedings of the 1985 National Conference on Standards and Guidelines for Cardiopulmonary Resuscitation and Emergency Cardiac Care. Circulation 1986; 74(Suppl IV):IV-1-153.

3.   Eisenberg MS, Hallstrom AP, Bergner L. Long-term survival after out-of-hospital cardiac arrest. N Engl J Med 1982;306:1340-1343.

4.   Eisenberg MS, Copass MK, Hallstrom AP, et al. Treatment of out-of-hospital cardiac arrests with rapid defibrillation by emergency medical technicians. N Engl J Med 1980;302:1379-1382.

5.   Stults KR, Brown DD, Schug VL, Bean JA. Prehospital defibrillation performed by emergency medical technicians in rural communities. N Engl J Med 1984;310:219-223.

6.   Weaver WD, Cobb LA, Copass MK, Hallstrom AP. Ventricular defibrillation: A comparative trial using 175J and 320J shocks. N Engl J Med 1983;307:1101-1106.

7.   Kerber RE. Energy requirements for defibrillation. Circulation 1986;74(Suppl IV):IV-117-119.

8.   Stempien A, Katz AM, Messineo FC. Calcium and cardiac arrest. Ann Int Med 1986;105:603-606.

9.   Hughes WG, Ruedy JR. Should calcium be used in cardiac arrest? Am J Med 1986;81:285-296.

10. Thompson BM, Steuven HS, Tonsfeldt DJ, et al. Calcium: Limited indications, some danger. Circulation 1986;74(Suppl IV):IV-90-93.

11. Dembo DH. Calcium in advanced life support. Crit Care Med 1981;9:358-359.

12. Bishop RL, Weisfeldt ML. Sodium bicarbonate administration during cardiac arrest. JAMA 1976;235:506-509.

13. Jaffe AS. Cardiovascular pharmacology I. Circulation 1986; 74(Suppl IV): IV-70-74.

14. Niemann JT, Criley JM, Rosborough JP, Niskanen RA, Alferness C. Predictive indices of successful cardiac resuscitation after prolonged arrest and experimental cardiopulmonary resuscitation. Ann Emerg Med 1985;14:521-528.

15. Smith TW, Butler VP, Haber E, et al. Treatment of life-threatening digitalis intoxication with digoxin-specific Fab antibody fragments. N Engl J Med 1982;307:1357-1362.

16. Wenger TL, Butler VP, Haber E, Smith TW. Treatment of 63 severely digitalis-toxic patients with digoxin-specific antibody fragments. J Am Coll Cardiol 1985;5(Suppl A):118A-123A.

17. Bass E. Cardiopulmonary arrest: Pathophysiology and neurologic complications. Ann Intern Med 1985;103:920-927.

18. Safar P. Cerebral resuscitation after cardiac arrest: A review. Circulation 1986;74(Suppl IV):IV-138-153.

19. Brain resuscitation clinical trial I study group. Randomized clinical study of thiopental loading in comatose survivors of cardiac arrest. N Engl J Med 1986;314:397-403.

Chapter 8

Interpretation of Arterial Blood Gases

Stephen S. Lefrak, M.D., and Stephen Liggett, M.D.

Arterial blood gas analysis is an indispensable and easily utilized tool for the evaluation of alveolar gas exchange and acid-base status. This chapter will review the interpretation of blood gases, stressing the cautions that need to be applied in using this information in the care of patients in the CCU.

Indications

Blood gas analysis should not be regarded as a routine test in patients admitted to the coronary care unit, although many patients will require such measurements. Arterial blood should be obtained for analysis whenever an acid-base disturbance is suspected, or whenever an abnormality of the respiratory system is present which would result in disordered alveolar gas exchange. Since significant abnormalities in alveolar ventilation, oxygenation, and acid-base status may exist but remain clinically undetectable, the threshold for obtaining an arterial blood gas should be rather low.

On the other hand, some caveats are in order. Although the absolute severity of any abnormality is important, the rapidity with which the disturbance has developed is of equal importance. Marked changes which are chronic are often well tolerated whereas smaller changes occurring rapidly may be fatal. Furthermore, arterial blood gas abnormalities are not diagnostic of specific diseases, but rather define physiologic processes and quantify abnormalities so that treatment may be effectively planned and the patient's course appropriately monitored. In this context, it should be stressed that oxygen therapy should not be withheld while obtaining arterial blood gases. Rather, the blood gas values should be utilized in guiding and refining oxygen therapy.

Alveolar Gas Exchange

The primary functions of the respiratory system are oxygenation of venous blood and elimination of carbon dioxide. Measurements of oxygen and carbon dioxide tensions in arterial blood are used to assess the adequacy and efficiency of alveolar gas exchange. In order to interpret this information properly, the physician must have an understanding of the concepts of alveolar ventilation, the alveolar air equation and alveolar-arterial pressure difference, and ventilation/perfusion matching.

Alveolar ventilation may be conceptualized as the volume of gas which reaches functioning (perfused and ventilated) lung tissue each minute. This volume is smaller than the total volume of gas respired (the minute ventilation), because some gas ventilates non-gas exchanging portions of the lungs and airways referred to as dead space. Adequacy of alveolar ventilation is reflected in the arterial pCO_2, which has a normal range of 35-45 mm Hg. Elevated pCO_2 indicates hypoventilation, while a low pCO_2 indicates hyperventilation. The pH (see below) is an indicator of whether the level of ventilation is appropriate to the acid-base status of the body and whether abnormalities of ventilation are acute or chronic. Commonly occurring disorders which produce alterations in the pCO_2 are listed in Table 8.1.

The adequacy of oxygenation is assessed using the arterial oxygen tension (p_aO_2) and saturation. In general, a p_aO_2 which produces 90% saturation of hemoglobin is sufficient. When the hemoglobin dissociation curve is normal, a p_aO_2 of 60 mm Hg will usually yield 90% saturation. However, it is apparent that a p_aO_2 of 60 mm Hg while breathing 100% oxygen indicates markedly abnormal lung function and alveolar oxygen exchange as compared with the same p_aO_2 on room air. To further evaluate oxygen transfer, the simplified alveolar air equation is used to calculate P_AO_2, the alveolar oxygen tension:

$$P_AO_2 = F_IO_2 \times (\text{Barometric pressure} - 47 \text{ mm Hg}) - p_aCO_2/R$$

where F_IO_2 = fraction of oxygen in inspired air, barometric pressure at sea level is assumed to be 760 mm Hg, 47 mm Hg is the partial pressure of water in the airways, p_aCO_2 is the arterial CO_2 tension, and R is the respiratory gas exchange ratio, usually assumed to be 0.8. As an example, assuming the patient is breathing room air ($F_IO_2 = 0.21$) and has a p_aCO_2 of 40 mm Hg,

$$p_AO_2 = 0.21 \times (760-47) - 40/0.8 = 100 \text{ mm Hg}$$

Note that p_AO_2, which reflects the maximum achievable arterial oxygen tension with "perfect" lung function, is dependent primarily on F_IO_2, less so on pCO_2 and R. Thus, moderate increases in pCO_2 (hypoventilation) or decreases in R (e.g. during hemodialysis) will not produce dangerous falls in arterial oxygen tension if alveolar gas exchange is initially normal. However, such perturbations can lead to serious hypoxemia in patients with already compromised oxygenation.

The difference between P_AO_2 and p_aO_2 is termed the alveolar-arterial oxygen difference or "A-a gradient", and is indicative of the efficiency of alveolar oxygen transfer. Under normal circumstances, this difference is small (≤ 15 mm Hg). Increases arise

Table 8.1
Common Etiologies of Hyperventilation and Hypoventilation

I. Hyperventilation ($pCO_2 < 35$ mm Hg)
    A. Metabolic acidosis with respiratory compensation
    B. Anxiety
    C. Central hyperventilation due to CNS disease
    D. Artificial respiration, mechanical ventilation
    E. Pulmonary embolus
    F. Acute airway obstruction
    G. Stiff lungs
    H. Hypoxia of any cause
    I. Sepsis
    J. Hyperthermia
    K. Hepatic failure with ammonia intoxication

II. Hypoventilation ($pCO_2 > 45$ mm Hg)
    A. Metabolic alkalosis with respiratory compensation
    B. Central hypoventilation
       1. CNS disease
       2. Opiates, barbiturates
       3. Myxedema
       4. Hypothermia
    C. Peripheral (neuromuscular) hypoventilation
       1. Amyotrophic lateral sclerosis
       2. Guillain-Barre syndrome
       3. Myasthenia gravis
       4. Muscular dystrophy
       5. C3-C5 quadriplegia
       6. Kyphoscoliosis
       7. Flail chest
       8. Muscular fatigue (e.g. in cardiogenic shock)
       9. Aminoglycosides, other drugs
    D. Intrinsic cardiopulmonary disease
       1. Asthma, COPD
       2. Pulmonary fibrosis
       3. Pulmonary edema
    E. Increased CO_2 production, inadequate excretion
       1. Overfeeding with high glucose solutions
       2. Severe shivering
       3. Metabolic acidosis without respiratory compensation
    F. Artificial respiration, mechanical ventilation

primarily as a result of ventilation/perfusion (V/Q) mismatching or
anatomic right-to-left shunting in the heart or lungs. Less commonly,
diffusion abnormalities may contribute to an increased A-a gradient.
V/Q mismatching implies that some areas of the lung are perfused but
not ventilated or vice-versa. In the former case, unoxygenated blood
is returned to the heart, resulting in a reduction in arterial oxygen
tension and a widened A-a gradient. In the latter case, there is an
increase in ventilatory dead space without a direct effect on

$p_a O_2$. Hypoxemia due to V/Q mismatching often responds readily to supplemental oxygen, whereas hypoxemia due to a right-to-left shunt is relatively resistant to supplemental oxygen and may require correction of the shunt, positive end-expiratory pressure breathing (PEEP), or inverse ratio ventilation.

In the presence of significant V/Q mismatching or right-to-left shunting, mixed venous (pulmonary arterial) oxygen saturation will also affect arterial oxygen tension because oxygen-poor blood becomes mixed with oxygenated blood. Thus, a mixed venous oxygen saturation of 50% would necessarily result in a lower arterial saturation than would a mixed venous saturation of 75%. This is of particular importance in the CCU, where low mixed venous saturation is commonly seen as a result of low cardiac output (Chapter 18). As a corollary, an improvement in cardiac output and mixed venous saturation can lead to increased arterial oxygenation without directly affecting pulmonary function. Also, since low mixed venous oxygenation may result from severe anemia, transfusion can improve oxygenation in some patients.

Oxygen Tension and Saturation

Oxygen saturation is the percent of hemoglobin carrying oxygen, whereas arterial oxygen tension is the partial pressure of oxygen dissolved in plasma. These two are normally closely linked by the sigmoid-shaped oxyhemoglobin dissociation curve, but it is important to note that oxygen saturation is the more physiologically meaningful measurement, since tissue oxygen uptake is dependent on oxygen release from hemoglobin, not plasma. The significance of this is illustrated by the example of carbon monoxide poisoning, in which the $p_a O_2$ remains normal while carbon monoxide displaces oxygen from hemoglobin, thus severely reducing oxygen availability to the tissues. In the blood gas laboratory, oxygen saturation may be measured directly or calculated from the $p_a O_2$ and pH by assuming a normal oxyhemoglobin dissociation curve. The physician should be aware of the technique used in the local institution, recognizing that calculated saturations are both less physiologic and less reliable.

With respect to the oxyhemoglobin saturation curve, several points are worth remembering. An arterial tension of 60 mm Hg, which normally corresponds to 90% saturation, occurs at the beginning of the flat upper portion of the curve (see Fig. 11.1). To achieve a higher saturation, a relatively large increment in $p_a O_2$ is needed, which may require exposing the patient to dangerous concentrations of oxygen. By contrast, below this point the curve becomes steep, and small changes in $p_a O_2$ result in larger changes in saturation. Therefore, small decrements in tension may cause rapid clinical deterioration which may respond to similarly small increments in $p_a O_2$. Normal mixed venous saturation (75%) corresponds to an oxygen tension of 40 mm Hg, and hemoglobin is normally 50% saturated at 28.6 mm Hg. Below this level, anaerobic metabolism and lactate production usually begin. Thus, it is desirable to maintain a mixed venous saturation of at least 50%. Finally, at an arterial oxygen tension of 20 mm Hg, the lower limit of oxygen transfer from blood to tissue is reached, and no further oxygen will be available for tissue utilization. It follows that under no circumstances should arterial oxygen tension be allowed to approach this level.

Acid-Base Equilibrium

A proper understanding of acid-base equilibrium is important in the management of CCU patients, since both acidosis and alkalosis are commonly associated with electrolyte disturbances, impaired oxygen transport, arrhythmias, and alterations in myocardial contractility. Although a thorough discussion of the factors affecting acid-base balance is beyond the scope of this manual, a few comments are in order. According to the Henderson-Hasselbach equation, hydrogen ion concentration is dependent on the ratio of pCO_2 to bicarbonate $[HCO_3]$. Blood pH, the negative log of $[H+]$, therefore reflects a balance between respiratory function, which controls pCO_2, and renal function, which controls $[HCO_3]$. Physiologic mechanisms always attempt to maintain pH within a narrow range, so that any perturbation of either respiratory or renal component will provoke a compensatory response designed to preserve acid-base homeostasis. Thus, the normal respiratory response to a fall in $[HCO_3]$ (i.e. metabolic acidosis) is hyperventilation, producing a compensatory fall in pCO_2, so that the ratio $pCO_2/[HCO_3]$ is maintained.

Table 8.2
Simple Acid-Base Disorders

Disorder	Primary change	Compensation	Range of compensation
Metabolic			
Acidosis	↓HCO_3	↓pCO_2	pCO_2 response slow but linear $pCO_2=(1.5 \times HCO_3) +8$ (±2) pCO_2=last 2 digits of pH
Alkalosis	↑HCO_3	↑pCO_2	pCO_2 response erratic pCO_2 ↑'s 0.6 Torr for each meq/L ↑ in HCO_3
Respiratory			
Acidosis	↑pCO_2	↑HCO_3	Acute: HCO_3 ↑'s 1 meq/L for each 10 Torr ↑ in pCO_2 Chronic: HCO_3 ↑'s 3.5 meq/L for each 10 Torr ↑ in pCO_2
Alkalosis	↓pCO_2	↓HCO_3	Acute: HCO_3 ↓'s 2 meq/L for each 10 Torr ↓ in pCO_2 Chronic: HCO_3 ↓'s 5 meq/L for each 10 Torr ↓ in pCO_2

Normal blood pH ranges from 7.35–7.45. A pH less than 7.35 is called acidemia, a pH in excess of 7.45 is termed alkalemia. Four primary derangements of acid-base balance are defined (Table 8.2). Metabolic acidosis occurs when $[HCO_3]$ falls below the normal range. Respiratory acidosis refers to an abnormally elevated pCO_2. Metabolic alkalosis is due to an elevated $[HCO_3]$, and respiratory alkalosis occurs when the pCO_2 is decreased. Under normal circumstances, a primary metabolic disturbance will lead to respiratory compensation and vice-versa, and the magnitude of the

Table 8.3
Common Causes of Acid-Base Disorders in the CCU

I. Metabolic acidosis
   A. Anion gap*
      1. Cardiogenic shock (or severe hypoperfusion)
      2. Sepsis
      3. Diabetic or alcoholic ketoacidosis
      4. Starvation
      5. Renal failure
   B. Non-anion gap
      1. Persistent diarrhea
      2. Renal tubular acidosis
      3. Renal failure

II. Metabolic alkalosis
   A. Volume contraction
   B. Hypokalemia
   C. Bicarbonate administration
   D. Persistent vomiting
   E. Nasogastric suction
   F. Secondary hyperaldosteronism

III. Respiratory acidosis
   A. Chronic obstructive lung disease
   B. Opiates, barbiturates
   C. Respiratory fatigue due to cardiogenic shock
   D. Pulmonary edema (cardiac or noncardiac)
   E. Inadequate mechanical ventilation

IV. Respiratory alkalosis
   A. Anxiety
   B. Hypoxia with increased respiratory drive
      (e.g. CHF, pulmonary embolus)
   C. Ventilator-induced hyperventilation
   D. Central nervous system disorders (central hyperventilation)
   E. Sepsis

*Anion gap = $[Na^+] - [Cl^-] - [HCO_3]$ (Normal range: 8–12 meq/L)

compensatory response is predictable (Table 8.2). When the degree of compensation is appropriate to the primary disturbance, a simple acid-base disorder is diagnosed; when it is not, a mixed acid-base disorder is present.

In most cases, acute disturbances in acid-base equilibrium can be readily diagnosed from the arterial pH and pCO_2. In general, respiratory compensation is relatively prompt, whereas metabolic compensation may take 24 hours or longer to develop. When chronic acid-base disorders (e.g. chronic obstructive lung disease, renal acidosis) or mixed acid-base problems are present, it may be more difficult to determine the cause of any acute change, and the reader is referred to standard texts for a more complete discussion.

In all cases, an attempt should be made to diagnose the primary etiology for any acute change in acid-base balance, since proper treatment should be directed at the underlying derangement. A common error, for example, is to administer bicarbonate to a patient with severe, respiratory acidosis and a pH of 7.10, when a moment's thought would make it apparent that intubation and mechanical ventilation would be more appropriate. On the other hand, in severe or mixed acid-base disturbances, treatment of both the metabolic and respiratory components may be required. Common causes of the four primary acid-base disorders are listed in Table 8.3.

FURTHER READING

1. Dantzker D, ed. Cardiopulmonary critical care. Grune & Stratton, Orlando, FL, 1986.

2. Filley G. Acid-base and blood gas regulation. Lea & Febiger, Philadelphia, 1971.

3. Narins RG, Emmett M. Simple and mixed acid-base disorders: A practical approach. Medicine 1980;59:161-187.

Chapter 9

Mechanical Ventilation in the Coronary Care Unit

Stephen Liggett, M.D., and Stephen S. Lefrak, M.D.

This chapter is not meant as an encyclopedic approach to mechanical ventilation, but rather will emphasize those aspects which apply to frequently encountered situations in the coronary care unit. There are many effects of mechanical ventilation on cardiac function, but we will provide only the most elementary discussion of these under the appropriate headings.

Although there are various types and brands of mechanical ventilators as well as multiple techniques employed in their use, it is important to remember that a mechanical ventilator is first and foremost a mechanical substitute for a patient's inspiratory muscles. Utilization and modification of the ventilator breathing circuit and supplemental oxygen concentration allow the clinician to supply higher concentrations of oxygen than can be supplied without an endotracheal tube, and to alter airway pressures and flow patterns. If one keeps in mind that ventilation and oxygenation, somewhat artificially separable, are the functions affected by mechanical ventilation, then ventilatory care of patients can be more readily understood.

In considering mechanical ventilation, it is helpful to think of it as a technique comprised of three stages: initiation, maintenance, and withdrawal.

Initiating Mechanical Ventilation

Mechanical ventilation is indicated in patients who are: 1) unable to maintain adequate alveolar gas exchange spontaneously, 2) in marked respiratory distress, or 3) in cardiogenic or severe septic shock. In essence these are patients who, in the first instance, demonstrate failure of either the respiratory bellows or lungs; or who, in the second and third instances, are at grave risk of developing bellows or lung failure.

The adequacy of alveolar gas exchange is evaluated by blood gas analysis, which is the accepted method of demonstrating respiratory failure. Commonly used blood gas criteria for intubation during acute respiratory failure in patients with previously normal gas exchange are: 1) a p_aO_2 of less than 55 mm Hg (or saturation less than 90%) despite supplemental oxygen, 2) a p_aCO_2 that is not adequate to maintain a blood pH of > 7.30. The latter may arise from either primary respiratory acidosis or an inability to compensate for metabolic acidosis (see Chapter 8).

Intubation is also indicated for severe respiratory distress regardless of gas exchange, especially in patients with compromised cardiac function. Useful clinical parameters include a respiratory rate greater than 35 breaths/min, paradoxical or alternating respiratory movements of the abdomen and chest, and accessory muscle use. These are especially ominous when accompanied by agitation, obtundation, diaphoresis, or marked abnormalities of the cardiovascular system. It should be emphasized that during respiratory distress, the respiratory muscles may account for as much as 30% of total oxygen uptake, compared to the normal 5%. The necessary increase in cardiac output markedly increases myocardial oxygen requirements. This development, obviously detrimental in patients with myocardial ischemia or limited cardiac reserve, may be alleviated by intubation and mechanical ventilation. Likewise, in cardiogenic shock mechanical ventilation may decrease blood flow requirements to respiratory muscles, thereby increasing systemic perfusion and alleviating lactic acidosis.

Patients with impending respiratory failure should be electively intubated under controlled circumstances. The procedure should be carried out in the least stressful manner in order to minimize further cardiopulmonary compromise. Thus, patients who require maintenance of an upright position should be intubated nasally with a 7.0-7.5 mm endotracheal tube (ETT). For those patients who can lie comfortably in a relatively supine position and in patients in full cardiopulmonary arrest, oral intubation is indicated. The oral route offers the advantages of direct visualization during insertion, use of a larger diameter ETT with a lower resistance to airflow, maintenance for longer periods of time without otitis media or sinusitis, and patient comfort. Regardless of the method of intubation, if time permits, sedation with an intravenous narcotic analgesic or benzodiazepine may provide for a less traumatic and better tolerated procedure. It should be noted that these agents may cause apnea and hypotension and should be administered only if the means of correcting such problems are available.

Proper ventilatory support during the acute phase of respiratory failure should provide adequate gas exchange and minimize the work of breathing. Initial ventilator settings should be tailored to the clinical setting and pre-intubation blood gases, but should generally include an F_IO_2 of 1.00 and a minute ventilation of 10-20 L/min (i.e. tidal volume of 10-15 cc/kg ideal body weight and assisted breaths of 10-20/min). If adequate gas exchange is not attained after intubation, one should consider the possibility of improper tube placement (esophageal or mainstem bronchus intubation), inadequate cuff inflation, traumatic rupture of the trachea, pneumothorax, inappropriate ventilator settings, or an improperly functioning ventilator. Substituting manual ventilation with a resuscitation bag and high flow oxygen will allow for troubleshooting the ventilator.

Even when acceptable gas exchange is attained, it is essential that the work of breathing be minimized during cardiac ischemia. This can be accomplished by appropriate sedation and proper choice of ventilator, ventilator settings, and mode of ventilation. When significant respiratory distress is not relieved by these measures, inducing skeletal muscle paralysis with pancuronium bromide (Pavulon) should be considered. This may also be considered during cardiogenic shock in order to minimize the shunting of blood to respiratory muscles. One must be completely familiar with pancuronium, as with any drug, before prescribing it; particularly noteworthy is its tendency to produce a tachycardia which may offset its other advantages in the cardiac patient. In addition, the paralyzed patient requires adequate sedation and must never be left unattended.

Maintenance of Mechanical Ventilation

A number of modes of ventilation are now available from a variety of commercial vendors. Different brands of ventilators can have markedly different properties while operating in the same mode; thus it is important to become familiar with the characteristics of the machines available at a particular institution.

The "mode" of ventilation refers to the mechanism employed to initiate a mechanically assisted breath. Controlled ventilation refers to inspiration which is independent of patient effort and is at a rate faster than the patient's spontaneous respiratory rate. In this mode all breaths are initiated by the ventilator, so that inspiratory muscle work, oxygen demand, and muscle blood flow are minimized--provided the patient is adequately synchronized with the ventilator. The reduction in work required for ventilation is the main advantage of this mode. Its main drawback is that the clinician must serve as the patient's respiratory center, since the patient cannot compensate for changes in respiratory drive by altering the respiratory rate. The clinician, therefore, must adjust this rate and monitor arterial carbon dioxide tension and pH frequently to avoid respiratory acidosis or alkalosis. Controlled ventilation is often used in patients who make no spontaneous inspiratory efforts, particularly those with drug overdoses or central nervous system injuries. It is particularly helpful in patients in whom one wishes to minimize respiratory work, such as those in cardiogenic shock or with other severe circulatory disorders. However, it frequently requires the use of sedation, and if respiratory drive is particularly strong, as in patients with stiff lungs, skeletal muscle paralysis may be required. Nonetheless, we favor the use of controlled ventilation in such patients, but insist on the safeguards mentioned previously, especially that paralyzed patients should never be left unattended.

Assist-Control Ventilation (ACV)

In this mode of mechanical ventilation, every inspiratory effort from the patient triggers delivery of a prescribed tidal volume. A "back-up" rate equivalent to about 75% of the total respiratory rate is also chosen in order to provide a minimally adequate minute ventilation if spontaneous initiation of mechanical breaths ceases. For example, if the total respiratory rate is 20/min, then the back-up rate is set at 15/min. Under these conditions, the patient never takes an unassisted breath and under appropriate circumstances the work of breathing may be minimal. The amount of patient-applied negative inspiratory pressure required to trigger the assisted breaths should be set at 2-5 cm H_2O. Tachypneic patients may continue to breathe rapidly despite adequate gas exchange and in this mode respiratory alkalosis may develop. Under these circumstances, sedation, a reduction in tidal volume, or a change in the mode of ventilation is required.

Intermittent Mandatory Ventilation (IMV)

This frequently used mode provides a prescribed number of machine-delivered breaths at a set tidal volume with the patient providing additional minute ventilation as needed. With most systems the unassisted breaths are accomplished when the patient's breathing triggers a demand valve in the ventilator, allowing the patient to inhale gas through the ventilator circuit. The work required for breathing may be quite high in some demand valve circuits and the increased oxygen uptake and need for an increase in cardiac output can result in deleterious cardiac ischemia. If the IMV mode is chosen, it is appropriate to keep the IMV rate high (i.e. few or no patient breaths) during the acute phase of respiratory failure in cardiac patients. Furthermore, while ventilatory support can be gradually decreased as the patient improves, it is generally not advisable to proceed with slow, step-wise reductions in the IMV rate below 8 machine breaths/min since patient effort can become considerable; rather, discontinuation of mechanical ventilation should be considered (see below).

Pressure Support Ventilation (PSV)

As a result of the increased respiratory work in demand valve IMV circuits, some manufacturers have added a mechanism which allows the clinician to pressurize the circuit to a selected plateau during each spontaneous breath. The ventilator provides this plateau pressure until a minimal inspiratory flow is reached. This pressure helps overcome the resistance in the tubing, demand valve and endotracheal tube, all of which may be considerable. In addition, this method allows the patient to determine the inspiratory time, flow rate, and tidal volume while the physician sets the airway pressure. The result is increased patient comfort and decreased respiratory work relative to demand valve IMV circuits. The initial pressure should be that which provides a tidal volume of 10-15 cc/kg body weight; this is tapered as the patient improves and is able to maintain tidal volume with a lower support pressure. PSV may be used with positive end-expiratory pressure (PEEP) and combined with IMV. We see little to recommend it as a mode of ventilation when compared to controlled or assist-controlled ventilation, especially in patients with severe circulatory dysfunction. However, it may be preferable to IMV at low rates of mechanically assisted breathing, and if IMV with a demand valve circuit is chosen as a weaning method, PSV may be useful in reducing work of breathing and subsequent inspiratory muscle fatigue.

Oxygenation and Mechanical Ventilation

Supplemental oxygen is provided in order to keep the p_aO_2 above 60 mm Hg (saturation $\geq$ 90%) and, when available, the mixed venous $pO_2 \geq$ 35 mm Hg (saturation $\geq$ 55%). Initially, oxygen is supplied at F_IO_2 = 1.00, but shortly thereafter efforts to decrease the F_IO_2 to the lowest amount necessary should be made since oxygen toxicity is imminent at high F_IO_2 levels. At times, a low F_IO_2 may be difficult to achieve in patients with severe pulmonary edema. Although it is unclear what constitutes a "safe" F_IO_2, as a general guideline positive end-expiratory pressure (PEEP) should be used when adequate oxygenation cannot be achieved with an F_IO_2 of < 50%.

PEEP facilitates oxygenation by improving the ventilation-perfusion ratio in terminal respiratory units that collapse at low distending airway pressures. Typically, PEEP is increased in 2-5 cm H_2O increments with reassessment of oxygenation and oxygen requirements via blood gas analysis or oximetry. PEEP may decrease cardiac output by decreasing venous return to the right heart, but this is not usually a problem at levels below 12 cm H_2O. In addition, the pulmonary artery occlusive pressure, which is measured with atmospheric pressure as zero reference, may be artifactually elevated with PEEP, although again this is usually not significant at levels below 12 cm H_2O. PEEP may be used with any of the modes discussed above. Criteria for determining the optimal level of PEEP remain undefined. However, the guiding principle for the application of PEEP in the CCU is to decrease the F_IO_2 to non-toxic levels while avoiding decreases in cardiac output and oxygen transport. Maximizing or maintaining the mixed venous oxygen saturation at 50% or greater is also a desirable goal in patients with impaired cardiovascular systems.

Positive end-expiratory pressure may be present even though PEEP has not intentionally been initiated, and without positive pressure appearing on the pressure manometer at end-exhalation. This has been called "intrinsic" or "auto PEEP." It arises as a result of shortened expiratory time, high airway resistance, or elevated minute ventilation, and may be detected by occluding the exhalation valve at end-expiration. It is most likely to occur in patients with severe obstructive airways disease in addition to cardiac disease, but it may be seen in patients with pulmonary edema requiring minute ventilations in excess of 20 liters. Intrinsic PEEP may result in erroneous pulmonary artery occlusive pressure readings, decreased cardiac output, increased work of breathing and, theoretically, barotrauma. Therefore, this phenomenon should be searched for and quantitated in appropriate patients at risk, and the ventilatory pattern should be adjusted accordingly.

In the patient with diffuse lung disease and marked resistance to oxygenation, various modifications of ventilatory modes and techniques have been advocated. Most of these are experimental and are not required in the management of patients with cardiovascular problems. Inverse ratio ventilation, which is usually applied under pressure control, is a recently developed mode which is receiving increasing attention. This mode of ventilation prolongs inspiratory time to obtain inspiratory/expiratory ratios greater than 1:1 and at times as high as 4:1. The usefulness of this maneuver remains to be demonstrated. However, the potential for severe cardiovascular compromise resulting from the marked increase in mean intrathoracic pressure is real. This risk, and the rare need for exceptional measures to oxygenate patients with cardiogenic pulmonary edema, suggest that inverse ratio ventilation should not be applied to patients with respiratory failure secondary to cardiovascular disease.

Discontinuation of Mechanical Ventilation

Pre-requisites for discontinuation of mechanical ventilation are appropriate muscle strength and endurance, adequate ventilatory drive, and satisfactory oxygenation. While assessing these factors is often relatively straightforward in patients who have had rapid resolution of respiratory failure, it is prudent to follow the checklist provided in Table 9.1 prior to discontinuing mechanical ventilation.

Table 9.1
Checklist for Discontinuation of Mechanical Ventilation

1) Satisfactory resolution of the underlying process which has produced the need for mechanical ventilation
2) Adequate mental status
3) p_aO_2 > 60 mm Hg, F_IO_2 $\leq$ 0.5, PEEP $\leq$ 5 cm H_2O
4) p_aCO_2 similar to baseline and adequate to maintain normal pH
5) Spontaneous minute ventilation < 10 L/min, maximum voluntary ventilation at least twice minute ventilation
6) Spontaneous respiratory rate < 25/min with a normal pattern
7) Vital capacity > 10-15 cc/kg or peak inspiratory pressure more negative than -25 mm Hg
8) Adequate cardiac output; stable hemodynamics and cardiac rhythm

We stress that the first criterion in the table is the most important. When the physiologic disturbance that has resulted in the need for mechanical ventilation has improved, the patient will be capable of assuming spontaneous breathing. Although this seems self-evident, it is puzzling how often it is ignored; consequently, the removal of ventilatory support becomes difficult. Our approach is to vigorously pursue the underlying physiologic abnormality and, when the patient is maximally improved, then to consider discontinuing ventilatory support.

The ultimate criterion for discontinuing mechanical ventilation is the patient's ability to comfortably maintain unassisted spontaneous ventilation, normal vital signs, and adequate gas exchange while still intubated. A carefully monitored trial of spontaneous ventilation lasting at least 30 minutes should be performed, preferably with the "T" piece in place. Mechanical ventilation should be reinstituted if dyspnea, angina, or other symptoms develop, or if there is a marked increase in respiratory rate or heart rate, a deterioration in gas exchange, or a change in the general status of the patient.

If the patient cannot tolerate the "T" tube trial, or demonstrates ventilator-dependency in other ways, then gradual removal from ventilatory support may be indicated. This process, often called weaning, can be carried out in several ways. Not every patient needs to be weaned; in fact, most do not. The most common causes of failure to wean in the coronary care unit are: 1) cardiac failure, 2) excess work of breathing, and 3) respiratory muscle fatigue. Less common causes include respiratory muscle weakness, increased carbon dioxide production, and failure of respiratory drive.

Cardiac failure may be exacerbated by attempts at removal from ventilatory support because intrathoracic positive pressure may ameliorate left ventricular dysfunction in several ways. Especially noteworthy are its ability to decrease left ventricular afterload, right and left ventricular preload, and oxygen uptake; these effects may be life-saving in patients with cardiac dysfunction. As a result, some patients with abnormal ventricular function, valvular heart disease, or ischemia may be unable to maintain spontaneous breathing without positive pressure ventilatory support. Accordingly, ventricular function must be optimized in such patients, and the use of intravenous inotropic agents and/or vasodilators is frequently required during the weaning process.

Work of breathing must be minimized by improving airway function, using appropriately sized endotracheal tubes, decreasing secretions, and minimizing extravascular lung water. Respiratory muscle fatigue, like other muscle fatigue, results from an imbalance of substrate supply and demand. It is therefore critical to: 1) decrease the afterload to the inspiratory muscles (decrease work of breathing); 2) improve delivery of substrate by improving cardiac function and oxygenation; and 3) maintain adequate nutrition and appropriate serum concentrations of key elements such as phosphorous, calcium, potassium, and magnesium. Occasionally, use of aminophylline as an inotrope for the diaphragm should be considered. Respiratory muscle weakness may result from underlying neurological disease or from drugs such as aminoglycosides or xylocaine which may exert an adverse effect on the neuromuscular junction. This may be sufficient to impair weaning in patients with other severe abnormalities.

Increased carbon dioxide production is an uncommon problem in the CCU, since it usually results from administration of hyperalimentation in excess of caloric requirements, especially if a large proportion of the calories are provided as glucose. If hyperalimentation is undertaken, we recommend that about half the non-protein calories be provided as lipid. Metabolic measurements may be taken to avoid excess caloric intake. Inadequate ventilatory drive may result from drug-induced respiratory depression or metabolic alkalosis, which should be treated vigorously. Other causes of decreased respiratory drive (e.g.hypothyroidism) are less common in the CCU but should not be overlooked.

In the difficult-to-wean patient the aforementioned obstacles to successful weaning should be considered and treated as necessary. Otherwise, weaning may be accomplished by providing the patient with progressively longer periods of time on the "T" tube or by use of IMV. With "T" tube weaning, periods up to one hour of spontaneous breathing are interspersed with equal periods of mechanically assisted breathing. The patient is allowed to sleep with mechanical support for about eight hours each night. Eventually the patient is completely withdrawn from ventilatory support. IMV may be used in a similar manner with the number of mechanically assisted breaths being gradually decreased and the patient's clinical and arterial blood gas response periodically evaluated. If a demand valve circuit is used, pressure support ventilation (see above) may be useful in decreasing the work of breathing. Support should be provided during the night to allow the patient to sleep. PSV is then gradually reduced to 2-3 cm H_2O, at which point the patient may be extubated.

Complications During Mechanical Ventilation

The major complications resulting directly from mechanical ventilation are: 1) malplacement or other dysfunction of the endotracheal tube, 2)ventilator failure, 3) disconnection between the patient and the ventilator, and 4) critical intolerance of increased airway pressure, the basis of positive pressure ventilation. Other complications occurring in critically ill patients include gastrointestinal bleeding and nutritional defects, but these will not be discussed here.

A cuffed endotracheal tube is required to mechanically ventilate a patient with positive pressure. If the tube is placed nasally, sinus drainage may be impaired. Not infrequently this results in sinusitis manifested as fever without an obvious source. Sinus films may be required to confirm the diagnosis. In addition, the endotracheal tube, in spite of its cuff, allows aspiration and impairs pulmonary defense mechanisms. Thus, nosocomial pneumonia is a frequent complication of prolonged intubation, although patients with this complication usually have additional risk factors as well.

Meticulous application of sterile airway care and suctioning is mandatory. Trauma to the upper airway, either during intubation or from inappropriate cuff inflation, is a major concern. Low pressure - high volume cuffs have decreased the incidence of tracheomalacia, but proper technique in ensuring a minimal leak remains critical. Vocal cord damage is not uncommon and glottic edema or ulceration occurs frequently. Therefore, following extubation patients should be examined for stridor by auscultation over the larynx. If present, inhalation of racemic epinepherine may reverse edema but reintubation may be necessary. Tracheostomy may avoid some laryngeal complications, but this has not been clearly established. We utilize tracheostomy to make the patient more comfortable, provide a larger airway, and to allow the patient to eat. This decision is usually made when it appears that an endotracheal tube will be necessary for longer than one week.

Ventilator malfunction is now unusual. However, if breathing difficulty develops during mechanical ventilation, the patient should be removed from the ventilator and ventilated with a resuscitation bag and supplemental oxygen. The ventilator may then be evaluated by respiratory therapy personnel. Disconnection from the ventilator should also be rare, and low pressure and volume alarms should be in place to alert the staff of this potential disaster. These are no substitute for constant vigilance by the nursing staff. This is especially critical in paralyzed patients; it is mandatory to have attendants continuously at the bedside of such individuals.

Increased airway pressure can cause barotrauma or hemodynamic alterations. Barotrauma may be manifested as pneumothorax, mediastinal emphysema, subcutaneous emphysema, or rarely, pneumoperitoneum. Pneumothorax is almost always life-threatening in ventilated patients and requires immediate insertion of a thoracostomy tube connected to closed drainage or suction. Mediastinal and subcutaneous emphysema are not life-threatening but should alert the clinician to the possibility of subsequent pneumothorax. The hemodynamic compromise associated with increased intrathoracic pressure (see above) is almost always related to decreased preload. Hypotension usually responds to volume expansion, although if blood pressure falls to critical levels vasoactive drugs may be necessary. Hyponatremia is seen more frequently in patients who are mechanically ventilated. Restriction of free water is frequently effective in correcting this. Increased secretion of antidiuretic hormone is one postulated mechanism; altered renal handling of solute and water may also occur. Increased intrathoracic pressure may produce changes in blood flow to regions of the kidney, liver, and splanchic bed. The physiologic importance of these alterations is unclear.

Finally, increased intrathoracic pressure may produce a decrease in cerebral perfusion pressure, particularly if systemic arterial pressure is reduced, intracranial pressure is elevated, or intracranial compliance is decreased. This occurs commonly with head injuries but is rare in the CCU.

FURTHER READING

1. Dupuis YG. Ventilators: Theory and clinical practice.   C. V.
   Mosby Co, St. Louis, 1986.

2. Morganroth ML, ed. Mechanical ventilation. Clin Chest Med 1988;
   9(1):1-173.

3. Natanson C, Shelhamer JH, Parrillo JE. Intubation of the trachea
   in the critical care setting.   JAMA 1985;253:1160-1165.

4. Smith BE, Hanning CD.   Advances in respiratory support.   Br J
   Anaesth 1986;58:138-150.

Chapter 10

Diagnosis and Early Management

Diagnosis of Acute Myocardial Infarction

The three cardinal features of acute myocardial infarction (MI) are a history of ischemic chest pain of at least 30 minutes duration, typical ECG changes which evolve over several days, and elevations of serum enzymes in a characteristic pattern. Classically, the diagnosis of acute MI has rested on the presence of at least two of the three cardinal features. More recently, it has become apparent that a large percentage of patients with MI have either atypical symptoms or clinically "silent" infarcts, and that the ECG is often non-diagnostic as well, particularly when the circumflex coronary artery is involved or when there is a non-Q wave MI. By contrast, studies in the 1960s and 1970s demonstrated that specific patterns of creatine kinase (CK) and lactic dehydrogenase (LDH) isoenzyme elevations provide a highly sensitive and specific means for diagnosing acute MI (1-4). Thus, serial enzyme and isoenzyme determinations have emerged as the "gold standard" for establishing the diagnosis.

Several important drawbacks in present enzymatic methods for diagnosing acute MI are worth noting. Foremost among these is that diagnostic serum enzyme changes frequently do not appear until several hours after the onset of coronary occlusion. Not only does this limit the utility of these tests in patients presenting to the emergency room soon after the onset of symptoms (5-7), but acute intervention decisions for limitation of infarct size (Chapters 11-14), must often be made without the benefit of enzyme determinations. Fortunately, in the subgroup of patients with large infarcts who are most likely to benefit from acute intervention, the history and ECG are usually diagnostic.

A second problem with cardiac enzymes has to do with the interpretation of marginally abnormal values, particularly in the setting of non-diagnostic symptoms and ECG findings. Most laboratories now quantify both total CK and the MB isoenzyme. In the appropriate clinical setting, if the total CK is elevated and the MB fraction exceeds 6%, myocardial cell necrosis is very likely (7). However, if the total CK is not elevated or the MB fraction is in the range of 3-6%, the diagnosis is less certain. Heller et al (8) reported that 65% of patients with suspected MI and normal total CK but elevated MB-CK met other criteria for infarction. These authors suggest that these findings, which occur more frequently in elderly patients, should be considered indicative of myocardial damage (8). MB levels < 3% of the total CK are usually considered normal. Similarly, elevation of the total LDH with a reversed isoenzyme 1:2 ratio (i.e. LDH1 ≧ LDH2) is a reliable indicator of acute infarction, but less pronounced changes may be more difficult to interpret.

A third potential difficulty is the problem of "false-positive" enzyme elevations (Tables 10.1 and 10.2) (7). Many of the entities associated with false positivity can be readily differentiated from acute MI by obtaining serial enzymes and assessing the time course of enzymatic changes (Figure 10.1). A question which arises frequently is the effect of prolonged CPR and electrical cardioversion on enzyme determinations. In general, both of these maneuvers may produce modest elevations in total CK which are most likely due to skeletal muscle injury. In most cases, the effect on MB-CK is minimal unless repetitive high-energy electrical shocks are delivered. Finally, in evaluating total CK levels, it is important to recognize that muscle mass is an important factor determining baseline values. Thus, men tend to have higher CKs than women, elderly patients have lower CKs, and blacks have higher CKs than Caucasians (9).

In light of these considerations, it is apparent that the proper diagnosis of acute MI rests on a detailed clinical history, serial ECGs, and a careful analysis of both the magnitude and pattern of enzymatic changes. Despite these tools, the accuracy of the diagnosis still remains in doubt in a small percentage of patients.

Before leaving this section, one other issue bears comment. This is the problem of confirming a diagnosis of acute MI in a patient presenting more than 48 hours after symptom onset with non-diagnostic ECG changes. As shown in Figure 10.1, CKs and transaminase levels may already have returned to normal, so that the LDH 1:2 ratio provides the best chance for enzymatic confirmation. In this situation, as well as in others in which the diagnosis remains uncertain, an echocardiogram or radionuclide angiogram may be helpful if wall motion abnormalities are identified. Thallium scintigraphy may also demonstrate a fixed perfusion defect compatible with an infarct, but its age cannot be determined. Technetium-99m pyrophosphate scanning exhibits 80-90% sensitivity and specificity in diagnosing acute transmural infarction, but it is only 40-50% sensitive for small, non-Q wave MIs (10). In addition, the scan may not be able to distinguish small infarcts from unstable angina or other conditions. Also, since maximum sensitivity occurs 36-72 hours after the onset of infarction followed by gradual resolution of abnormal uptake over 7-10 days (11), the test is frequently not helpful in diagnosing small infarcts in those patients presenting late. Thus, pyrophosphate scanning has a limited role in the diagnosis of acute MI in patients admitted to the CCU. It may, however, be useful in evaluating patients following cardiac surgery (12).

Table 10.1
Causes of "False Positive" Elevations of MB-CK*

A. Technical factors
   1. Spillover of MM-CK
   2. Atypical CK variant

B. Myocardial source
   1. Myocarditis
   2. Pericarditis
   3. Myocardial trauma
   4. Cardiac surgery

C. Systemic illness with cardiac involvement
   1. Muscular dystrophy
   2. Hypothermia or hyperthermia
   3. Reye's syndrome
   4. Collagen vascular disease, esp. systemic lupus erythematosus
   5. Rocky Mountain spotted fever
   6. Polymyositis

D. Peripheral source
   1. Myositis
   2. Rhabdomyolysis
   3. Vigorous exercise
   4. Prostate surgery
   5. Cesarian section
   6. Gastrointestinal surgery
   7. Splenic infarction
   8. Severe skeletal muscle trauma
   9. Chronic alcoholism
   10. Tumors

E. Miscellaneous
   1. Renal failure
   2. Hypothyroidism
   3. Subarachnoid hemorrhage
   4. Severe burns

* Adapted from Lee TH, Goldman L. Serum enzyme assays in the
  diagnosis of acute myocardial infarction. Ann Intern Med
  1986;105:224. Used with permission.

Table 10.2
Causes of Reversed LDH1:LDH2 Ratio

1. Acute myocardial infarction
2. Acute renal cortical infarction
3. Pernicious anemia
4. Sickle cell crisis
5. Hemolysis of any cause

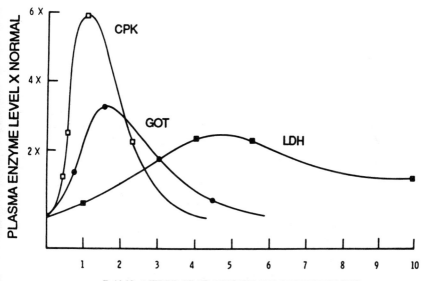

Figure 10.1.   Time course of enzyme changes following acute myocardial infarction.   CPK: creatine kinase; GOT: glutamate oxaloacetic transaminase; LDH, lactic dehydrogenase.   From Hearse DJ. Myocardial enzyme leakage.   J Mol Med 1977;2:185.   Used with permission.

Early Management

The principal goals of the early CCU phase of acute myocardial infarction are to: 1)   relieve chest pain, dyspnea, and anxiety; 2)   stabilize hemodynamics and minimize complications; and 3)   limit myocardial infarct size.   The management of chest pain is discussed in Chapter 4.   Supplemental oxygen and diuretics should be administered as indicated for dyspnea.   Morphine and benzodiazepines are useful for reducing anxiety.   Management of hemodynamic problems and other complications are discussed in detail in subsequent chapters. Finally, as it is now well established that the cumulative extent of myocardial damage is the most potent predictor of both short and long-term prognosis, it is essential that the early management of acute MI be oriented towards limitation of infarct size, particularly in patients presenting within the first few hours of infarct onset. Limitation of infarct size encompasses both measures designed to salvage ischemic myocardium and the avoidance of agents or procedures which might increase oxygen demand, such as inotropic agents or other drugs which may increase heart rate (e.g., nifedipine, hydralazine). Fever should be treated promptly with aspirin or acetaminophen. Blood pressure should be normalized and the heart rate should be controlled if possible. The next four chapters will review the current status of interventions designed to limit infarct size. It should be recognized, however, that this is a rapidly evolving field, and information presented here may already be out-of-date by the time this manual appears in press.

REFERENCES

1. Wagner GS, Roe CR, Limbird LE, Rosati RA, Wallace AG. The importance of identification of the myocardial-specific isoenzyme of creatinine phosphokinase (MB form) in the diagnosis of acute myocardial infarction. Circulation 1973;47:263-269.

2. Roberts R, Gowda KS, Ludbrook PA, Sobol BE. Specificity of elevated serum MB creatine phosphokinase activity in the diagnosis of acute myocardial infarction. Am J Cardiol 1975;36:433-437.

3. Vasudevan G, Mercer DW, Varat MA. Lactic dehydrogenase isoenzyme determination in the diagnosis of acute myocardial infarction. Circulation 1978;57:1055-1057.

4. Grande P, Christiansen C, Pedersen A, Christensen MS. Optimal diagnosis of acute myocardial infarction: A cost-effectiveness study. Circulation 1980;61:723-728.

5. Lee TH, Cook EF, Weisberg M, Sargent RK, Wilson C, Goldman L. Acute chest pain in the emergency room: Identification and examination of low-risk patients. Arch Intern Med 1985;145:65-69.

6. Lee TH, Weisberg MC, Cook EF, Daley K, Brand DA, Goldman L. Evaluation of creatine kinase and creatine kinase-MB for diagnosing myocardial infarction. Arch Intern Med 1987;147:115-121.

7. Lee TH, Goldman L. Serum enzyme assays in the diagnosis of acute myocardial infarction. Ann Intern Med 1986;105:221-233.

8. Heller GV, Blaustein AS, Wei JY. Implications of increased myocardial isoenzyme activity in the presence of normal serum creatine kinase activity. Am J Cardiol 1983;51:24-27.

9. Black HR, Quallich H, Gareleck CB. Racial differences in serum creatine kinase levels. Am J Med 1986;81:479-487.

10. Holman BL, Wynne J. Infarct avid (hot spot) myocardial scinti-graphy. Radiol Clin North Am 1980;18:487-499.

11. Berger HJ, Zaret BL. Nuclear cardiology. N Engl J Med 1981; 305:799–807 and 855–865.

12. Platt MR, Parkey RW, Willerson JT, Boute FJ, Shapiro W, Sugg WL. Technetium stannous pyrophosphate myocardial scintigrams in the recognition of myocardial infarction in patients undergoing coronary artery revascularization. Ann Thorac Surg 1976; 21:311–317.

Chapter 11

Limitation of Myocardial Infarct Size

It is estimated that 1.2–1.5 million acute MIs occur annually in the United States. Of these, approximately 30% are "silent" or clinically unrecognized, and an additional 10–15% of patients suffer arrhythmic death before ever reaching the hospital. Thus, 800,000 patients are hospitalized each year with a diagnosis of acute MI. Residual myocardial function, which correlates inversely with infarct size, is the most important determinant of short and long-term prognosis as well as functional status in patients surviving the first few hours of acute infarction (1,2). For this reason, in the past 20 years there has been considerable research effort expended in developing strategies for decreasing infarct size in the hope of reducing early and late mortality and improving functional class (3). However, in contrast to arrhythmic deaths, which have been dramatically reduced by the widespread availability of emergency medical services and coronary care units, until recently there has been little proof that ischemic myocardium could be effectively salvaged in humans with acute MI.

Acute MI occurs when there is a sustained imbalance between myocardial oxygen supply and demand, usually of at least 20–30 minutes duration. Theoretically, infarct size may be reduced by improving oxygen supply (e.g. by direct reperfusion, improved collateral flow, or enhanced oxygen delivery), decreasing myocardial oxygen demand (by reducing heart rate or altering loading characteristics), or by modifying the tissue response to ischemic injury. In addition, it has been shown that myocardial damage is usually complete within 6 hours after the onset of infarction, so that, in general, 6 hours is the maximum time during which any intervention may be expected to favorably affect infarct size. Furthermore, the more rapidly an intervention is initiated, the larger is the potential salutory effect (4–7). Thus, the importance of instituting treatment to limit MI size as quickly as possible cannot be overemphasized. Delays of as little as 30 minutes will result in a substantial loss of benefit.

Table 11.1 lists some of the interventions studied for limitation of infarct size. At present, only thrombolytic therapy and intravenous beta blockade have been shown to reduce infarct size and improve prognosis in the clinical setting. These two treatments are discussed in detail in the next two chapters. The remainder of this chapter will review some of the other approaches.

Table 11.1
Interventions for Limitation of Infarct Size

I. Measures to improve oxygen supply

   A. General measures
      1. Correct hypoxemia
      2. Correct alkalosis
      3. Correct anemia

   B. Improve collateral flow
      1. Nitroglycerin
      2. Other vasodilators

   C. Inotropic agents

   D. Revascularization
      1. Thrombolysis
      2. Angioplasty
      3. Coronary bypass surgery

II. Measures to reduce oxygen demand

   A. General measures
      1. Maintain normothermia
      2. Control blood pressure
      3. Alleviate anxiety

   B. Pharmacologic agents
      1. Beta blockers
      2. Nitroglycerin
      3. Calcium channel blockers
      4. Other vasodilators

   C. Intra-aortic balloon counterpulsation

III. Alteration of tissue response to ischemia; metabolic factors

   A. Calcium channel blockers
   B. Hyaluronidase
   C. Glucocorticoids
   D. Non-steroidal anti-inflammatory drugs
   E. Glucose-insulin-potassium
   F. Anti-oxidants

General Measures

In years past, the goal of early acute MI management was to make the patient comfortable and allow the heart to rest. In recent years, there has been increased emphasis on aggressive intervention, but the importance of prior conventional wisdom should not be overlooked.

Oxygen supply to the ischemic tissue may be enhanced in several ways. Arterial oxygen saturation should be maintained at 90% or greater by administration of supplemental oxygen. Optimal arterial pH is 7.35-7.40; alkalosis shifts the oxyhemoglobin saturation curve to the left, thereby inhibiting oxygen release (Fig. 11.1), while acidosis interferes with myocardial contractility. Serum hemoglobin concentration is an important determinant of arterial oxygen content, and severe anemia may exacerbate ischemia. In general, a hemoglobin of > 10 g/dl is desirable, and transfusion is indicated if the hemoglobin is < 8 g/dl.

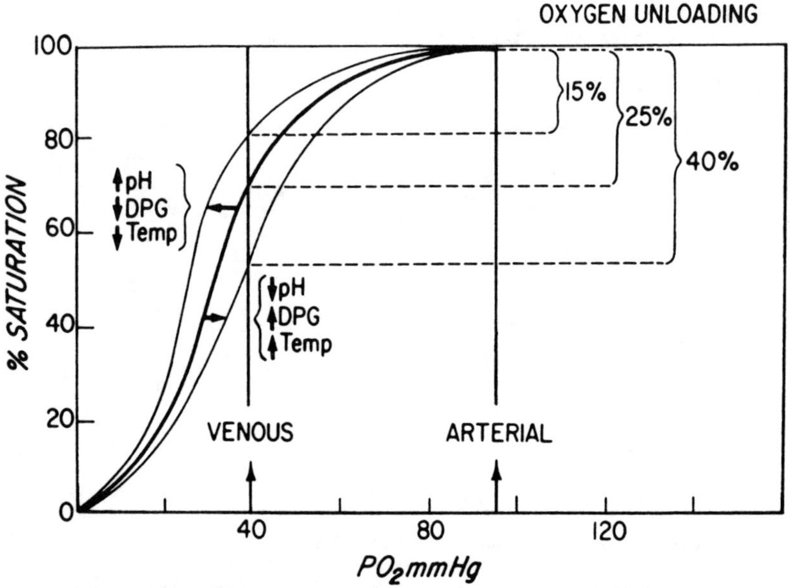

Figure 11.1. Oxyhemoglobin dissociation curve of normal blood. DPG: 2,3-diphosphoglycerate. From Bunn HF. Pallor and anemia. In: Isselbacher KJ, et al, eds. Harrison's principles of internal medicine, 9th ed. McGraw-Hill Book Co, New York, 1980:266. Used with permission.

Fever increases oxygen demand by increasing the metabolic rate, while at the same time shifting the oxygen saturation curve to the right. The net effect on the oxygen supply/demand ratio is unfavorable, so that fever should be suppressed with aspirin or acetaminophen. Hypertension increases oxygen demand by increasing afterload, while hypotension diminishes coronary perfusion pressure. Optimally, blood pressure should be maintained in the normal range. Rapid reduction of the blood pressure should be avoided, however, since this may compromise coronary blood flow. Finally, the anxiety and resultant sympathetic arousal associated with acute infarction should be minimized with the judicious use of analgesics, anxiolytics, and beta blockers.

Nitroglycerin and Other Vasodilators

Nitroglycerin decreases myocardial oxygen demand by reducing preload, and also improves oxygen supply through direct coronary vasodilation and by increasing collateral blood flow. At one time, nitroglycerin was thought to be contraindicated in acute MI because of its potential for causing hypotension, reflex tachycardia, and a coronary steal syndrome. Current data do not support the concept of nitroglycerin–induced coronary steal, but marked hypotensive responses and reflex tachycardia can occur, particularly in patients with reduced left ventricular preload as a result of hypovolemia or right ventricular infarction. However, with the availability of transcutaneous and intravenous delivery systems, nitroglycerin can be administered safely in most patients with acute MI.

Several studies have now been published evaluating the use of intravenous nitroglycerin for limiting infarct size (8-10). The results have been generally favorable but not completely conclusive, intravenous nitroglycerin cannot be recommended for routine use in acute MI at this time. Nonetheless, nitroglycerin is quite useful in the management of persistent ischemic chest pain, hypertension, and pulmonary congestion, and we maintain a relatively low threshold for its use at our institution. Blood pressure should be monitored carefully during nitroglycerin infusion, and the reduction in mean arterial pressure should not exceed 10 mm Hg, nor should the fall in systolic pressure exceed 20 mm Hg during the first 6 hours of MI.

Several properties of nitroprusside make it less desirable than nitroglycerin in the early hours of acute MI. Nitroprusside causes intrapulmonic shunting which may lead to a fall in oxygen saturation (nitroglycerin does this to a lesser degree), and it may produce a coronary steal by shunting blood away from the ischemic zone to nonischemic areas (11). In addition, hypotension and reflex tachycardia may be more pronounced than with nitroglycerin. The drug should therefore not be used in the early phase of acute MI (12). However, nitroprusside may be useful in the management of post-MI congestive heart failure, in low output states associated with a high pulmonary artery occlusive pressure (13), and in the management of acute mitral regurgitation or ventricular septal rupture (Chapter 20). Other vasodilatators, including angiotensin converting enzyme inhibitors, have not been adequately studied in the acute setting.

Calcium Antagonists

Experimentally, calcium antagonists have been shown to limit infarct size by improving coronary blood flow, decreasing oxygen demand, and inhibiting the detrimental effects of calcium influx into the ischemic myocytes. Unfortunately, clinical trials of calcium blockers have been disappointing.

Three studies evaluating the acute administration of nifedipine have now been reported (Table 11.2); in each case, there was either no benefit or a trend toward adverse outcome in nifedipine-treated patients. These findings may be due to adverse effects of this agent on heart rate (reflex tachycardia) and blood pressure (hypotension). Thus, nifedipine should be avoided in the early phase of acute MI.

Table 11.2
Randomized Trials of Nifedipine in Acute MI

| | N | % Change in Nifepidine Patients Relative to Placebo | | |
		Infarct Prevention	MI Size	Mortality
Muller[14]	171	0%	0%	↑7.9%*
Sirnes[15]	227	↓6.1%+	↑8.7%+	0%
Wilcox[16]	4488	0%	--	↑0.5%+

*p < .05   +not significant

Initial results with verapamil were encouraging (17,18), but in the only large scale trial reported to date, verapamil was associated with increased early mortality, primarily due to a higher incidence of congestive heart failure and cardiogenic shock (19). Thus, verapamil should also be avoided in the early hours of acute MI. On the other hand, this study reported a lower mortality in verapamil-treated patients between 3 weeks and 6 months, suggesting a benefical effect of this agent in secondary prevention following acute MI.

Diltiazem reduces infarct size in animals but has not been adequately studied in humans. It has been shown to reduce early re-infarction in patients presenting with initial non-Q wave MI (20). In patients with acute MI who require a calcium channel blocker, diltiazem may be preferrable to nifedipine or verapamil because it has fewer hemodynamic effects and a more favorable side-effect profile.

Metabolic Agents

Hyaluronidase reduces experimental infarct size, presumably by improving nutrient delivery to the ischemic tissue, but clinical trials have failed to demonstrate significant benefit (21,22). Glucocorticoids reduce edema and inflammation in the infarct zone but adversely affect infarct healing (23), particularly when administered in high doses (24).   Non-steroidal anti-inflammatory agents may limit MI size through similar mechanisms, but may retard healing and contribute to myocardial rupture (25).   In addition, some of these agents may decrease coronary blood flow by increasing coronary vascular tone (26).   Glucose is the primary energy source in ischemic myocytes, and glucose-insulin-potassium infusions could theoretically inhibit or delay cell death by increasing glucose availability. However, clinical studies using this combination are inconclusive (27).   Oxygen-free radicals are generated by ischemic tissue and accelerate necrosis, but there is currently little data that anti-oxidants such as superoxide dismutase, allopurinol, and vitamin E can effectively alter the course of infarction in humans.   Thus, none of these metabolic agents can be recommended for routine use in acute MI at this time.

Miscellaneous

In patients with low cardiac output, inotropic agents may improve coronary blood flow (by increasing cardiac output) and decrease oxygen demand by reducing wall stress and pre-load.   On the other hand, these agents increase myocardial oxygen consumption by increasing contractility and, in the case of sympathomimetic agents, by increasing heart rate.   Such agents are useful in the management of congestive heart failure (Chapter 17), but should usually be avoided during the first 6 hours of infarction if possible.

Intra-aortic balloon (IABP) counterpulsation reduces myocardial work while enhancing coronary blood flow and increasing cardiac output (Chapter 37).   Although useful in the management of cardiogenic shock and other post-infarction complications, the IABP has not been shown to limit infarct size (28).

REFERENCES

1.   Sanz G, Castaner A, Betriu A, et al. Determinants of prognosis in survivors of myocardial infarction. N Engl J Med 1982; 306:1065-1070.

2.   The Multicenter Postinfarction Research Group.   Risk stratification and survival after myocardial infarction.   N Engl J Med 1983;309:331-336.

3.   Rude RE, Muller JE, Braunwald E. Efforts to limit the size of myocardial infarcts.   Ann Intern Med 1981;95:736-761.

4.   Schwarz F, Schuler G, Katus H, et al.   Intracoronary thrombolysis in acute myocardial infarction: Duration of ischemia as a major determinant of late results after recanalization.   Am J Cardiol 1982;50:933-937.

5. Davies GJ, Chierchia S, Maseri A. Prevention of myocardial infarction by very early treatment with intracoronary strepto- kinase. N Engl J Med 1984;311:1488-1492.

6. Mathey DG, Sheehan FH, Schofer J, Dodge HT. Time from onset of symptoms to thrombolytic therapy: A major determinant of myocardial salvage in patients with acute transmural infarction. J Am Coll Cardiol 1985;6:518-525.

7. Koren G, Weiss AT, Hasin Y, et al. Prevention of myocardial damage in acute myocardial ischemia by early treatment with intravenous streptokinase. N Engl J Med 1985;313:1384-1389.

8. Bussman WD, Passek D, Seidel W, Kaltenbach M. Reduction of CK and CK-MB indexes of infarct size by intravenous nitroglycerin. Circulation 1981;63:615-622.

9. Flaherty JT, Becker LC, Bulkley BH, et al. A randomized prospective trial of intravenous nitroglycerin in patients with acute myocardial infarction. Circulation 1983;68:576-588.

10. Jaffe AS, Geltman EM, Tiefenbrunn AF, et al. Reduction of infarct size in patients with inferior infarction with intravenous glyceryl trinitrate. Br Heart J 1983;49:452-460.

11. Mann T, Cohn PF, Holman BL, Green LH, Markis JE, Phillips DA. Effect of nitroprusside on regional myocardial blood flow in coronary artery disease. Circulation 1978;57:732-738.

12. Chiariello M, Gold HK, Leinbach RC, Davis MA, Maroko PR. Comparison between the effects of nitroprusside and nitroglycerin on ischemic injury during acute myocardial infarction. Circulation 1976;54:766-773.

13. Cohn JN, Franciosa JA, Francis GS, et al. Effect of short-term infusion of sodium nitroprusside on mortality rate in acute myocardial infarction complicated by left ventricular failure. N Engl J Med 1982;306:1129-1135.

14. Muller JE, Morrison J, Stone PH, et al. Nifedipine therapy for patients with threatened and acute myocardial infarction: A ran- domized, double-blind, placebo-controlled comparison. Circula- tion 1984;69:740-747.

15. Sirnes PA, Overskeid K, Pederson TR, et al. Evolution of infarct size during the early use of nifedipine in patients with acute myocardial infarction: The Norwegian nifedipine multicenter trial. Circulation 1984;70:638-644.

16. Wilcox RG, Hampton JR, Banks DC, et al. Trial of early nifedipine treatment in patients with suspected myocardial infarction (the TRENT Study). Br Heart J 1986;55:506. (Abstr)

17. Bussman WD, Seher W, Gruengras M. Reduction of creatine kinase and creatine kinase—MB indexes of infarct size by intravenous verapamil. Am J Cardiol 1984;54:1224–1230.

18. Heikkila J, Nieminen MS. Effects of verapamil in patients with acute myocardial infarction: Hemodynamics and function of normal and ischemic left ventricular myocardium. Am Heart J 1984;107:241–247.

19. Danish Multicenter Study Group on Verapamil in Myocardial Infarction. Verapamil in acute myocardial infarction. Am J Cardiol 1984; 54(Suppl E):24E–28E.

20. Gibson RS, Boden WE, Theroux P, et al. Diltiazem and reinfarction in patients with non-Q-wave myocardial infarction. N Engl J Med 1986;315:423–429.

21. MILIS Study Group. Hyaluronidase therapy for acute myocardial infarction: Results of a randomized, blinded, multicenter trial. Am J Cardiol 1986;57:1236–1243.

22. Julian DG, Pentecost BL, Simpson JM, Smith RH, Codigan PJ, Petri MP. Intravenous hyaluronidase in suspected acute myocardial infarction. Circulation 1985;72(Suppl III):III–222. (Abstr)

23. Bulkley BH, Roberts WC. Steroid therapy during acute myocardial infarction: A cause of delayed healing and ventricular aneurysm. Am J Med 1974;56:244–250.

24. Hammerman H, Kloner RA, Hale S, Schoen FJ, Braunwald E. Dose-dependent effects of short-term methylprednisolone on myocardial infarct extent, scar formation, and ventricular function. Circulation 1983;68:446–452.

25. Silverman HS, Pfeifer MP. Relation between use of anti-inflammatory agents and left ventricular free wall rupture during acute myocardial infarction. Am J Cardiol 1987;59:363–364.

26. Friedman PL, Brown EJ, Gunther S, et al. Coronary vaso-constrictor effect of indomethacin in patients with coronary artery disease. N Engl J Med 1981;305:1171–1175.

27. Rogers WJ, McDaniel HG, Mantle JA, Rackley CE. Prospective randomized trial of glucose-insulin-potassium: Effects on hemodynamics, short and long-term survival. J Am Coll Cardiol 1983;1:628. (Abstr)

28. Flaherty JT, Becker LC, Weiss JL, et al. Results of a randomized prospective trial of intra-aortic balloon counterpulsation and intravenous nitroglycerin in patients with acute myocardial infarction. J Am Coll Cardiol 1985;6:434–446.

Chapter 12

Thrombolytic Therapy

Although thrombolytic agents were first used in patients with acute myocardial infarction in the 1950s, intensive clinical investigation did not begin until the 1980s, after De Wood et al (1) conclusively demonstrated an 85-90% incidence of total thrombotic coronary occlusion in patients undergoing coronary angiography within 6 hours of onset of acute transmural infarction. Numerous studies showing beneficial effect of early reperfusion on mortality and left ventricular function have now been published (2-20). Based on these reports, in November, 1987 the Food and Drug Administration licensed intravenous streptokinase and tissue plasminogen activator (TPA) for use in acute MI. This chapter will summarize some of the major clinical trials involving these agents, outline protocols for their use, and briefly discuss some of the commonly asked questions about thrombolytic therapy. It should be noted that knowledge in this area is proliferating rapidly, and guidelines for using thrombolytic agents are likely to evolve as new data become available.

Clinical Trials

Effect on Mortality and Ventricular Function

There have now been 9 large, prospective randomized trials evaluating the effect of early thrombolytic treatment on mortality (Table 12.1). Six of these trials involved streptokinase (either intracoronary or intravenous), two involved tissue plasminogen activator (TPA), and one used anisoylated plasminogen-streptokinase activator complex (APSAC). All trials showed a reduction in early mortality in treated patients; in all but one trial, the difference was statistically significant. Furthermore, this survival benefit appears to be maintained for at least 1 year (5,6,14,15,17). In the recent ISIS-2 trial, aspirin was independently associated with a reduction in mortality, and the combination of aspirin plus streptokinase was superior to either agent alone (15). Similarly, TPA together with aspirin may be more beneficial than TPA alone (16,20). Studies have also shown that patients treated with streptokinase, TPA, or APSAC have improved left ventricular function as compared with controls. The absolute magnitude of improvement in ejection fraction ranges from 2-9% and is highly dependent on time to treatment. At present, these three agents appear comparable in their ability to salvage myocardium, improve ventricular function, and reduce mortality.

Table 12.1
Effect of Thrombolytic Therapy on Early Mortality

	Route/Agent	N	Mortality (%) Control	Treatment	Difference	Ref
Western Washington	ICSK	250	11.2	3.7	-67%	4,5
Netherlands	IC+IVSK	533	11.7	5.9	-50%	9
GISSI	IVSK	11806	13.0	10.7	-18%	8,14
ISAM	IVSK	1741	7.1	6.3	-11%	11
New Zealand	IVSK	219	12.9	2.5	-81%	13
AIMS	IVAPSAC	1004	12.2	6.4	-47%	17
ISIS-2	IVSK	17187	12.0	9.2	-23%	15
ASSET	IVTPA	5011	9.8	7.2	-26%	16
ECSG	IVTPA	721	5.7	2.8	-51%	20

ICSK: intracoronary streptokinase, IVSK: intravenous streptokinase,
IVTPA: intravenous tissue plasminogen activator, IVAPSAC: intravenous
anisoylated plasminogen-streptokinase activator complex

Clinical Course and Complications

The GISSI trial (8), ISIS-2 (15), and ASSET (16), by virtue of
their size (Table 12.1), provide the best available data on the
hospital course and incidence of complications following
administration of intravenous streptokinase or TPA. Table 12.2
summarizes adverse reactions in these trials. The incidence of major
bleeding (i.e., requiring transfusion) is quite low and, although the
studies cannot be strictly compared, bleeding does not appear to be
less frequent with TPA despite the fact that it induces a less intense
systemic "lytic" state. Minor allergic reactions to streptokinase
occur infrequently, and anaphylaxis is very rare; allergic reactions
to TPA have not been reported. Drug-induced hypotension also occurs
in 3-10% of patients treated with streptokinase. This complication,
which occurs with increasing frequency at infusion rates exceeding 500
U/kg/min, usually responds to a reduction in the rate of administration, but may require initiation of a vasopressor agent.

The incidence of other non-fatal events (e.g., ventricular
arrhythmias or CHF) varies in the different trials, but in general
patients receiving thrombolytic therapy tend to have a more favorable
course with fewer complications. Of particular note is that although

Table 12.2
Adverse Reactions to Thrombolytic Therapy*

	GISSI (N=5860)	ISIS-2 (N=8592)	ASSET (N=2512)
Major bleeding	0.3%	0.5%	1.4%
Minor bleeding	3.7%	3.5%	6.3%
Allergic reactions	2.3%	4.4%	0
Anaphylaxis	0.1%	0	0
Hypotension	3.0%	10.0%	NR
Stroke	1.1%	0.7%	1.1%
Intracerebral hemorrhage	NR	0.1%	0.3%

NR = not reported

* Intravenous streptokinase in GISSI and ISIS-2 (Ref. 8,15); intravenous TPA in ASSET (Ref. 16)

clinical reinfarction occurred twice as often in streptokinase-treated patients in the GISSI trial (8), the addition of aspirin in ISIS-2 decreased the reinfarction rate to the same level as in the control group (2%). In ASSET, the reinfarction rate with TPA and short-term heparin was similar to that seen with heparin alone (4%).

Patient Selection

In general, patients with potentially large infarcts who present very early in the course of infarction are most likely to benefit from interventional therapy. Traditional teaching has been that patients successfully reperfused within 2 hours of coronary occlusion will receive maximum benefit, those treated from 2-4 hours still receive substantial benefit, from 4-6 hours benefit is probably limited to selected subgroups, and beyond 6 hours benefit is likely to be small. Although this wisdom has recently been questioned by the publication of ISIS-2 (15), in which patients treated up to 24 hours with a combination of aspirin and streptokinase had a reduction in mortality, it is still true that the time from symptom onset to clinical presentation is among the most important factors influencing the likelihood of achieving significant myocardial salvage. Thus, this factor should continue to play an important role in patient selection. However, with ISIS-2 it is also clear that selected patients may benefit from treatment even after 6 hours.

Subgroup analyses of the major trials have failed to identify a population of patients who do not benefit from thrombolytic therapy. Thus, age, sex, infarct location, specific cardiac risk factors, and prior cardiac history cannot be used as sole selection criteria when evaluating a patient for thrombolytic therapy. Rather, the potential benefits and risks must be assessed in each patient individually. To this end, the following caveats should be kept in mind. First, the potential for benefit correlates directly with the amount of myocardium still in jeopardy at the time thrombolytic therapy is initiated. Therefore, the longer treatment is delayed, the less likely is the patient to benefit. In addition, since anterior MIs and MIs involving multiple anatomic territories on ECG tend to be larger than inferior and lateral infarcts, the potential for benefit is also greater. Combining these factors, it follows that a patient with a large anterior MI with CHF presenting at 5 hours after symptom onset may be a good candidate for thrombolysis, whereas a patient with a small, uncomplicated, inferior MI presenting at the same time is less likely to receive significant benefit. Age is another factor worthy of note. The package inserts for both streptokinase and TPA specify age greater than 75 years as a relative contraindication to thrombolytic therapy, and a small, retrospective study indicated a higher incidence of complications in patients over 75 years of age (21). In the GISSI trial (8), mortality was lower in patients over 75 years receiving streptokinase, but not significantly so. On the other hand, there was no increase in complications in this age group, which included 592 patients treated with streptokinase. In ISIS-2 (15), a significant reduction in mortality was seen with treatment in patients 70 years or older. However, the magnitude of benefit was less than in younger patients, and the results in patients over 75 years were not reported separately. In ASSET (16), patients older than 75 years were excluded, so that the safety and efficacy of TPA in the very elderly has not been tested. On the other hand, the greatest benefit in this trial was seen in patients 66-75 years of age. In summary, the value of thrombolytic therapy in patients over 75 years of age has not been proven, but with careful selection it is likely that some patients will benefit. Therefore, age per se should not be considered a contraindication to thrombolytic therapy.

Choice of Thrombolytic Agent

At this writing, streptokinase, urokinase, and recombinant TPA are available for use in the United States. It seems likely that anisoylated plasminogen-streptokinase activator complex (APSAC; anistreplase) will be approved in the near future. Each of these agents has potential advantages and disadvantages compared with the others, so that at present there is no consensus as to which is the "preferred" thrombolytic agent for use in acute MI (22,23).

Two randomized trials comparing intravenous TPA and streptokinase have now been published (24,25). In both trials, the reperfusion rate was higher with TPA (70% vs. 55% and 62% vs. 31%). The incidence of major complications, including bleeding, was similar with both drugs, although there was less fibrinogen depletion with TPA. Despite these factors, existing data suggest that streptokinase and TPA have comparable effects on ventricular function and mortality and are associated with a similar risk of bleeding complications (Tables 12.1 and 12.2). In contrast, the cost of streptokinase is substantially less than TPA (< $200/1.5 million units vs. > $2000/100mg).

Intracoronary urokinase and streptokinase have comparable efficacy in achieving reperfusion, but urokinase causes less fibrinogen depletion and may reduce bleeding complications (26,27). Experience with urokinase in acute MI is limited, the drug is expensive, and it is not approved for intravenous use in acute MI at this time. APSAC improves ventricular function and reduces mortality (17), and has the additional advantage of administration by bolus injection rather than continuous infusion (28). The role of this agent in the treatment of acute MI remains to be seen.

Protocols for Use of Thrombolytic Agents

The decision to administer a thrombolytic agent to a patient with acute myocardial infarction must always be based on a careful assessment of the potential risks versus benefits. In general, the most important factors to consider are: (1) time elapsed since onset of infarction; (2) estimated extent of salvageable myocardium; and (3) risk of bleeding. Clearly, the earlier thrombolysis can be achieved, the more likely is the patient to benefit. Patients with large MIs, as judged by the extent of ECG changes and clinical criteria such as heart rate, blood pressure, and presence of pulmonary congestion, are also more likely to obtain significant myocardial salvage. Although no absolute guidelines can be given as to who should receive thrombolytic therapy, the approach outlined in Tables 12.3-12.5 is in keeping with current practice at most institutions.

Following initiation of thrombolytic therapy, patients should be observed closely for evidence of reperfusion and signs of bleeding or other adverse reactions. Clinical signs of reperfusion include a decrease in chest pain, return of ST segment shifts toward baseline,

Table 12.3
Indications for Thrombolytic Therapy

    1. Acute onset of chest pain or other ischemic symptoms within 6 hours of presentation*

AND

    2. Electrocardiographic evidence of acute MI, as indicated by ST segment elevation or depression in 2 or more contiguous leads, or by the presence of "hyperacute" T-waves.[+]

*   Recent evidence suggests that some patients presenting more than 6 hours after symptom onset may also benefit from thrombolytic therapy (15).

[+]   Other causes of ST segment changes and T-wave abnormalities, such as intraventricular conduction defects, left ventricular hypertrophy, and pericarditis, should be excluded. The presence of Q-waves does not preclude thrombolytic therapy.

Table 12.4
Contraindications to Thrombolytic Therapy

1. Absolute
   a. Active, uncontrollable bleeding
   b. Recent major surgery or trauma (< 10 days)
   c. Recent cerebrovascular event (< 2 months)
   d. Intracranial neoplasm
   e. Known hemorrhagic diathesis
   f. Severe uncontrolled hypertension (BP ≥ 200/120)
   g. Pregnancy

2. Relative*
   a. Active peptic ulcer disease
   b. Chronic cerebrovascular disease
   c. Diabetic hemorrhagic retinopathy
   d. Recent prolonged cardiopulmonary resuscitation
   e. Recent minor surgical procedure (such as organ biopsy)
   f. Active endocarditis
   g. Intramyocardial thrombus
   h. Persistent moderate hypertension (BP ≥ 180/110)
   i. Age ≥ 75 years
   j. Recent puncture of non-compressible vessel
   k. Any other condition predisposing to excessive bleeding
   l. Advanced unrelated illness
   m. Allergy to specific agent

*Potential risk must be weighed carefully against
potential benefit.

reperfusion arrhythmias, hemodynamic stabilization, rapid evolution of
ECG changes, and an early peaking of the CK and CK-MB (within 18 hours
of symptom onset) due to the enzymes being "washed out" of the
ischemic zone. Although one or more of these findings is usually seen
following successful thrombolysis, reperfusion may occur in their
absence. Reperfusion arrhythmias typically occur 15 minutes to 2
hours after recanalization, and most commonly consist of frequent
ventricular premature beats, accelerated idioventricular rhythm, or
short runs of ventricular tachycardia. In inferior infarcts,
bradycardia and A-V nodal block may occur. Reperfusion arrhythmias
are usually self-limited and require no specific therapy, but
occasionally ventricular fibrillation or profound bradycardia
requiring aggressive treatment may occur. Major bleeding may occur up
to 48 hours after completion of therapy, and is more common in
patients maintained on heparin following thrombolysis. Treatment of
major bleeding consists of discontinuation of anti-coagulants and
administration of blood products as needed to maintain an adequate
hemoglobin level (usually ≥ 10 g/dl) and reverse the hemostatic
defect. Hypotension during streptokinase infusion should prompt a
reduction in the infusion rate. Other major complications from
thrombolytic therapy are infrequent.

Table 12.5
Suggested Protocols for Use of Thrombolytic Agents

I. General measures prior to initiation of therapy

    A. Admission blood work, urinalysis, stool for occult blood
    B. Begin continuous ECG monitoring
    C. Minimum of one free-flowing intravenous line
    D. Lidocaine 75-100 mg IV followed by continuous infusion*
    E. Aspirin 160 mg, chewed or swallowed
    F. Heparin 5000 U by bolus injection[+]

II. Streptokinase

    A. Hydrocortisone 100 mg IV bolus*
    B. Diphenhydramine 50 mg IV bolus*
    C. 1.5 million units intravenous streptokinase by continuous infusion over 60 minutes
    D. Reduce infusion rate if hypotension develops
    E. Consider smaller dose for patients $\geq$ 75 years of age

III. Tissue plasminogen activator (total dose 100 mg)

    A. 10 mg IV bolus over 2 minutes
    B. 50 mg by continuous infusion over 60 minutes
    C. 40 mg by continuous infusion over 120 minutes (20 mg/hr)
    D. For patients < 65 kg, a total dose of 1.5 mg/kg should be used

IV. Following thrombolytic therapy

    A. Heparin to maintain PTT 1.5-2.5 X control[+]
    B. Aspirin 160-325 mg/day
    C. Monitor closely for evidence of reperfusion, bleeding, other adverse effects
    D. Further cardiac evaluation as clinically indicated

* Optional

[+] Although most centers use heparin, the specific dosage and timing vary widely.

    Effective thrombolysis with myocardial salvage produces a region of myocardium which remains in ischemic jeopardy due to persistence of the underlying atherosclerotic plaque. Patients are thus at increased risk for re-infarction during follow-up (5,6,8). For this reason, early catheterization and evaluation for possible angioplasty or bypass surgery may be advisable. However, the precise role and appropriate timing of these procedures remain undefined (Chapter 14).

REFERENCES

1. DeWood MA, Spores J, Notske R, et al. Prevalence of total occlusion during the early hours of transmural myocardial infarction. N Engl J Med 1980;303:897-902.

2. Anderson JL, Marshall HW, Bray BE, et al. A randomized trial of intracoronary streptokinase in the treatment of acute myocardial infarction. N Engl J Med 1983;308:1312-1318.

3. Smalling RW, Fuentes F, Matthews MW, et al. Sustained improvement in left ventricular function and mortality by intracoronary streptokinase administration during evolving myocardial infarction. Circulation 1983;68:131-138.

4. Kennedy JW, Ritchie JL, Davis KB, Fritz JK. Western Washington randomized trial of intracoronary streptokinase in acute myocardial infarction. New Engl J Med 1983;309:1477-1482

5. Kennedy JW, Ritchie JL, Davis KB, Stadius ML, Maynard C, Fritz JK. The Western Washington randomized trial of intracoronary streptokinase in acute myocardial infarction: A 12-month follow-up report. N Engl J Med 1985;312:1073-1078.

6. Simoons ML, Serruys PW, vanden Brand M. Improved survival after early thrombolysis in acute myocardial infarction. Lancet 1985;II:578-581.

7. Koren G, Weiss AT, Hasin Y, et al. Prevention of myocardial damage in acute myocardial ischemia by early treatment with intravenous streptokinase. N Engl J Med 1985;313:1384-1389.

8. Gruppo Italiano per lo studio della streptochinasi nell'infarto miocardico (GISSI). Effectiveness of intravenous thrombolytic treatment in acute myocardial infarction. Lancet 1986;I:397-402.

9. Simoons ML, Serruys PW, vanden Brand M, et al. Early thrombolysis in acute myocardial infarction: Limitation of infarct size and improved survival. J Am Coll Cardiol 1986;7:717-728.

10. Serruys PW, Simoons ML, Suryapranata H, et al. Preservation of global and regional left ventricular function after early thrombolysis in acute myocardial infarction. J Am Coll Cardiol 1986;7:729-742.

11. The I.S.A.M. Study Group. A prospective trial of intravenous streptokinase in acute myocardial infarction (I.S.A.M.). N Engl J Med 1986;314:1465-1471.

12. Sheehan FH, Braunwald E, Canner P, et al. The effect of intravenous thrombolytic therapy on left ventricular function: A report on tissue-type plasminogen activator and streptokinase from the thrombolysis in myocardial infarction (TIMI Phase I) trial. Circulation 1987;75:817-829.

13. White HD, Norris RM, Brown MA, et al. Effect of intravenous streptokinase on left ventricular function and early survival after acute myocardial infarction. N Engl J Med 1987;317:850-855.

14. Gruppo Italiano per lo studio della streptochinasi nell'infarto miocardico (GISSI). Long-term effects of intravenous thrombolysis in acute myocardial infarction: A final report of the GISSI study. Lancet 1987;II:871-874.

15. ISIS-2 (Second International Study of Infarct Survival) Collaborative Group. Randomised trial of intravenous streptokinase, oral aspirin, both, or neither among 17,187 cases of suspected acute myocardial infarction: ISIS-2. Lancet 1988;II:349-360.

16. Wilcox RG, von der Lippe G, Olsson CG, et al. Trial of tissue plasminogen activator for mortality reduction in acute myocardial infarction. Anglo-Scandinavian Study of Early Thrombolysis (ASSET). Lancet 1988;II:525-530.

17. AIMS Trial Study Group. Effect on intravenous APSAC on mortality after acute myocardial infarction: preliminary report of a placebo-controlled clinical trial. Lancet 1988;I:545-549.

18. Guerci AD, Gerstenblith G, Brinker JA, et al. A randomized trial of intravenous tissue plasminogen activator for acute myocardial infarction with subsequent randomization to elective coronary angioplasty. N Engl J Med 1987;317:1613-1618.

19. National Heart Foundation of Australia Coronary Thrombolysis Group. Coronary thrombolysis and myocardial salvage by tissue plasminogen activator given up to 4 hours after onset of myocardial infarction. Lancet 1988;I:203-208.

20. Van de Werf F, Arnold A. Intravenous tissue plasminogen activator and size of infarct, left ventricular function, and survival in acute myocardial infarction. Br Med J 1988;297:1374-1379.

21. Lew AS, Hod H, Cercek B, Shah PK, Ganz W. Mortality and morbidity rates of patients older and younger than 75 years with acute myocardial infarction treated with intravenous streptokinase. Am J Cardiol 1987;59:1-5.

22. Sherry S. Recombinant tissue plasminogen activator (rt-PA): Is it the thrombolytic agent of choice for an evolving acute myocardial infarction? Am J Cardiol 1987;59:984-989.

23. Rich MW. TPA: Is it worth the price? Am Heart J 1987; 114:1259-1261.

24. Verstraete M, Bernard R, Borg M, et al. Randomized trial of intravenous recombinant tissue-type plasminogen activator versus intravenous streptokinase in acute myocardial infarction. Lancet 1985;I:842-847.

25. Chesebro JH, Knatterud G, Roberts R, et al. Thrombolysis in myocardial infarction (TIMI) trial, Phase I: A comparison between intravenous tissue plasminogen activator and intravenous streptokinase. Circulation 1987;76:142-154.

26. Tennant SN, Dixon J, Venable TC, et al. Intracoronary thrombolysis in patients with acute myocardial infarction: Comparison of the efficacy of urokinase with streptokinase. Circulation 1984;69:756-760.

27. Mathey DG, Schafer J, Sheehan FH, Becker H, Tilsner V, Dodge HT. Intravenous urokinase in acute myocardial infarction. Am J Cardiol 1985;55:878-882.

28. Marder VJ, Rothbard RL, Fitzpatrick PG, Francis CW. Rapid lysis of coronary artery thrombi with anisoylated plasminogen: streptokinase activator complex. Ann Intern Med 1986;104:304-310.

Chapter 13

Intravenous Beta Blockade

Beta adrenergic blockade decreases myocardial oxygen demand by lowering heart rate and blood pressure and reducing myocardial contractility. When administered early in the course of acute MI, beta blockers diminish ischemia in the "border zone" surrounding the central area of necrosis, thereby limiting infarct size. Other beneficial effects include a favorable redistribution of blood flow to the subendocardium (the most poorly perfused region of the heart), and a reduction in the heart's vulnerability to sustained ventricular tachyarrhythmias through inhibition of the pro-arrhythmic effect of local catecholamines and by elevation of the ventricular fibrillation threshold.

Although the potential for myocardial salvage is not as great as with thrombolytic agents, several controlled trials have documented reductions in enzymatically estimated infarct size ranging from 15-40% with both cardioselective and non-selective beta blockers (1-8). These studies have also shown significant reductions in serious ventricular and supraventricular arrhythmias, length of hospital stay, re-infarction rate, and early and late mortality. In addition, patients with unstable angina receiving intravenous beta blockade are less likely to progress to acute MI.

Indications and Contraindications

Any patient presenting with prolonged ischemic chest pain (or other ischemic symptoms) with or without associated ECG changes should be considered a potential candidate for intravenous beta blockade. This would include patients with acute MI, unstable angina, recurrent chest pain following infarction, or other unstable coronary syndromes.

Contraindications to intravenous beta blockade are listed in Table 13.1. Mild bradycardia, mild congestive heart failure, and chronic obstructive lung disease without active wheezing are not absolute contraindications to beta blockade, but close observation (and in some cases a reduction in dosage) is warranted in these situations. Since patients previously taking a beta blocker may gain additional benefit from a further reduction in heart rate, such patients remain suitable candidates for intravenous therapy. However, beta blockers should be used cautiously in patients receiving verapamil, particularly if left ventricular dysfunction is also present.

Table 13.1
Contraindications to Intravenous Beta Blockade

Heart rate < 45/min
Systolic blood pressure < 100 mm Hg
PR interval ≥ 0.24 seconds
Heart block greater than first degree
Severe left ventricular dysfunction
Moderate or severe congestive heart failure
  (pulmonary rales ≥10 cm from lung bases)
Evidence of tissue hypoperfusion or shock
Active wheezing or history of bronchospasm
Pregnancy
Prior major adverse reaction to beta blockade

Dosage and Administration

In the United States, metoprolol is the only intravenous beta
blocker currently approved for use in acute MI. Table 13.2 outlines
the recommended protocol for this agent. Patients 75 years of age or
older and those with congestive heart failure or ventricular dysfunction may benefit from a reduction in both the intravenous and oral
doses. Similarly, patients who develop mild adverse reactions during
intravenous loading should be started on a lower dose of the oral drug.

Management of Adverse Reactions

Using the above guidelines for patient selection and dosing, over
90% of patients will tolerate the full intravenous loading dose. Late
adverse reactions (cardiac and non-cardiac) will necessitate
discontinuation of treatment in an additional 15-30% of patients.

During the IV loading phase, mild bradycardia and hypotension are
the most common adverse effects. Asymptomatic bradycardia requires no
specific treatment unless there is hemodynamic compromise. More
severe bradycardia (heart rate < 40/min) usually responds to atropine
0.5-1.0 mg IV. Similarly, asymptomatic mild hypotension (systolic
blood pressure 80-90 mm Hg) can be managed conservatively by placing
the patient in the Trendelenburg (head down) position and by
cautiously administering fluids (in the absence of heart failure).
Hemodynamically compromising bradycardia and hypotension are less
common, but require more aggressive measures which may include
temporary pacing or use of an inotropic agent or vasopressor.
Significant hypotension associated with congestive heart failure may
require insertion of a pulmonary artery catheter to guide therapy.

Congestive heart failure may occur either early or late in the
hospital course. When mild, diuretics should be administered while
continuing beta blockade. With more severe CHF, beta blockade should
be discontinued. Severe or refractory CHF requires an investigation
into its etiology (Chapter 17), and is usually best managed using

Table 13.2
Protocol for Intravenous Metoprolol in Acute Ischemia

1. Metoprolol 5 mg IV bolus q 2 minutes x 3 doses* (Total 15 mg)

                            THEN

2. Metoprolol 50 mg p.o. q 6 hours for 48 hours, beginning 15
    minutes after completion of intravenous loading

                            THEN

3. Metoprolol 100 mg p.o. q 12 hours for long-term maintenance

4. Monitor heart rate, blood pressure, and cardiac rhythm
    closely during the intravenous infusion

5. Reduce dose or discontinue therapy for:

    a. Severe bradycardia (heart rate < 40/min)
    b. Hypotension (systolic blood pressure < 90 mm Hg)
    c. Progressive PR interval prolongation or PR ≥ 0.26 seconds
    d. Heart block greater than first degree
    e. Increased dyspnea or bronchospasm
    f. Worsening CHF not readily controlled with diuretics
    g. Evidence of tissue hypoperfusion
    h. Other major adverse reaction

* Boluses of 2.5 mg at 2-5 minute intervals up to a total dose of 15 mg
  may be given in patients at increased risk for adverse reactions

inotropic and vasodilator therapy guided by hemodynamic monitoring.

    Advanced heart block warrants discontinuation of metoprolol. If
there is hemodynamic compromise, atropine 0.5-1.0 mg should be
administered intravenously and repeated if necessary. If this
treatment is insufficient, isoproterenol or a pacemaker may be needed
(Chapter 15). Bronchospasm also requires discontinuation of beta
blockade. Administration of aminophylline or other bronchodilators
may be necessary. Other side effects, including central nervous
system complaints, gastrointestinal disturbances, skin rash, etc.
occur infrequently but may require a reduction in dosage, a change to
an alternate agent, or discontinuation of beta blocker therapy.

                Combined Use of Beta Blockers and Thrombolytic Agents

    Theoretically, the combination of a beta blocking agent to reduce
myocardial oxygen demand and a thrombolytic agent to improve oxygen
supply might be expected to result in enhanced myocardial salvage.
Experimental data support this hypothesis (9), and preliminary results
from Phase IIB of the thrombolysis in myocardial infarction (TIMI)

trial indicate that early administration of intravenous metoprolol reduces reinfarction and mortality in patients treated with TPA.

REFERENCES

1. Hjalmarson A, Elmfeldt D, Herlitz J, et al. Effect on mortality of metoprolol in acute myocardial infarction. Lancet 1981; II:823-827.

2. Herlitz J, Elmfeldt D, Hjalmarson A, et al. Effect of metoprolol on indirect signs of the size and severity of acute myocardial infarction. Am J Cardiol 1983;51:1282-1288.

3. Ryden L, Ariniego R, Arnman K, et al. A double-blind trial of metoprolol in acute myocardial infarction. Effects on ventricular tachyarrhythmias. N Engl J Med 1983;308:614-618.

4. The MIAMI Trial Research Group. Metoprolol in acute myocardial infarction (MIAMI). A randomized placebo-controlled international trial. Eur Heart J 1985;6:199-226.

5. Yusuf S, Sleight P, Rossi P, et al. Reduction in infarct size, arrhythmias, and chest pain by early intravenous beta blockade in suspected acute myocardial infarction. Circulation 1983;67(Suppl I):I-32-41.

6. ISIS-1 (First International Study of Infarct Survival) Collaborative Group. Randomized trial of intravenous atenolol among 16,027 cases of suspected acute myocardial infarction. ISIS-1. Lancet 1986;II:57-66.

7. The International Collaborative Study Group. Reduction of infarct size with the early use of timolol in acute myocardial infarction. N Engl J Med 1984;310:9-15.

8. Peter T, Norris RM, Clarke ED, et al. Reduction of enzyme levels by propranolol after acute myocardial infarction. Circulation 1978;57:1091-1095.

9. Van de Werf F, Vanhaecke J, Jang IK, Flameng W, Collen D, DeGeest H. Reduction in infarct size and enhanced recovery of systolic function after coronary thrombolysis with tissue-type plasminogen activator combined with beta-adrenergic blockade with metoprolol. Circulation 1987;75:830-836.

FURTHER READING

1. Yusuf S, Peto R, Lewis J, Collins R, Sleight P. Beta blockade during and after myocardial infarction. An overview of the randomized trials. Prog Cardiovasc Dis 1985;27:335-371.

Chapter 14

Acute Angioplasty and Bypass Surgery

Although early thrombolysis results in significant myocardial salvage and an improved prognosis, recurrent ischemia and infarction can occur due to the presence of a residual high grade stenosis or thrombogenic atherosclerotic plaque (1). Acute angioplasty and bypass surgery offer the possibility of more complete revascularization either alone or in conjunction with other interventions. In this chapter, the current status of these procedures in the early phase of acute infarction is reviewed.

Percutaneous Transluminal Coronary Angioplasty (PTCA)

Several small studies have demonstrated that emergency PTCA with or without concomitant thrombolytic therapy can be performed with an acceptable level of safety in the early hours of acute MI and results in significant myocardial salvage (2-8). In a randomized trial comparing PTCA to intracoronary streptokinase, recanalization rates were comparable but the residual coronary stenosis was significantly less in the PTCA group (8). There was also greater improvement in global and regional ventricular function in the PTCA group, although this could in part reflect a shorter symptom duration prior to treatment. The subsequent hospital course was similar in both groups.

Although the above data indicate a possible role for emergency PTCA in acute MI, this strategy has two major drawbacks: (1) the inherent delay in achieving reperfusion may result in a loss of myocardial salvage, and (2) the technique is not widely available. On the other hand, PTCA is likely to play an important role in managing residual stenosis following successful thrombolysis, and possibly in patients in whom thrombolytic therapy is contraindicated or unsuccessful.

An important consideration is the timing of PTCA following intravenous thrombolytic therapy. In three independent, multicenter trials, immediate PTCA following TPA was associated with significant complications but did not enhance myocardial salvage or improve outcome (9-11). Thus, emergent PTCA following thrombolytic therapy cannot be recommended as a general treatment strategy at this time. However, as noted above it is likely that selected patients will benefit from this approach. Our policy at present is to perform acute angiography and PTCA (if indicated) on hemodynamically unstable patients and on those with either contraindications to thrombolytic therapy or persistent pain and ST segment elevation following attempted thrombolysis. Most other patients undergo elective catheterization 3-10 days later, sooner if chest pain recurs.

Coronary Bypass Surgery

Two large series of emergency coronary bypass surgery for acute myocardial infarction have now been reported (12,13). Both studies demonstrated excellent early and late survival, particularly in selected subgroups. However, neither series was randomized and there could have been a selection bias (14). In addition, as with PTCA, surgery results in important time delays and is not widely available on an emergency basis. Thus, the primary role of surgery in acute MI is in the management of mechanical complications (Chapter 20), and in selected patients with persistent ischemia despite conventional therapy (14). Rarely, patients with cardiogenic shock unrelated to mechanical complications may benefit from emergency surgery (15,16).

REFERENCES

1. Schaer DH, Ross AM, Wasserman AG. Reinfarction, recurrent angina, and reocclusion after thrombolytic therapy. Circulation 1987; 76(Suppl II):II-57-62.

2. Meyer J, Merx W, Schmitz H, et al. Percutaneous transluminal coronary angioplasty immediately after intracoronary streptolysis of transmural myocardial infarction. Circulation 1982;66:905-913.

3. Hartzler GO, Rutherford BD, McConahoy DR, et al. Percutaneous transluminal coronary angioplasty with and without thrombolytic therapy for treatment of acute myocardial infarction. Am Heart J 1983;106:965-973.

4. Hartzler GO, Rutherford BD, McConahay DR. Percutaneous transluminal coronary angioplasty: Application for acute myocardial infarction. Am J Cardiol 1984;53:117C-121C.

5. Gold HK, Cowley MJ, Palacios IF, et al. Combined intracoronary streptokinase infusion and coronary angioplasty during acute myocardial infarction. Am J Cardiol 1984;53:122C-125C.

6. Papapietro SE, MacLean W, Stanley A, et al. Percutaneous transluminal coronary angioplasty after intracoronary streptokinase in evolving acute myocardial infarction. Am J Cardiol 1985;55:48-53.

7. Prida XE, Holland JP, Feldman RL, et al. Percutaneous transluminal coronary angioplasty in evolving acute myocardial infarction. Am J Cardiol 1986;57:1069-1074.

8. O'Neill W, Timmis GC, Bourdillon PD, et al. A prospective randomized clinical trial of intracoronary streptokinase versus coronary angioplasty for acute myocardial infarction. N Engl J Med 1986;314:812-818.

9. Topol EJ, Califf RM, George BS, et al. A randomized trial of immediate versus delayed elective angioplasty after intravenous tissue plasminogen activator in acute myocardial infarction. N Engl J Med 1987;317:581-588.

10. Simoons ML, Arnold AER, Betriu A, et al. Thrombolysis with tissue plasminogen activator in acute myocardial infarction: no additional benefit from immediate percutaneous coronary angioplasty. Lancet 1988;I:197-203.

11. The TIMI Research Group. Immediate vs delayed catheterization and angioplasty following thrombolytic therapy for acute myocardial infarction. TIMI IIA results. JAMA 1988;260:2849-2858.

12. DeWood MA, Spores J, Berg R, et al. Acute myocardial infarction: A decade of experience with surgical reperfusion in 701 patients. Circulation 1983;68(Suppl II):II-8-16.

13. Phillips SJ, Zeff RH, Skinner JR, Toon RS, Grignon A, Kongtahworn C. Reperfusion protocol and results in 738 patients with evolving myocardial infarction. Ann Thorac Surg 1986;41:119-125.

14. Jones EL. Surgical revascularization during acute evolving myocardial infarction. Circulation 1987;76(Suppl III):III-146-148.

15. Laks H, Rosenkranz E, Buckberg GD. Surgical treatment of cardiogenic shock after myocardial infarction. Circulation 1986;74(Suppl III):III-11-16.

16. Guyton RA, Arcidi JM, Langford DA, Morris DC, Liberman HA, Hatcher CR. Emergency coronary bypass for cardiogenic shock. Circulation 1987;76(Suppl V):V-22-27.

Chapter 15

Arrhythmias and Conduction Disturbances

As shown in Table 15.1, a wide range of arrhythmias and conduction disturbances may complicate acute myocardial infarction (1-7). The general approach to arrhythmia diagnosis and management is outlined in chapters 5-7; the present chapter will focus on selected issues in the acute MI setting.

Table 15.1
Incidence of Arrhythmias and Conduction Disturbances Complicating Acute Myocardial Infarction

Sinus bradycardia	14-28%
Sinus tachycardia	20-53%
Atrial premature contractions	10-57%
Atrial fibrillation or flutter	13-28%
Supraventricular tachycardia	0-4%
Ventricular premature contractions	33-71%
Accelerated idioventricular rhythm	9-13%
Ventricular tachycardia	4-28%
Ventricular fibrillation	3-10%
Right bundle branch block	5-8%
Left bundle branch block	2-7%
Second degree A-V block, Type I	4-10%
Second degree A-V block, Type II	0.5-2%
Complete heart block	4-8%
Asystole	1-5%

Ventricular Premature Contractions (VPCs)

VPCs occur in a high percentage of patients in the first few hours of acute MI, and the frequency of VPCs correlates inversely with the serum potassium level (8). Early data indicated that frequent VPCs, salvos, and R-on-T beats might be a harbinger of more malignant arrhythmias (1), and it was suggested that prophylactic treatment of these "warning arrhythmias" might decrease the incidence of primary ventricular fibrillation (2). Subsequently, several randomized trials demonstrated a reduction in the occurrence of primary ventricular fibrillation in patients treated with lidocaine (4,5). However, such treatment is associated with a significant incidence of central nervous system and gastrointestinal side effects. In addition, primary ventricular fibrillation in the CCU virtually always responds to prompt defibrillation (9), and although hospital mortality tends to be higher in patients with primary ventricular fibrillation (9,10), this does not appear to be attributable to the arrhythmia per se (9). Furthermore, late mortality and functional status among patients resuscitated from ventricular fibrillation do not differ from patients without ventricular fibrillation (11-13). Finally, it has been shown that warning arrhythmias, including R-on-T VPCs, are poor predictors of progression to sustained ventricular tachyarrhythmias, and that approximately 50% of ventricular fibrillation episodes occur in the absence of warning arrhythmias (14-19). For these reasons, the routine use of prophylactic lidocaine has been questioned (9,19,20).

Despite the above considerations, prevention of cardiac arrest due to ventricular fibrillation seems a desirable goal. We therefore use "prophylactic" lidocaine in selected patients who present with definite evidence of transmural infarction by ECG or enzyme criteria and who do not have a contraindication to using this agent. Relative contraindications include age over 70 and significant congestive heart failure or hepatic insufficiency. Prior allergic reaction to lidocaine is an absolute contraindication. The dosage is 1 mg/kg by bolus injection repeated after 10-15 minutes and followed by a 2-3 mg/min continuous infusion. The dose is reduced in patients at increased risk of toxicity, and lidocaine levels are monitored routinely (see Chapter 2). As the incidence of primary ventricular fibrillation decreases markedly after the first few hours of MI (20), prophylactic lidocaine is discontinued within 24-48 hours.

Accelerated Idioventricular Rhythm (AIVR)

AIVR occurs in approximately 10% of patients with acute MI and with approximately equal frequency in anterior and inferior infarctions (3). It is also commonly seen during reperfusion following thrombolytic therapy. The mechanism of this arrhythmia is thought to be enhanced automaticity of Purkinje fibers. In most cases, AIVR is self-limited, does not produce hemodynamic compromise, and requires no specific therapy. However, since ventricular tachycardia and fibrillation occur more frequently in patients with AIVR (3,21), some experts recommend anti-arrhythmic therapy when AIVR occurs in the acute MI setting. Our policy is not to treat AIVR unless it is associated with hemodynamic compromise (due to loss of normal A-V synchrony) or progresses to more serious arrhythmias. Since AIVR may simulate an accelerated ventricular escape rhythm (3), a satisfactory supraventricular or paced rhythm must be present prior to suppresion of AIVR in order to avoid profound bradycardia.

Ventricular Tachycardia (VT) and Ventricular Fibrillation (VF)

Paroxysmal VT is common in the first 24 hours after acute MI and is usually self-limited, although it may progress to VF. As with

VPCs, there is a close inverse correlation between the incidence of VT and the serum potassium level (8). Since sustained VT increases oxygen demand while diminishing supply, prompt treatment is indicated in the early phase of acute MI, and usually consists of electrical cardioversion (Chapter 33) using an initial energy level of 20-50 joules. Hemodynamically stable patients may be given a brief trial of lidocaine, but if the tachycardia does not respond within 10-15 minutes, electrical cardioversion should be performed. Following reversion of VT, the serum potassium level should be maintained in the range of 4.0-5.0 meq/L, and prophylactic antiarrhythmic therapy with lidocaine or procainamide should be initiated for 24-48 hours.

VT late in the hospital course (more than 3-5 days after admission) usually occurs in the setting of significant left ventricular dysfunction and is associated with increased late mortality (22-24). To date, empiric anti-arrhythmic therapy has not been shown to alter prognosis, but this is a subject of ongoing investigation. The role of electrophysiologic testing in defining high-risk patients and guiding therapy is also being studied. Optimal management of these patients is currently unknown; however, patients with decreased left ventricular function (ejection fraction < 0.40) and either sustained ventricular tachycardia or frequent episodes of non-sustained VT probably warrant anti-arrhythmic therapy.

As discussed in Chapter 6, VF complicating acute MI may be primary, secondary, or late, and the prognosis varies depending on the type. The peak incidence of primary VF is in the first hour of MI (20). It occurs with equal frequency in inferior and anterior infarctions and is the leading cause of pre-hospital mortality. Primary VF is uncommon after 6 hours and rare more than 12 hours after the onset of infarction (20). As discussed above (section on VPCs), primary VF responds readily to prompt defibrillation, and although it is associated with increased hospital mortality, late morbidity and mortality among hospital survivors are not affected.

Secondary VF usually occurs in the setting of severe left ventricular dysfunction and cardiogenic shock and is associated with a poor prognosis. Late VF also occurs in patients with left ventricular dysfunction and has an intermediate prognosis. Patients with anterior infarctions complicated by persistent sinus tachycardia, atrial fibrillation, or bundle branch block are at increased risk for late VF. Treatment is best guided by electrophysiologic testing and may consist of anti-arrhythmic drugs, surgery, and/or insertion of an anti-tachycardia device. The acute management of VF includes prompt defibrillation, correction of any precipitating factors, and institution of anti-arrhythmic therapy (see Chapters 6 and 7).

Conduction Disturbances

Bundle branch block (BBB), whether new or pre-existing, is associated with increased hospital and late mortality, but this risk appears to be due to the extent of myocardial damage and the occurrence of ventricular tachyarrhythmias rather than to BBB per se (25). Table 15.2 summarizes the association between BBB and high degree A-V block and its effect on early and late mortality (26,27).

Table 15.2
Bundle Branch Block in Acute Myocardial Infarction: Progression to High Degree Block and Effect on Mortality*

	Progression to High Degree A-V Block (%)	Hospital Mortality (%)	Total 12-month Mortality (%)
LBBB	13	21	48
RBBB	14	25	42
RBBB + LAFB	27	28	44
RBBB + LPFB	29	43	58
Alternating BBB	44	40	70

* Adapted from Hindman MC, Wagner GS, JaRo M, et al. The clinical significance of bundle branch block complicating acute myocardial infarction. Circulation 1978;58:683-684. Used by permission of the American Heart Association, Inc.

In the study by Hindman et al. (Table 15.2), patients with BBB had anterior infarction in 63% of cases, inferoposterior MI in 18%, lateral MI in 1%, and indeterminant location in 18%. Hospital mortality was twice as high in patients with BBB as in patients without BBB, regardless of MI location. Patients with new BBB associated with either PR interval prolongation or bilateral BBB (e.g., RBBB + LAFB) were at greater risk for progression to high-degree block (27). The rate of progression of isolated right or left BBB to high degree A-V block was relatively low in this series; other reports have indicated a higher risk (25).

Isolated first degree A-V block (PR interval > 0.20 sec), Mobitz Type I second degree A-V block, and complete heart block with a narrow QRS junctional escape rhythm usually occur in the setting of an inferior or posterior infarction, are often self-limited, and require no specific treatment in the absence of hemodynamic compromise. In patients with anterior infarcts and BBB, first degree or second degree A-V block with a Wenckebach structure may represent advanced infranodal block warranting aggressive management (Chapter 16). Mobitz Type II second degree A-V block or complete heart block with a wide complex ventricular escape rhythm may herald the sudden onset of profound bradycardia or asystole; temporary pacing is advisable, although there is little evidence that this maneuver improves survival.

The diagnosis and treatment of other bradyarrhythmias are discussed in Chapters 5-7, and specific indications for temporary pacemaker insertion are outlined in the next chapter. Permanent pace-

makers are indicated for patients with persistent high degree A-V
block or complete heart block after MI, and should be inserted prior
to hospital discharge (28). The role of permanent pacing in patients
with transient high degree A-V block or with trifascicular block
remains controversial (28-30).

REFERENCES

1. Julian DG, Valentine PA, Miller GG. Disturbances of rate, rhythm
   and conduction in acute myocardial infarction. Am J Med 1964;
   37:915-927.

2. Lown B, Fakhro AM, Hood WB, Thorn GW. The coronary care unit.
   New perspectives and directions. JAMA 1967;199:188-198.

3. Lichstein E, Ribas-Meneclier C, Gupta PK, Chadda KD. Incidence
   and description of accelerated ventricular rhythm complicating
   acute myocardial infarction. Am J Med 1975;58:192-198.

4. DeSilva RA, Hennekens CH, Lown B, Casscells W. Lignocaine
   prophylaxis in acute myocardial infarction: An evaluation of
   randomized trials. Lancet 1981;II:855-858.

5. Lie KI, Wellens HJ, van Capelle FJ, Durrer D. Lidocaine in the
   prevention of primary ventricular fibrillation. N Engl J Med
   1974;291:1324-1326.

6. Godman MJ, Lassers BW, Julian DG. Complete bundle branch block
   complicating acute myocardial infarction. N Engl J Med
   1970;282:237-240.

7. Mullins CB, Atkins JM. Prognosis and management of ventricular
   conduction blocks in acute myocardial infarction. Mod Concepts
   Cardiovasc Dis 1976;45:129-134.

8. Nordrehaug JE, Johannessen KA, von der Lippe G. Serum potassium
   concentration as a risk factor of ventricular arrhythmias early in
   acute myocardial infarction. Circulation 1985;71:645-649.

9. Carruth JE, Silverman ME. Ventricular fibrillation complicating
   acute myocardial infarction: Reasons against the routine use of
   lidocaine. Am Heart J 1982;104:545-550.

10. Volpi A, Maggioni A, Franzosi MG, Pampallona S, Mauri F, Tognoni
    G. In-hospital prognosis of patients with acute myocardial
    infarction complicated by primary ventricular fibrillation. N
    Engl J Med 1987;317:257-261.

11. Geddes JS, Adgey AAJ, Pantridge JF. Prognosis after recovery from
    ventricular fibrillation complicating ischemic heart disease.
    Lancet 1967;II:273-275.

12. Kushnir B, Fox KM, Tomlinson IW, Portal RW, Aber CP. Primary ventricular fibrillation and resumption of work, sexual activity, and driving after first acute myocardial infarction. Br Med J 1975;4:609-611.

13. Tofler GH, Stone PH, Muller JE, et al. Prognosis after myocardial infarction complicated by ventricular fibrillation. Circulation 1986;74(Suppl II):II-304. (Abstr)

14. Lie KI, Wellens HJJ, Downar E, Durrer D. Observations on patients with primary ventricular fibrillation complicating acute myocardial infarction. Circulation 1975;52:755-759.

15. deSoyza N, Meacham D, Murphy ML, Kane JJ, Doherty JE, Bisset JK. Evaluation of warning arrhythmias before paroxysmal ventricular tachycardia during acute myocardial infarction in man. Circulation 1979;60:814-818.

16. El-Sherif N, Myerburg RJ, Scherlag BJ, et al. Electrocardiographic antecedents of primary ventricular fibrillation: Value of the R-on-T phenomenon in myocardial infarction. Br Heart J 1976;38:415-422.

17. Roberts R, Ambos HD, Loh CW, Sobel BE. Initiation of repetitive ventricular depolarizations by relatively late premature complexes in patients with acute myocardial infarction. Am J Cardiol 1978;41:678-683.

18. Harrison DC. Should lidocaine be administered routinely to all patients after acute myocardial infarction? Circulation 1978;58:581-584.

19. Dunn HM, McComb JM, Kinney CD, et al. Prophylactic lidocaine in the early phase of suspected myocardial infarction. Am Heart J 1985;110:353-362.

20. O'Doherty M, Taylor DI, Quinn E, Vincent R, Chamberlain DA. Five hundred patients with myocardial infarction monitored within one hour of symptoms. Br Med J 1983;286:1405-1408.

21. DeSoyza N, Bissett JK, Kane JJ, Murphy ML, Doherty JE. Association of accelerated idioventricular rhythm and paroxysmal ventricular tachycardia in acute myocardial infarction. Am J Cardiol 1974;34:667-670.

22. Anderson KP, DeCamilla J, Moss AJ. Clinical significance of ventricular tachycardia (3 beats or longer) detected during ambulatory monitoring after myocardial infarction. Circulation 1978;57:890-897.

23. Bigger JT, Weld FM, Rolnitzky LM. Prevalence, characteristics, and significance of ventricular tachycardia (three or more complexes) detected with ambulatory electrocardiographic recording in the late hospital phase of acute myocardial infarction. Am J Cardiol 1981;48:815-823.

24. Kleiger RE, Miller JP, Thanavaro S, Province MA, Martin TF, Oliver GC. Relationship between clinical features of acute myocardial infarction and ventricular runs 2 weeks to 1 year after infarction. Circulation 1981;63:64-70.

25. Fisch GR, Zipes DP, Fisch C. Bundle branch block and sudden death. Prog Cardiovasc Dis 1980;23:187-224.

26. Hindman MC, Wagner GS, JaRo M, et al. The clinical significance of bundle branch block complicating acute myocardial infarction. 1. Clinical characteristics, hospital mortality, and one-year follow-up. Circulation 1978;58:679-688.

27. Hindman MC, Wagner GS, JaRo M, et al. The clinical significance of bundle branch block complicating acute myocardial infarction. 2. Indications for temporary and permanent pacemaker insertion. Circulation 1978;58:689-699.

28. Frye RL, Fisch C, Collins JJ, et al. Guidelines for permanent cardiac pacemaker implantation, May, 1984. J Am Coll Cardiol 1984;4:434-442.

29. Ritter WS, Atkins JM, Blomqvist CG, Mullins CB. Permanent pacing in patients with transient trifascicular block during acute myocardial infarction. Am J Cardiol 1976;38:205-208.

30. Ginks WR, Sutton R, Winston DH, Leatham L. Long-term prognosis after acute anterior infarction with atrioventricular block. Br Heart J 1977;39:186-189.

Chapter 16

Temporary Pacemakers

Edward C. Miller, M.D.

Questions concerning indications for temporary transvenous pacemakers and problems related to their function arise frequently in the CCU. This chapter focuses on the use of temporary pacemakers in the acute MI setting. Chapter 35 reviews modes of pacing, techniques of pacemaker insertion, and complications related to their use.

Indications

In general, temporary pacemaker insertion is indicated in the treatment of sustained or recurrent symptomatic bradyarrhythmias associated with hemodynamic compromise, and in situations where there is known to be a high risk of such bradyarrhythmias. Additional indications include the treatment of torsade de pointes ventricular tachycardia, recurrent sustained monomorphic VT, and selected supraventricular tachycardias. Atropine and/or isoproterenol may be indicated prior to inserting a pacemaker (Chapter 6).

In most situations, a standard ventricular demand pacemaker is adequate. In some patients, e.g. those with markedly decreased ventricular compliance or right ventricular infarction, preservation of normal A-V synchrony may result in improved hemodynamics. In these cases, an A-V sequential pacemaker should be considered.

Acute Myocardial Infarction (Fig. 16.1)

Inferior MI

Sinus bradycardia and AV nodal conduction disturbances (1° A-V block, Mobitz Type I 2° A-V block, and complete heart block with a narrow QRS junctional escape) are commonly seen in inferior infarction. Factors contributing to their development include heightened vagotonia (the Bezold-Jarisch reflex), ischemia involving the sinus or A-V nodal arteries, medications, and edema of the nodes themselves. In most cases, severe bradyarrhythmias are accompanied by a junctional escape rhythm and respond readily to atropine. Therefore, prophylactic temporary pacing is not necessary. In contrast, sustained or recurrent bradycardia associated with hemodynamic compromise recalcitrant to atropine warrants temporary pacemaker insertion. New bundle branch block is uncommon in inferior MI and may signify ischemia at a distance or pre-existing conduction system disease; continued close observation is usually justified.

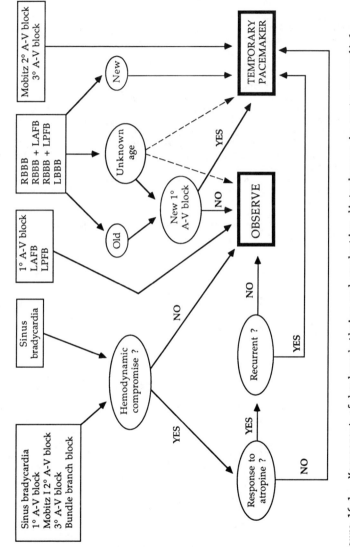

Figure 16-1. Management of bradyarrhythmias and conduction disturbances in acute myocardial infarction.

In many cases, bradyarrhythmias occurring in association with inferior infarcts resolve within 24-48 hours; occasionally, they may persist for 7-14 days. Permanent pacemaker implantation is rarely required. Resolution of bradyarrhythmias and hemodynamic stabilization portend a favorable long-term prognosis.

Anterior MI

Conduction disturbances in anterior MI result from injury to the His bundle or bundle branches supplied by proximal septal branches of the left anterior descending artery. Since the level of block is below the A-V junction (i.e. infranodal), pharmacologic intervention is less effective and subsidiary ventricular escape mechanisms are less reliable for preserving hemodynamic stability. As in inferior MI, any sustained bradyarrhythmia associated with hemodynamic compromise is an indication for temporary pacemaker insertion. Mobitz Type II second degree A-V block often progresses to complete heart block, and prophylactic pacemaker insertion is indicated even when its duration is very brief.

New isolated left anterior fascicular block (LAFB) is common in acute anterior infarction but usually does not progress to complete heart block and does not require pacemaker insertion. New right bundle branch block, with or without associated axis deviation (i.e., LAFB or LPFB), carries a relatively high risk for progression to complete heart block; temporary pacemaker insertion is warranted. Pacemaker insertion in new left bundle branch block is somewhat controversial, but most experts now favor its use. New isolated left posterior fascicular block is rare, and there are insufficient data on which to base a recommendation.

In the absence of new conduction system disease, pre-existing bundle branch block probably does not warrant pacemaker insertion. On the other hand, pre-existing bundle branch block associated with new PR interval prolongation is grounds for a prophylactic pacemaker.

Although the above guidelines represent a reasonable and accepted approach, it is important to recognize that the majority of patients with anterior infarction who progress to complete heart block have suffered extensive myocardial damage. Most patients will die due to pump failure, mechanical complications, or refractory arrhythmias. Thus, the number of patients with anterior MI for whom prophylactic pacemaker insertion is truly a life-saving maneuver is small.

Other Indications for Temporary Pacemaker Insertion

Pulmonary artery catheterization occasionally induces right bundle branch block due to trauma of the intraventricular septum (more common from femoral approach). If pre-existing left bundle branch block is present, complete heart block may ensue. Thus, prophylactic pacemaker insertion should be considered in this situation.

Overdrive pacing is effective in treating recurrent torsade de pointes ventricular tachycardia associated with prolonged QT interval, and is the treatment of choice in the acute phase of this syndrome. The initial rate should be 90-120/min with further increases if the arrhythmia persists. Rarely, recurrent sustained monomorphic VT is treated with temporary overdrive, underdrive, or burst pacing while effective alternative therapy is being developed.

Frequent symptomatic bradyarrhythmias associated with acute or chronic A-V block, carotid hypersensitivity, or sick sinus syndrome may require temporary pacemaker insertion while awaiting cessation of drug therapy or permanent pacemaker implantation.

Finally, very rapid atrial or burst pacing is effective in treating supraventricular tachycardia or atrial flutter. Pacing is rarely needed for conversion of these arrhythmias, but is an alternative to direct current cardioversion.

Troubleshooting

Failure to Sense

Normal pacemaker function consists of two components: sensing and capturing. Sensing is the ability to detect intrinsic myocardial electrical activity. The standard temporary ventricular pacemaker responds to sensed events by inhibiting the output channel. The sensitivity level or threshold is adjusted so that spontaneous ventricular depolarizations (QRSs) are sensed, but extraneous electrical activity (e.g. muscle artifact, T-waves) is ignored. Capture refers to the ability of the pacemaker to generate an electrical impulse sufficient to depolarize the heart and produce a contraction.

Failure to sense occurs when the pacemaker fires at the programmed rate with apparent disregard for the native QRS (Fig. 16.2). Pacemaker spikes seen on or shortly following (< .04 msec) the QRS do not constitute failure to sense because there may be a slight delay from the onset of electrical systole to the time the beat is sensed by the pacemaker and the output current is inhibited.

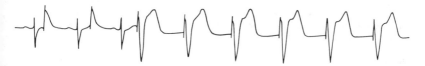

Figure 16.2. Failure to sense. Inappropriate pacemaker artifact is seen following native QRS at beginning of strip. After the third native beat, the pacemaker captures the ventricle resulting in an R-on-T phenomenon. Note that the first two pacer spikes occur during the refractory period and do not represent failure to capture.

Frequent failure to sense in an otherwise functioning pacemaker should first be managed by decreasing the pacemaker sensitivity threshold. If this is ineffective, converting the bipolar electrode system to a unipolar configuration by grounding the positive (proximal) electrode to the skin will usually improve sensitivity. This is accomplished by disconnecting the positive terminal of the pacemaker box and attaching it to a standard ECG patch electrode on the chest wall using an alligator clip. If sensitivity is still a problem, repositioning the pacemaker may be necessary.

Failure to Capture

Capture depends on the integrity of the pacemaker power supply and electrodes and the delivery of sufficient energy to the electrode tip in contact with the endocardium to depolarize the myocardium and produce a contraction. The minimum energy capable of reliably inducing capture is the output threshold.

Failure to capture is diagnosed when the pacemaker fires appropriately but fails to capture the ventricle (i.e., no QRS is inscribed following the pacemaker artifact; Fig. 16.3). Failure to capture is occasionally misdiagnosed when the pacemaker artifact falls during the refractory period; this may in fact represent failure to sense (Fig. 16.2).

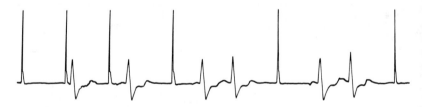

Figure 16.3.   Failure to capture.   Multiple pacemaker artifacts are seen, but none are followed by a pacemaker-induced QRS.

Isolated failure to capture can first be treated by slowly increasing the current output on the pacemaker box. Current requirements in excess of 5-6 milliamps generally indicate improper positioning of the catheter tip or electrical failure due to battery depletion or lead fracture.

Failure to Fire

Failure to fire refers to the absence of appropriate pacemaker output spikes at the desired rate. The pacemaker box should be checked to see that it is turned on, the battery is charged, and the output current setting is correct. Oversensing (i.e., sensing of T-waves or muscle artifact) may produce apparent failure to fire;

thus, the sensing threshold should be tested and increased if necessary. Oversensing can often be diagnosed by observing the sensing needle or light on the pacemaker box, and correlating it with electrical activity seen on the ECG monitor. If these maneuvers fail to correct the problem, the pacing wire should be repositioned or replaced.

Pacemaker-Induced Arrhythmias

Pacemaker-induced arrhythmias usually occur during insertion or manipulation of the electrode, and may include atrial or ventricular premature beats, atrial fibrillation, or ventricular tachycardia or fibrillation. Serious rhythm disturbances require withdrawal of the pacemaker; if this does not produce resolution, appropriate treatment should be instituted (Chapters 6-7). Once the pacemaker is in stable position, ventricular premature beats may still be seen, but this is usually a transient problem which resolves within several hours. Less commonly, sustained ventricular arrhythmias due to R-on-T phenomenon (Fig. 16.2), positional changes, or persistent ventricular irritability will require pacemaker repositioning; anti-arrhythmic drugs are rarely effective in this setting.

FURTHER READING

1. Austin JL, Preis LK, Crampton RS, Beller GA, Martin RP. Analysis of pacemaker malfunction and complications of temporary pacing in the coronary care unit. Am J Cardiol 1982;49:301-306.

2. Brown RW, Hunt D, Sloman JG. The natural history of atrioventricular conduction defects in acute myocardial infarction. Am Heart J 1969;78:460-466.

3. Dreifus LS, Michelson EL, Kaplinsky E. Bradyarrhythmias: Clinical significance and management. J Am Coll Cardiol 1983; 1:327-338.

4. Gann D, Balachandran PK, Sherif NE, Samet P. Prognostic significance of chronic versus acute bundle branch block in acute myocardial infarction. Chest 1975;67:298-303.

5. Godman MJ, Lassers BW, Julian DG. Complete bundle branch block complicating acute myocardial infarction. N Engl J Med 1970; 282:237-240.

6. Hindman MC, Wagner GS, JaRo M, et al. The clinical significance of bundle branch block complicating acute myocardial infarction. Circulation 1978;58:679-699.

7. Hollander G, Nadiminti V, Lichstein E, Greengart A, Sanders M. Bundle branch block in acute myocardial infarction. Am Heart J 1983;105:738-743.

8. Hynes JK, Holmes DR, Harrison CE. Five year experience with temporary pacemaker therapy in the coronary care unit. Mayo Clinic Proc 1983;58:122-126.

9. Jones ME, Terry G, Kenmure ACF. Frequency and significance of conduction defects in acute myocardial infarction. Am Heart J 1977;94:163-67.

10. Lie KI, Wellens HJJ, Schuilenberg RM, et al. Factors influencing prognosis of bundle branch block complicating acute anteroseptal myocardial infarction. The value of His bundle recordings. Circulation 1974;50:935-941.

11. Mark AL. The Bezold-Jarisch reflex revisited: Clinical implications of inhibiting reflexes originating in the heart. J Am Coll Cardiol 1983;1:90-102.

12. Mullins CB, Atkins JM. Prognosis and management of ventricular conduction blocks in acute myocardial infarction. Mod Concepts Cardiovasc Dis 1976;45:129-133.

13. Nimetz AA, Schubrooks SJ, Hutter AM, et al. The significance of bundle branch block during acute myocardial infarction. Am Heart J 1975;90:439-444.

14. Norris RM. Heart block in posterior and anterior myocardial infarction. Br Heart J 1969;31:352-356.

15. Rotman M, Wagner GS, Wallace AG. Bradyarrhythmias in acute myocardial infarction. Circulation 1973;45:703-722.

16. Rotman M, Wagner GS, Waugh RA. Significance of high degree atrioventricular block in acute posterior myocardial infarction. The importance of clinical setting and mechanisms of block. Circulation 1973;47:257-262.

17. Scheinman M, Brenman B. Clinical and anatomic implications of intraventricular conduction blocks in acute myocardial infarction. Circulation 1972;46:753-760.

18. Sutton R, Davies M. The conduction system in acute myocardial infarction complicated by heart block. Circulation 1968;38:987-992.

19. Waugh RA, Wagner GS, Haney TL, et al. Immediate and remote prognostic significance of fascicular block during acute MI. Circulation 1973;47:765-775.

20. Zoll PM, Zoll RH, Falk RH, Clinton JE, Eitel DR, Antman EM. External noninvasive temporary cardiac pacing: Clinical trials. Circulation 1985;71:937-944.

Chapter 17

Hypoperfusion, Congestive Heart Failure, and Shock

Hemodynamic disturbances complicate the course of one-half to two-thirds of patients with acute myocardial infarction and, as a general rule, short-term prognosis correlates closely with the severity of the hemodynamic impairment (1-4). In 1976, Forrester et al. (4) demonstrated the prognostic value of classifying patients according to four hemodynamic subsets, and the close correlation between outcome based on clinical criteria and that based on the results of invasive hemodynamic monitoring with a flow-directed balloon-tipped pulmonary artery catheter (Table 17.1). In this chapter, the management of hypoperfusion, congestive heart failure, and shock will be discussed.

Table 17.1
Mortality Rates in Clinical and Hemodynamic Subsets[+]

Subset	Pulmonary Congestion*	Peripheral Hypoperfusion**	% Mortality Clinical	% Mortality Hemodynamic
I	-	-	1	3
II	+	-	11	9
III	-	+	18	23
IV	+	+	60	51

* Pulmonary wedge pressure ≥ 18 mm Hg
**Cardiac index ≤ 2.2 liters/min/M^2

[+] Reprinted with permission from Forrester JS, Diamond G, Chatterjee K, Swan HJC. Medical therapy of acute myocardial infarction by application of hemodynamic subsets. N Engl J Med 1976;295:1361.

Hypoperfusion

Hypotension is defined by a blood pressure below a certain absolute level (e.g., 90 mm Hg systolic). Hypoperfusion occurs when there is inadequate blood flow to meet tissue demands; if the condition is not rapidly corrected, organ dysfunction occurs. Since hypotension can occur without hypoperfusion (e.g., in a healthy young woman), and hypoperfusion can occur despite a "normal" blood pressure (e.g., in a previously hypertensive patient or in a patient with marked activation of the adrenergic nervous system), to avoid confusion the term hypotension will not be used in this discussion. Causes of hypoperfusion are shown in Table 17.2.

Table 17.2
Causes of Hypoperfusion in Acute MI

Cardiac

        Severe left ventricular dysfunction
        Right ventricular infarction
        Persistent or recurrent ischemia
        Tachyarrhythmias
        Bradyarrhythmias
        Mechanical complications
            Left ventricular aneurysm or pseudoaneurysm
            Ventricular septal defect
            Papillary muscle dysfunction or rupture
        Pericardial effusion
        Chronic valvular heart disease, esp. aortic stenosis

Non-cardiac

        Hypovolemia, relative or absolute
        Vagal reaction
        Sepsis
        Pulmonary embolus
        Medications
            Vasodilators
            Beta blockers
            Calcium channel blockers (esp. verapamil)
            Anti-arrhythmic agents
            Narcotics
            Sedatives and tranquilizers

In acute MI, hypoperfusion usually indicates a low cardiac output state, with a cardiac index $\leq$ 2.2 L/min/M^2 (4). Clinical signs may include fatigue, altered mental status, oliguria, cool or clammy skin, diaphoresis, tachycardia, decreased blood pressure with a low pulse pressure, and pre-renal azotemia. The treatment of hypoperfusion is dependent on the cause and the severity of hemodynamic compromise. Since hypoperfusion may exacerbate myocardial ischemia, prompt treatment is indicated, especially in the early hours of acute MI.

In the absence of evidence for pulmonary congestion, initial treatment should consist of placing the patient in the Trendelenburg (head down) position and administering intravenous fluids cautiously while observing carefully for signs of left heart failure. Chest pain and arrhythmias should be managed as previously described (Chapters 4 and 15). Potentially offending medications should be withdrawn or

minimized   until   the   disturbance   is   corrected.   A   careful
cardiovascular examination should be performed to elicit signs of a
mechanical complication (Chapter 21) or underlying valvular heart
disease, such as aortic stenosis. Patients who have undergone
invasive procedures or who have received systemic anticoagulation or
thrombolytic therapy should be checked for pulsus paradoxus, and if
pericardial tamponade is suspected, an emergency echocardiogram should
be obtained. Right ventricular infarction should be considered in
patients with inferior MIs, and managed as outlined in Chapter 19.
Vagal reactions usually respond to atropine 0.5–1.0 mg IV (repeated if
necessary) and supportive care.

In patients who do not respond to the above measures or in whom
congestive heart failure is also present, pulmonary artery
catheterization is indicated. Blood gases should be analyzed for
evidence of a left to right shunt, and the pulmonary artery occlusive
pressure (PAOP) tracing should be carefully inspected for the presence
of an abnormal v-wave, usually indicating acute mitral regurgitation.
The right-sided pressures should be analyzed for evidence of right
ventricular infarction (Chapter 19). If the mean PAOP is ≤ 15 mm Hg
in the presence of a low cardiac index, volume expansion to achieve a
PAOP of 18–20 mm Hg is indicated. If the PAOP is already greater than
18 mm Hg, addition of an inotropic agent is warranted (see below).

Occasionally, the hemodynamic data will fail to confirm a low
cardiac output state. If an echocardiogram or radionuclide angiogram
indicates adequate ventricular function, a non-cardiac cause of hypoperfusion (e.g. sepsis, pulmonary embolus) should be considered.

Congestive Heart Failure (CHF)

The prognostic significance of CHF complicating acute MI has long
been recognized (2), and the modified Killip classification, based on
clinical assessment of ventricular function on admission to the CCU,
has been widely used to estimate infarct severity and hospital
mortality (Table 17.3). Although current treatment strategies have
reduced the mortality of patients in Killip Classes I–III, the
prognosis of patients with cardiogenic shock remains poor.

The pathophysiology of CHF in patients with acute MI may involve
systolic contractile dysfunction, decreased compliance (diastolic
dysfunction), or a combination of systolic and diastolic abnormalities. Occasionally, a pre-existing valvular lesion, most commonly
mitral regurgitation or aortic stenosis, will contribute to the
development of CHF. Less frequently, mechanical complications such as
papillary muscle dysfunction or a ventricular septal defect will be
the cause of CHF. New onset atrial or ventricular tachyarrhythmias
(less commonly bradyarrhythmias) may also precipitate CHF. Medications, particularly beta blockers, calcium antagonists, and anti-
arrhythmic agents, may precipitate or exacerbate CHF in patients with
already compromised ventricular function. In all of these situations,
excess fluid administration may contribute to the development of CHF.

Table 17.3
Modified Killip Classification: Clinical Assessment of Ventricular
Function*

Killip Class	Patients N (%)	Mortality (%)
I: No rales, no S_3	81 (33)	6
II: Rales over < 50% of lungs or S_3	96 (38)	17
III: Rales over > 50% of lungs	26 (10)	38
IV: Cardiogenic shock	47 (19)	81

* Adapted from Killip T, Kimball JT. Treatment of myocardial infarction in a coronary care unit. Am J Cardiol 1967;20:459. Used with
permission.

The goals of CHF treatment include correction or modification of
the underlying pathophysiology, relief of pulmonary congestion,
improving myocardial contractile performance, and providing effective
systemic and regional blood flow to meet tissue demands. Patients
should be placed at bed rest and given supplemental oxygen to maintain
an arterial oxygen saturation of at least 90%. In severe cases, this
may require endotracheal intubation and mechanical ventilation
(Chapters 8-9). A careful cardiac examination should be performed,
paying particular attention to any new murmurs which might suggest a
mechanical complication. Potentially offending medications should be
minimized or withdrawn. Chest pain, when present, should be managed
with morphine and/or nitroglycerin as discussed in Chapter 4. Both of
these agents promptly and effectively reduce left ventricular preload
and are therefore useful in the acute management of CHF. Arrhythmias
should be managed as outlined in Chapter 15.

Medical therapy specific for CHF consists of diuretics,
vasodilators, and inotropic agents. Proper use of these agents is
dependent on the etiology, severity, and timing of CHF in relation to
the onset of infarction. In patients with mild to moderate CHF
(Killip Class II) who are otherwise stable, treatment with a diuretic
such as intravenous furosemide in doses of 20-80 mg (repeated as
necessary) is usually sufficient. Many Killip Class III patients will
also respond satisfactorily to aggressive diuresis with or without
concomitant vasodilator therapy. Patients with more advanced heart
failure or pulmonary edema who do not respond readily to conservative
therapy should undergo pulmonary artery catheterization. Appropriate
blood samples and pressure tracings should be obtained to exclude
mechanical complications. The hemodynamic data can then be used to
guide therapy (Table 17.4). (Caution: Hemodynamic data should never

Table 17.4
Suggested Guidelines for Managing Hemodynamic Disturbances in Acute MI*

Systolic BP (mm Hg)	PAOP (mm Hg)	Cardiac Index (L/min/M^2)	Suggested Treatment
≥ 110	≤ 15	≥ 2.5	Normal; observe
< 110	≤ 15	< 2.5	Cautious fluid administration
≥ 110	> 15	≥ 2.5	Diuretic if CHF present
≥ 110	> 15	< 2.5	Diuretic; consider inotrope or vasodilator
< 110	> 15	< 2.5	Inotropic agent; vasodilator and diuretic if tolerated
< 90	> 18	< 2.2	Inotropic agent; consider intra-aortic balloon

*These guidelines should be used in conjunction with clinical data and an assessment of the probable cause of the hemodynamic disturbance.

be taken as "absolute" and should be used only in the clinical context of the individual patient. Also, pulmonary artery catheterization is not a substitute for, nor does it preclude, a careful clinical assessment of the etiology and severity of the hemodynamic impairment).

The selection of an inotropic agent or vasodilator as initial therapy in patients with severe CHF unresponsive to diuretics is controversial. However, during the first 6-12 hours of acute MI, a vasodilator is preferable to a sympathomimetic agent, since the latter may increase oxygen demand and exacerbate ischemia. Intravenous nitroglycerin is a rational choice because it is safe and effective. The dose should be titrated to achieve a reduction in mean arterial pressure of 5-10% or a decrease in the systolic pressure of 10-20 mm Hg. Nitroprusside and nifedipine may have adverse effects when given early in acute MI (5,6), and other vasodilators, including converting enzyme inhibitors, have not been adequately studied. If the response to diuretics and nitroglycerin is insufficient, amrinone may be added. The role of digoxin in this setting is unclear (7,8).

Killip Class III CHF which persists for more than 6-12 hours after the onset of infarction may be treated with inotropic agents or vasodilators, alone or in combination. Converting enzyme inhibitors are effective oral vasodilating agents, and the combination of nitrates and hydralazine provide a suitable alternative. In more severe cases, treatment should include either intravenous nitroglycerin or nitroprusside (5). In selecting an inotropic agent, dobutamine and amrinone have comparable hemodynamic effects, but dobutamine has a much shorter half-life (2 min vs 4-6 hr), which allows for easier titration and rapid elimination should adverse effects occur. Dobutamine is also substantially more effective than digoxin (7) and is also preferable to dopamine in the absence of hypotension (9,10). The usual dose of dobutamine is 5-10 mcg/kg/min (Appendix D). Modest additional benefit may be obtained with doses up to 20 mcg/kg/min; doses above 20 mcg/kg/min usually do not result in further hemodynamic improvement. Patients continued on dobutamine for longer than 72 hours may require an increase in dosage due to the development of tolerance (11).

Shock

Shock is an advanced state of hemodynamic impairment in which a prolonged imbalance between tissue nutrient supply and demand leads to severe multiorgan dysfunction. Cardiogenic shock complicating acute MI is usually due to necrosis of 40% or more of left ventricular mass (12). Despite advances in hemodynamic monitoring and pharmacotherapy, mortality from cardiogenic shock due to pump failure remains high, exceeding 75%. Other causes of cardiogenic shock include mechanical complications (rupture of the ventricular septum, papillary muscle, or free wall) and massive right ventricular infarction. In patients with pre-existing aortic or mitral valve disease, acute MI may lead to shock in the absence of extensive myocardial damage. In addition, marked intravascular volume contraction, sepsis, pulmonary embolus, or tension pneumothorax may masquerade as cardiogenic shock. In the absence of severe left ventricular dysfunction, shock complicating acute MI is amenable to aggressive medical or surgical therapy. It is therefore imperative that all potentially treatable causes of shock be evaluated in a systematic fashion.

The clinical manifestations of cardiogenic shock include signs of both severe hypoperfusion with peripheral vasoconstriction and concomitant CHF. Cardiac auscultation should be performed frequently, since a new or changing murmur would suggest a ventricular septal defect or papillary muscle rupture (Chapter 21). An assessment of ventricular function should be obtained promptly. Bedside echocardiography is extremely valuable in this regard, since it enables evaluation of global ventricular performance and also permits visualization of the mitral and aortic valves, ventricular aneurysms, right ventricular function, and pericardial effusions. Urgent pulmonary artery catheterization should be performed, and blood gases analyzed to exclude an oxygen "step-up." The PAOP tracing should be carefully inspected for an abnormal v-wave, and the hemodynamic data should be reviewed to determine whether there is evidence of hypovolemia or right ventricular infarction. Finally, if the cardiac index is not < 2.0 L/min/M^2 (in the absence of a VSD), the diagnosis of cardiogenic shock is suspect, and other disorders should be considered.

Patients with cardiogenic shock should be intubated and placed on controlled mechanical ventilation to minimize cardiac work and ensure adequate oxygenation and ventilation (Chapters 8-9). Placing the patient in the head-down (Trendelenburg) position improves venous return from the lower extremities and helps maintain cerebral perfusion. Agitated patients may require sedation with anxiolytic agents or narcotics. Inotropic therapy should be initiated, and an arterial catheter inserted to monitor blood pressure changes. In severely hypotensive patients, dopamine or norepinephrine may be preferable to dobutamine, and in some patients combination therapy with dobutamine and either dopamine or amrinone may be beneficial (13,14). Intra-aortic balloon counterpulsation (Chapter 37) should be considered in any patient with cardiogenic shock due to a potentially reversible cause. However, IABP is not indicated in patients with irreversible severe global left ventricular dysfunction unless cardiac transplantation is available (15). In patients with mechanical complications of acute MI, urgent consultation with a cardiovascular surgeon should be obtained, and arrangements made for cardiac catheterization if indicated.

The prognosis in any patient with cardiogenic shock is poor, but the above guidelines should help prevent errors in misdiagnosing potentially treatable causes of shock, and allow expeditious intervention in those patients who may benefit from aggressive therapy.

REFERENCES

1. Peel AAF, Semple T, Wang I, Lancaster WM, Doll JLG. A coronary prognostic index for grading the severity of infarction. Br Heart J 1962;24:745-760.

2. Killip T, Kimball JT. Treatment of myocardial infarction in a coronary care unit. Am J Cardiol 1967;20:457-464.

3. Norris RM, Brandt PWT, Caughey DE, Lee AJ, Scott PJ. A new coronary prognostic index. Lancet 1969;I:274-278.

4. Forrester JS, Diamond G, Chatterjee K, Swan HJC. Medical therapy of acute myocardial infarction by application of hemodynamic subsets. N Engl J Med 1976;295:1356-1362 & 1404-1413.

5. Cohn JN, Franciosa JA, Francis GS, et al. Effect of short-term infusion of sodium nitroprusside on mortality rates in acute myocardial infarction complicated by left ventricular failure. N Engl J Med 1982;306:1129-1135.

6. Muller JE, Morrison J, Stone PH, et al. Nifedipine therapy for patients with threatened and acute myocardial infarction: A randomized, double-blind, placebo-controlled comparison. Circulation 1984;69:740-747.

7. Goldstein RA, Passamani E, Roberts R. A comparison of digoxin and dobutamine in patients with acute infarction and cardiac failure. N Engl J Med 1980;303:846–850.

8. Marchionni N, Pini R, Vannucci A, et al. Hemodynamic effects of digoxin in acute myocardial infarction in man: A randomized controlled trial. Am Heart J 1985;109:63–69.

9. Maekawa K, Liang C, Hood WB. Comparison of dobutamine and dopamine in acute myocardial infarction. Circulation 1983; 67:750–759.

10. Keung ECH, Siskind HJ, Sonnenblick EH, Ribner HS, Schwartz WJ, LeJemtel TH. Dobutamine in acute myocardial infarction. JAMA 1981;245:144–146.

11. Unverferth DV, Blanford M, Kates RE, Leier CV. Tolerance to dobutamine after a 72 hour continuous infusion. Am J Med 1980; 69:262–266.

12. Page DL, Caulfield JB, Kastor JA, DeSanctis RW, Sanders CA. Myocardial changes associated with cardiogenic shock. N Engl J Med 1971;285:133–137.

13. Richard C, Ricome JL, Rimailho A, Bottineau G, Auzepy P. Combined hemodynamic effects of dopamine and dobutamine in cardiogenic shock. Circulation 1983;67:620–626.

14. Gage J, Rutman H, Lucido D, LeJemtel TH. Additive effects of dobutamine and amrinone on myocardial contractility and ventricular performance in patients with severe heart failure. Circulation 1986;74:367–373.

15. Scheidt S, Wilner G, Mueller H, et al. Intra-aortic balloon counterpulsation in cardiogenic shock. N Engl J Med 1973; 288:979–984.

Chapter 18

Invasive Hemodynamic Monitoring

Edward C. Miller, M.D.

Techniques for invasive hemodynamic monitoring evolved from methods originally developed to assess cardiac performance in the cardiac catheterization laboratory. Advances in technology, most notably the introduction of the balloon-tipped, flow-directed "Swan-Ganz" pulmonary artery catheter in 1970, now permit serial measurements of intracardiac pressures and various hemodynamic parameters, and hemodynamic monitoring has become a standard tool for managing critically ill patients. This chapter will review the indications for hemodynamic monitoring, interpretation of hemodynamic data, and troubleshooting pulmonary artery catheters. A discussion of available equipment and the technique of pulmonary artery catheterization is provided in Chapter 34.

Indications

The most common indications for hemodynamic monitoring in the CCU are hypoperfusion and congestive heart failure complicating acute myocardial infarction. Pulmonary artery (PA) catheters are also used in managing patients with hemodynamic dysfunction arising from other cardiac and noncardiac causes (e.g., cardiomyopathy, pericardial disease, septic shock, adult respiratory distress syndrome). Patients with refractory congestive heart failure requiring intravenous inotropic agents and vasodilators are best managed with a pulmonary artery catheter to monitor and guide therapy. Other indications include: major cardiac surgery; non-cardiac surgery in patients with decompensated heart failure, unstable angina, or recent myocardial infarction; diagnosis of intracardiac shunts, pericardial tamponade or constriction, or pulmonary hypertension; cardiovascular instability in critically ill patients with primary respiratory, renal, hepatic, infectious, or endocrine disease; intractable angina with hemodynamic instability; suspected acute mitral regurgitation or ventricular septal perforation; and assessment of intravascular volume status and cardiac performance in marginally compensated patients in whom this information would significantly affect therapy. Regardless of the original indication for pulmonary artery catheterization, the need for continued hemodynamic monitoring should be reassessed daily.

Interpretation of Hemodynamic Data

Normal Physiology and Waveforms

The normal resting right atrial (RA) pressure waveform contains a, c, v, and h waves corresponding to pressure crests, and x, x', and y descents following the a, c, and v waves respectively (Fig. 18.1). The a-wave represents the rise in RA pressure caused by atrial contraction in late diastole, and occurs immediately following atrial depolarization (P-wave on the ECG). Atrial relaxation then causes a fall in the RA pressure, manifested by the x-descent. With the onset of ventricular systole, the tricuspid valve is thrust closed, resulting in a small rise in the RA pressure (c-wave). As systole continues, the tricuspid anulus is pulled downward and toward the apex, producing a fall in RA pressure (x'-descent). In late systole, passive filling of the RA by blood from the vena cavae again causes the RA pressure to rise (v-wave), and when the tricuspid valve opens in early diastole, rapid emptying of the atrium is accompanied by a fall in pressure (y-descent). Passive filling during mid-diastole produces a gradual common rise in the RA and right ventricular (RV) pressure (h-wave) which is terminated by the next atrial contraction (a-wave).

RIGHT HEART PRESSURES

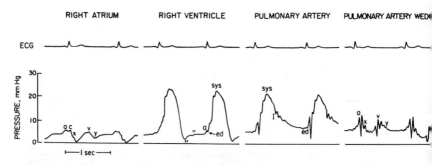

Figure 18.1. Normal hemodynamic waveforms. (ed: end diastole, I: incisura, RF: rapid filling, SF: slow filling, sys: systole). Reproduced with permission from Grossman W, Barry WH. Cardiac catheterization. In: Braunwald E, ed. Heart disease. A textbook of cardiovascular medicine, 3rd ed. W.B. Saunders Co, Philadelphia, 1988:250.

In mid- and late-diastole, when the tricuspid valve is open and the rapid ventricular filling phase is complete, RA and RV pressures are identical, and the h-wave, a-wave, and early x-descent are manifest on both pressure waveforms. With the onset of ventricular contraction, RV pressure exceeds RA pressure (resulting in tricuspid valve closure) but not pulmonary artery (PA) pressure (pulmonic valve remains closed). This isovolumetric contraction results in a sudden rapid rise in the RV pressure which then exceeds PA pressure, causing the pulmonic valve to open and permitting forward ejection of blood to occur. As ejection continues, RV and PA systolic pressures equalize and the RV pressure begins to fall. At end-systole, the PA pressure again exceeds the RV pressure causing the pulmonic valve to close. The RV then undergoes an isovolumetric relaxation period marked by a rapid fall in RV pressure. When RV pressure falls below RA pressure, the tricuspid valve opens and the rapid filling phase begins.

Rapid ejection of blood into the pulmonary artery in early systole causes the PA pressure to rise rapidly, and the PA waveform follows the RV waveform until pulmonic valve closure. At this point, elastic recoil of the pulmonary artery against a closed pulmonic valve produces a notch on the descending portion of the PA waveform known as the incisura (Fig. 18.1). The PA pressure then continues a gradual decline until end diastole is reached and ejection again occurs.

Characteristics of the left atrial (LA), left ventricular (LV), and systemic arterial pressure waveforms are similar to those of the RA, RV, and PA respectively. The pulmonary artery occlusive pressure (PAOP; also called the "wedge" pressure) is obtained by inflating the balloon while the catheter tip is positioned in a proximal branch of the pulmonary artery. Forward blood flow carries the balloon distally, resulting in occlusion of one of the smaller branches of the PA. The PA exit port of the catheter, being distal to the balloon, is thus shielded from the PA pressure, and pressure recordings at this point reflect pressure changes in the distal circulation, i.e. the pulmonary veins and left atrium. Thus, the PAOP waveform (Fig. 18.1) reflects the left atrial pressure (in the absence of disease in the pulmonary veins), which in turn reflects the left ventricular pressure during diastole (in the absence of mitral stenosis). Note, however, that transmission of left atrial pressure changes back through the pulmonary veins and capillaries to the catheter tip results in a phasic delay of about 0.25 seconds in the pressure recordings. In addition, the low amplitude c and h waves are frequently obscured. Finally, in patients on PEEP in whom intra-alveolar pressure exceeds left atrial pressure, the wedge recording may reflect the end-expiratory alveolar pressure rather than the left heart pressures.

The normal waveforms described above are subject to a number of other influences aside from the effects of the cardiac cycle itself. Inspiration causes a fall in intrathoracic pressure which is also reflected as a fall in intracardiac pressures. By convention, pressure measurements are made at end-expiration during normal quiet breathing. Positional changes also affect intracardiac pressures (e.g. pressures fall with standing due to decreased venous return); standardized recordings are thus taken with the patient supine and with the transducer at the level of the RA or in the mid-axillary

line. During exercise, pressures normally rise modestly, so ideally
patients should be at rest for 15-30 minutes before pressure
recordings are made. Finally, numerous pathologic conditions affect
intracardiac pressures; the next section will briefly discuss those
relevant to the CCU.

Pathophysiology and Abnormal Waveforms

Normal hemodynamic values are listed in Table 18.1 and Appendix
C. Common etiologies of various abnormalities in the pressure
waveforms are shown in Table 18.2. As is apparent, any given
abnormality must be interpreted in light of the specific clinical
setting, as there is no hemodynamic finding that is "pathognomonic" of
a single disease process.

RA pressures may be elevated due to RV failure, decreased RV
compliance, pericardial disease, or tricuspid valve disease. A-waves,
corresponding to atrial contraction, are absent in atrial
fibrillation, increased when RV diastolic pressure is increased (often
due to decreased RV compliance), and in tricuspid stenosis (during
sinus rhythm). In A-V dissociation, atrial contraction occurs
randomly during the cardiac cycle resulting in a-waves of varying
intensity, including giant ("cannon") a-waves when the atrium
contracts against a closed tricuspid valve. A v-wave exceeding the
a-wave by 5 mm Hg or more, or exceeding the mean RA pressure by 10 mm
Hg or more indicates rapid filling of the atrium beyond its capacity.
This most commonly occurs with new or worsening tricuspid
insufficiency. In chronic tricuspid regurgitation the atrium becomes
greatly enlarged and compliant, and is able to accept a large volume
of blood without a marked increase in pressure. In this situation,
the v-wave may be unremarkable despite severe tricuspid insufficiency.

As discussed earlier, the y-descent represents rapid atrial
emptying in early diastole. In pericardial tamponade, the RV is
compressed by pericardial fluid under pressure. The atrium is unable
to empty rapidly, and this is manifested by a marked attenuation or
even absence of the y-descent. In pericardial constriction and
restrictive cardiomyopathy, the RV is not compressed as in tamponade,
and there is a large gradient in early diastole between the elevated
RA pressure and the low RV pressure. This results in very rapid
atrial emptying and a rapid fall in RA pressure, manifested by a
prominent y-descent. However, as a result of the constrictive
physiology, the ventricle is soon unable to receive any more blood,
and the RV diastolic pressure plateaus. This combination of a rapid
y-descent followed by an abrupt rise and mid-to-late diastolic plateau
produces the so-called "square root sign" in the RV pressure tracing.
This finding is typical of constrictive pericarditis, but may also be
seen with restrictive cardiomyopathy or right ventricular infarction.

During normal inspiration, negative intrathoracic pressure causes
increased blood return to the heart and a fall in jugular venous
pressure. In the presence of constrictive physiology, this blood is

Table 18.1
Normal Resting Hemodynamic Values*

Pressures (mm Hg)	a-wave	v-wave	systolic	end diastolic	mean
Right atrium	2-10	2-10			2-8
Right ventricle			15-30	2-8	
Pulmonary artery			15-30	4-12	8-18
PAOP/left atrium	3-15	3-12			3-12
Left ventricle			100-140	3-12	
Systemic arterial			100-140	60-90	70-105

Oxygen consumption index (ml/min/M^2)	110-150
Arteriovenous O_2 content difference (ml/L)	30-50
Cardiac index (L/min/M^2)	2.6-4.2
Stroke volume index (ml/M^2)	30-65

Resistances (dyne-sec/cm^5)

Pulmonary vascular	40-150
Systemic vascular	800-1500

* Adapted from Grossman W, Barry WH. Cardiac catheterization. In: Braunwald E, ed. Heart disease. A textbook of cardiovascular medicine, 3rd ed. W.B. Saunders Co, Philadelphia, 1988:250.

unable to enter the ventricle, the RA also fills rapidly, and the blood backs up into the vena cavae and jugular veins, producing Kussmaul's sign (inspiratory expansion of the jugular veins). In pericardial tamponade, RV filling during mid-diastole is compromised to a lesser degree because the intraventricular septum bows to the left. With inspiration, this bowing becomes more pronounced and actually compromises LV filling. This leads to a reduction in left ventricular stroke volume and a fall in cardiac output. This inspiratory fall in cardiac output is manifested clinically by pulsus paradoxus (inspiratory decline in arterial systolic pressure in excess of 10 mm Hg during quiet breathing).

Another hemodynamic finding often associated with pericardial disease is equalization of end-diastolic pressures in the RA, RV, PA, LA (or PAOP), and LV. This is, however, a non-specific finding which can also be seen in cardiomyopathy, chronic pulmonary disease, and RV infarction. Equalization of pressures is thus compatible with pericardial disease, but additional confirmation is required (e.g., echocardiography). By contrast, the absence of equalization in euvolemic patients reliably excludes constrictive pericarditis.

Table 18.2
Common Etiologies of Abnormal Cardiac Pressure Waveforms

Abnormality	Pathophysiology	Examples
Increased mean RA pressure	RV failure	Pulmonary hypertension of any cause, RV infarct, cardiomyopathy, tricuspid disease, pericardial disease, congenital heart disease
	Decreased RV filling rate	
Decreased mean RA pressure	Decreased preload	Hypovolemia
Increased a-wave in RA	Decreased RV filling rate	Elevated RV diastolic pressure of any cause, decreased RV compliance, tricuspid stenosis
Absent a-wave in RA	Diminished atrial contraction	Atrial fibrillation, hyperkalemia
Variable a-wave in RA	A-V dissociation	Multiple causes (see Chapter 6)
Prominent v-wave in RA	Augmented atrial filling	Tricuspid regurgitation, acute left to right shunt at atrial level
Prominent y-descent in RA	Rapid atrial emptying	Constrictive pericarditis, restrictive cardiomyopathy, RV infarct
Absent y-descent in RA	Poor atrial emptying	Pericardial tamponade
Increased RV systolic pressure	RV pressure overload	Pulmonary hypertension (any cause), pulmonic stenosis
Increased RV diastolic pressure	RV failure	Pulmonary hypertension, RV infarct, cardiomyopathy, pericardial disease
	Decreased RV compliance	
RV "square root sign"	Rapid filling to plateau	Constrictive pericarditis, restrictive cardiomyopathy, RV infarct
Increased PA systolic and mean pressures	Pulmonary hypertension	Primary pulmonary or pulmonary vascular disease, left heart failure, mitral valve disease
Increased PA diastolic pressure PA diastolic-PAOP < 5 mm Hg	Elevated left heart pressures	LV failure, mitral valve disease
PA diastolic-PAOP < 5 mm Hg	Pulmonary vascular disease	Primary pulmonary hypertension Chronic lung disease
Increased mean PAOP	LV failure	LV systolic dysfunction, aortic or mitral valve disease, decreased LV compliance, volume overload
	Decreased LV filling rate	
Decreased mean PAOP	Decreased preload	Hypovolemia, severe RV failure
Increased a-wave in PAOP	Decreased LV filling rate	Increased LV diastolic pressure, decreased LV compliance, mitral stenosis
Prominent v-wave in PAOP	Augmented LA filling	Mitral regurgitation, acute intracardiac shunt
Equalization of RA, RV, PA, and PAOP diastolic pressures	Multiple	Pericardial disease, cardiomyopathy RV infarct, pulmonary disease

Elevated RV systolic pressure is usually a compensatory response to pulmonary hypertension, but can also be seen in pulmonic stenosis. Causes of RV diastolic pressure elevation are similar to those discussed for increased mean RA pressure, with the exception of tricuspid stenosis. Severe RV dysfunction (e.g. due to massive RV infarction) may produce a narrow RV pulse pressure.

Pulmonary arterial hypertension is usually due to chronic lung disease, pulmonary vascular disease (including pulmonary embolus), or left atrial hypertension caused by left-sided myocardial or valvular dysfunction. Pulmonary artery end-diastolic pressure is normally equal to LA end-diastolic pressure and can be used as a surrogate PAOP if the balloon cannot be successfully "wedged." If the PA end diastolic pressure is consistently > 5 mm Hg higher than the PAOP, intrinsic lung disease or pulmonary vascular disease is suggested; pulmonary vascular resistance will usually be elevated as well.

As mentioned earlier, the PAOP is usually a reliable indicator of LA pressure and, in the absence of mitral stenosis, LV diastolic pressure. Alterations in the PAOP waveform are caused by conditions on the left side of the heart similar to those on the right side which produce corresponding changes in the RA pressure. A v-wave > 10 mm Hg above the mean PAOP excluding the v-wave usually connotes significant mitral regurgitation. Acute ventricular septal perforation produces a sudden augmentation of blood flow to the LA (via the pulmonary veins) and is a less frequent cause of an abnormal v-wave. Incomplete "wedging" of the catheter can also mimic an elevated v-wave.

Proper interpretation of the mean PAOP can be accomplished only in conjunction with relevant clinical data. This is because the magnitude of changes in the PAOP are as important as the absolute pressure reading. To illustrate, consider two patients with a moderately elevated PAOP of 20 mm Hg. The first is a previously healthy man with an acute MI complicated by congestive heart failure. The PAOP reflects an abrupt rise from a previously normal value, producing pulmonary vascular congestion and requiring treatment with a diuretic. In the second case, a patient with severe ischemic cardiomyopathy is hospitalized with congestive heart failure and vigorously diuresed until pre-renal azotemia develops. The PAOP of 20 mm Hg reflects a fall from a previous baseline of 30 mm Hg. The value may be below the patient's optimal filling pressure for maximizing cardiac output, and the patient is more likely to benefit from volume administration than continued diuresis. Thus, the PAOP should not be viewed as an absolute number, but should be interpreted in the context of whether the value is appropriate for optimal hemodynamic performance in the specific clinical setting. It is also worth remembering that modest increases in the PAOP will improve cardiac performance even in normal individuals, since the increased preload augments stroke volume via the Frank-Starling mechanism. In normal patients, cardiac output is maximal at a PAOP of 15-18 mm Hg. In patients with cardiac disease, even higher values may be beneficial, as noted in the example above. One implication of this is that in a patient with low cardiac output and a PAOP < 15-18 mm Hg, fluid administration may improve cardiac output by increasing preload to a more optimal level.

Oximetry

During initial placement of the PA catheter, blood gas samples should be obtained from the RA, RV, and PA in any patient with an unexplained murmur, suspected intracardiac shunt, or change in hemodynamic status post MI. A step-up in oxygen saturation in excess of 10% in moving from one chamber to the next indicates a left-to-right shunt at that level. Using standard equations, these data can also be used in conjunction with arterial blood gases to calculate the fraction of shunted blood.

In the absence of an intracardiac shunt, severe anemia, or marked arterial hypoxemia, the mixed venous oxygen saturation obtained from the PA provides a rough guide to the adequacy of cardiac performance. This is because tissues extract oxygen in proportion to their needs and the volume of blood delivered. Thus, in a low cardiac output state, a given tissue will extract a greater percentage of oxygen from the blood received than when cardiac output is normal. Venous blood returning to the system will therefore have a lower oxygen saturation, and this will be reflected in a lower mixed venous saturation as well. As a general guideline, recognizing that there is wide individual variation, a mixed venous saturation of 70% or greater corresponds to a normal cardiac output and adequate delivery of blood and oxygen to the tissues. A mixed venous saturation in the 60-70% range indicates mild hemodynamic impairment, 45-60% corresponds to moderate impairment (anaerobic metabolism begins to occur at this level; see Chapter 8), 30-45% represents severely reduced cardiac performance; and sustained saturations below 30% are not usually compatible with life.

Cardiac Output Determination

The PA catheter permits measurement of cardiac output by two independent techniques: the thermodilution method and the Fick method.

In the thermodilution method, 10 cc of saline at a known temperature (usually 0° C) are injected at a fixed rate into the proximal port of the catheter, and a subsequent temperature drop is sensed by the thermister at the catheter tip. The time course and magnitude of the temperature change are recorded on a computer which then calculates cardiac output. Intuitively, it should be apparent that temperature change correlates inversely with cardiac output, since the larger the volume of blood into which the injectate is diluted (i.e., the higher the cardiac output), the less pronounced will be the temperature change. The injection should be repeated at least 3 times, and when 3 recordings within 5-10% precision of each other are obtained, they are averaged to give the cardiac output. Note that the value obtained represents flow through the <u>right</u> side of the heart. Under normal circumstances, this equals the left-sided cardiac output. With a left-to-right shunt, right heart output will exceed left heart output by an amount equal to the volume of the shunt, and vice-versa for right-to-left shunts. With tricuspid insufficiency (less commonly pulmonic insufficiency), the apparent volume into which the injectate is diluted may be artifactually increased by the regurgitant flow. In these situations, the measured thermodilution cardiac output may not reflect the true systemic cardiac output, and caution must be used in interpreting the results. Other factors affecting the reliability of the thermodilution technique include the injection rate, injectate temperature, and technical problems with the equipment. This method also tends to overestimate the true cardiac output in very low flow situations.

The principles discussed earlier relating blood flow and oxygen extraction derive from the Fick equation for calculating cardiac output:

$$\text{Cardiac output (L/min)} = \frac{\text{Oxygen consumption (ml/min)}}{\text{A-V } O_2 \text{ content difference (ml/L)}}$$

Oxygen consumption can be measured using a Douglas bag or a Beckman metabolic cart, and the A-V O_2 difference (i.e., the difference in oxygen content between arterial and mixed venous blood) can be calculated from arterial and mixed venous blood samples and the patient's hemoglobin:

A-V O_2 diff (ml/L)=1.36(ml O_2/gm Hgb) X Hgb(gm/dl) X 10(dl/L) X

(arterial - mixed venous O_2 saturation)

In actual practice, oxygen consumption is often estimated as 125 or 130 ml O_2/min/M^2 (normal range = 110-150 ml O_2/min/M^2). Correcting for body surface area (BSA), the formula becomes:

$$\text{Cardiac index} = \frac{\text{Oxygen consumption index}}{\text{A-V } O_2 \text{ difference}}$$

As an example, assume: O_2 consumption index = 125 ml O_2/min/M^2, Hgb = 14.0 gm/dl, arterial O_2 saturation (from blood gas) = 95%, mixed venous O_2 saturation = 65%, and BSA = 1.8 M^2. Then,

$$\text{Cardiac index} = \frac{125}{1.36 \text{ X } 14.0 \text{ X } 10 \text{ X } (.95-.65)} = 2.2 \text{ L/min/}M^2; \text{ and}$$

Cardiac output = Cardiac index X BSA = 2.2 x 1.8 = 4.0 L/min

Note that this technique does not require a functioning PA catheter; only that blood can be obtained simultaneously from the PA port and a peripheral artery. Results obtained by this technique should be compared with the thermodilution method when the PA catheter is initially inserted, any time there is a significant change in hemodynamics, and whenever the thermodilution data do not fit the clinical picture. The two techniques should provide results that differ by no more than 15-20%. The Fick technique is preferable when cardiac output is very low and when an intracardiac shunt or significant tricuspid regurgitaton is suspected. The major disadvantage of the Fick method lies in the estimation of O_2 consumption, which can vary greatly with age, sex, body temperature, state of wellness, mechanical ventilation, and the use of vasopressors.

Hemodynamic Calculations

A variety of calculations can be performed utilizing the pressure and oximetric data obtained from the PA catheter in conjunction with the cardiac output, heart rate, and systemic blood pressure. It is important to recognize that the accuracy of all calculated data is wholly dependent on the accuracy of measured data used in the calculation. Thus, if the cardiac output is "wrong," all data calculated from the cardiac output (e.g. stroke volume, vascular resistances, etc) will also be wrong.

From the perspective of patient management, perhaps the two most useful hemodynamic calculations are the systemic and pulmonary vascular resistances, formulas for which are provided below. Formulas for other commonly performed calculations are given in Appendix B.

Systemic vascular resistance (SVR) =

$$\frac{(\text{Mean arterial pressure} - \text{mean RA pressure}) \times 80}{\text{Cardiac Output}}$$

(Normal range = 800-1500 dyne-sec/cm^5)

Pulmonary vascular resistance (PVR) =

$$\frac{(\text{Mean PA presure} - \text{mean PAOP}) \times 80}{\text{Cardiac Output}}$$

(Normal range = 40-150 dyne-sec/cm^5)

Note that vascular resistance is inversely related to cardiac output. If cardiac output falls (or is underestimated), the calculated SVR and PVR will rise (assuming the numerator remains constant). A common error is to assume that cardiac output has declined because SVR has gone up when in fact the converse is frequently the case.

Troubleshooting

Several difficulties may arise when using PA catheters; management of some of the more common problems is discussed below.

Continuous PAOP Tracing ("overwedging")

This generally indicates peripheral advancement of the catheter tip, which can be confirmed by chest x-ray (the tip should not extend more than 3-4 cm out from the hilum). Be sure the balloon is deflated and carefully flush the distal port. If a PA tracing does not appear, pull the catheter back 2-3 cm at a time, flushing after each adjustment, and recheck the waveform. If the catheter is withdrawn too rapidly, the tip may come back to the right ventricle (RV waveform appears). If this occurs, inflate the balloon with 1 cc of air and readvance into the PA. (Note: The latter maneuver should be performed only if a sterile sleeve is in place around the catheter.) If ventricular tachycardia develops during catheter manipulation, deflate the balloon and remove the catheter.

Over-damped Tracing

An over-damped waveform lacks normal high frequency components. Be sure the balloon is deflated, check the pressure tubing for small air bubbles (often at connection points), flush the entire system by hand, and recalibrate. If the tracing is still damped, the catheter is probably either twisted or the tip is positioned against a vessel wall. Carefully pull the catheter back 1-2 cm and inflate the balloon. If a proper tracing still does not appear, reflush and recalibrate the system. Occasionally, additional adjustment in the catheter position may be necessary.

Failure to Obtain PAOP (catheter won't "wedge")

This usually indicates that the catheter tip is not out far enough into the PA. Inflate the balloon with 1 cc of air, and have the patient take a deep breath while advancing the catheter 2-3 cm through a sterile sleeve. This procedure may need to be repeated several times. After a PAOP tracing has been obtained, deflate the balloon and check to see that the PA waveform reappears (i.e., the catheter is not "overwedged"). Occasionally, "failure to wedge" is due to rupture of the balloon, in which case injected air will not return to the syringe when the balloon is deflated. If the PAOP is critical to the patient's management, the catheter should be replaced. Less commonly, it may be difficult to distinguish the PAOP waveform from that of the PA. This is most common with tachycardias (esp. atrial fibrillation) and when there is a large v-wave. Usually, the situation can be clarified by obtaining a simultaneous dual channel recording of a surface ECG lead and the pressure waveform, remembering that the upstroke of the PA waveform occurs immediately after the QRS, while that of the v-wave occurs later in systole. Finally, in patients with severe pulmonary hypertension, it may not be possible to obtain a PAOP.

Inconsistent Readings

On occasion, pressure or hemodynamic data will be inconsistent or irreproducible. Be sure the patient and equipment are properly positioned, and there are no kinks in the catheter. Check for bubbles, flush and recalibrate the entire system, and repeat the desired measurements.

FURTHER READING

1. Boutros AR, Lee C. Value of continuous monitoring of mixed venous blood oxygen saturation in the management of critically ill patients. Crit Care Med 1986;14:132-134.

2. Connors AF, Castele RJ, Farhat NZ, Tomashefski JF. Complications of right heart catheterization: A prospective autopsy study. Chest 1985;88:567-572.

3. Daily EK, Schroeder JS. Hemodynamic waveforms. Exercises in identification and analysis. C. V. Mosby Co, St. Louis, 1983:277.

4. Damen J. Ventricular arrhythmias during insertion and removal of pulmonary artery catheters. Chest 1985;88:190-193.

5. Davies GG, Jebson PJR, Glasgow BM, Hess DR. Continuous Fick cardiac output compared to thermodilution cardiac output. Crit Care Med 1986;14:881-885.

6. Downes TR, Hackshaw BT, Kahl FR, et al. Frequency of large V waves in the pulmonary artery wedge pressure in ventricular septal defect of acquired (during acute myocardial infarction) or congenital origin. Am J Cardiol 1987;60:415-417.

7. Forrester JS, Diamond G, Chatterjee K, Swan HJC. Medical therapy of acute myocardial infarction by application of hemodynamic subsets. N Engl J Med 1976;295:1356-1362 & 1404-1413.

8. Forrester JS, Diamond GA, Swan HJC. Bedside diagnosis of latent cardiac complications in acutely ill patients. JAMA 1972; 222:59-63.

9. Gore JM, Alpert JS, Benotti JR, Kotilainen PW, Haffajee CI. Handbook of hemodynamic monitoring. Little, Brown & Company, Boston, 1985.

10. Iberti TJ, Benjamin E, Gruppi L, Raskin JM. Ventricular arrhythmias during pulmonary artery catheterization in the intensive care unit: Prospective study. Am J Med 1985;78:451-454.

11. Levin RI, Glassman E. Left atrial-pulmonary artery wedge pressure relation: Effect of elevated pulmonary vascular resistance. Am J Cardiol 1985;55:856-857.

12. Morris AH, Chapman RH, Gardner RM. Frequency of wedge pressure errors in the ICU. Crit Care Med 1985;13:705-708.

13. Moser KM, Spragg RG. Use of the balloon-tipped pulmonary artery catheter in pulmonary disease. Ann Intern Med 1983;98:53-58.

14. Myers ML, Austin TW, Sibbald WJ. Pulmonary artery catheter infections: A prospective study. Ann Surg 1985;201:237-241.

15. Okamoto K, Komatsu T, Kumar V, et al. Effects of intermittent positive-pressure ventilation on cardiac output measurements by thermodilution. Crit Care Med 1986;14:977-980.

16. Patel C, Laboy V, Venus B, Mathru M, Wier D. Acute complications of pulmonary artery catheter insertion in critically ill patients. Crit Care Med 1986;14:195-197.

17. Pizzarello RA, Turnier J, Padmanabhan VT, Goldman M, Tortolani A. Left atrial size, pressure and v-wave height in patients with isolated, severe, pure mitral regurgitation. Cathet Cardiovasc Diagn 1984;10:445-454.

18. Robin ED. The cult of the Swan-Ganz catheter: Overuse and abuse of pulmonary flow catheters. Ann Intern Med 1985;103:445-449.

19. Rowley KM, Clubb S, Smith GJ, Cabin HS. Right-sided infective endocarditis as a consequence of flow-directed pulmonary-artery catheterization. N Engl J Med 1984;311:1152-1156.

20. Russell RO, Mantle JA, Rogers WJ, Rackley CE. Current status of hemodynamic monitoring: Indications, diagnoses, complications. In: Rackley CE, ed. Critcal care cardiology. Cardiovascular clinics. F. A. Davis Company, Philadelphia, 1981:1-13.

21. Sharkey SW. Beyond the wedge: Clinical physiology and the Swan-Ganz catheter. Am J Med 1987;83:111-122.

22. Spodick DH. Physiologic and prognostic implications of invasive monitoring: Undetermined risk/benefit ratios in patients with heart disease. Am J Cardiol 1980;46:173-175.

23. Swan HJC, Ganz WW, Forrester JS, et al. Catheterization of the heart in man with use of a flow-directed balloon-tipped catheter. N Engl J Med 1970;283:447-451.

24. Weisel RD, Berger RL, Hechtman HB. Measurement of cardiac output by thermodilution. N Engl J Med 1975;292:682-684.

25. Weisse AB, Narang R, Haider B, Regan TJ. Right and left heart pressures in acute myocardial infarction. Cardiovasc Res 1973; 7:251-260.

Chapter 19

Right Ventricular Infarction

Blood flow to the right ventricular free wall is provided by right ventricular branches arising from the midportion of the right coronary artery. Although isolated infarction of the right ventricle (RV) is rare, RV involvement occurs in 20-45% of patients with inferoposterior MI (1), and it is hemodynamically significant in 10-20% (2).

Diagnosis

Hemodynamically important right ventricular infarction should be suspected in any patient with inferior MI complicated by hypotension or signs of right heart failure (Table 19.1). Kussmaul's sign (late inspiratory expansion of the internal jugular veins) is present in 63-100% of patients with significant RV infarction (3-5). Jugular venous distension is more variable, occurring in 29-88% of cases (3-5). The classic triad of hypotension, increased jugular venous pressure, and clear lung fields (6) occurs in only about 25% of patients (3), but defines a subgroup with more extensive right ventricular involvement. Other findings may include a prominent y-descent in the jugular venous pressure contour, a right-sided S_3 or S_4 gallop, or evidence of tricuspid regurgitation (2,4).

Electrocardiographic findings suggestive of acute RV infarction include ST segment elevation in leads V1-V2 or right precordial leads V3R-V4R in association with evidence of an inferior MI (7-9). Cardiac enzyme elevations in patients with substantial RV involvement are disproportionately high relative to the degree of left ventricular dysfunction (10). In the acute phase, echocardiography or nuclear angiography reveals a dilated RV with reduced ejection fraction. If indicated, technetium pyrophosphatase scanning may provide confirmatory evidence of RV infarction when performed within 24-72 hours of symptom onset (1,2).

Hemodynamics

Right ventricular infarction results in decreased compliance of the RV, altered right ventricular filling characteristics, and an increase in RV diastolic pressure. These changes are manifest clinically as a Kussmaul's sign and elevated central venous pressure. In patients with more extensive right ventricular infarction, forward stroke volume is reduced. In addition, left ventricular filling may

Table 19.1
Clinical Features of Right Ventricular Infarction

Physical findings
    Kussmaul's sign
    Elevated jugular venous pressure
    Hypotension
    Absence of pulmonary congestion

Diagnosis
    ECG: Inferior MI + ST elevation
       in V1, V2, V3R, V4R
    Echo or nuclear angiography: dilated RV with
       decreased ejection fraction
    PA catheter: Prominent y-descent,
       RAP > 10 mm Hg, RA pressure/PAOP > 0.8

Treatment options
    Volume loading
    Inotropic agents
    Vasodilators
    Atrial or A-V sequential pacing
    Intraaortic balloon pump

Complications
    Bradyarrhythmias or tachyarrhythmias
    Tricuspid regurgitation
    Septal, papillary muscle, or free wall rupture
    Right to left shunt
    Cardiogenic shock

be abnormal as a result of altered septal motion and concomitant left ventricular infarction. In concert, these complex hemodynamic changes result in a reduction in cardiac output and a fall in systemic arterial pressure. Bradycardia and A-V block (or atrial fibrillation) with loss of the atrial component of ventricular filling (atrial "kick") further compromise cardiac output and may lead to cardiogenic shock.

Based on the results of pulmonary artery catheterization, various hemodynamic criteria for the diagnosis of right ventricular infarction have been proposed (1,2). In the setting of an inferior MI, when the right atrial pressure is greater than 10 mm Hg, exceeds 80% of the PA occlusive pressure, and has a prominent y-descent (deeper than x-descent), right ventricular infarction is likely (2,11). Occasionally, volume loading is required before the typical hemodynamic features become manifest (3,5), but this maneuver is not recommended in the absence of hypotension (2). The pattern of "equalization" of left- and right-sided diastolic pressures may mimic constrictive pericarditis, restrictive cardiomyopathy, pericardial tamponade, or pulmonary hypertension of any cause. However, attention to the clinical setting and the results of non-invasive and invasive cardiac tests should reliably differentiate right ventricular infarction from these other conditions (12).

Treatment

In hemodynamically stable patients without evidence of organ hypoperfusion, no specific therapy is required. In hypotensive patients with clear lung fields, volume loading with intravenous saline at 100-300 cc/hr should be initiated. If this fails to increase blood pressure or if pulmonary congestion is present, a pulmonary artery catheter should be inserted to guide therapy. Patients with right atrial and PA occlusive pressures of less than 15 mm Hg may benefit from additional volume loading. However, if further increases in systemic and pulmonary venous pressure fail to produce an increase in cardiac output, inotropic therapy with dobutamine should be instituted (13). Intravenous nitroglycerin or nitroprusside may be added if severe low cardiac output state persists. Note, however, that these agents, as well as morphine and other venodilators, must be used with caution, since the reduction in preload may further compromise cardiac output.

As noted above, bradycardia, heart block, or atrial fibrillation may contribute to the hemodynamic impairment associated with RV infarction. Bradyarrhythmias unresponsive to atropine should be treated with a temporary pacemaker. In this setting, atrial or A-V sequential pacing is often superior to ventricular pacing (14) and should be strongly considered in patients with shock (15). Finally, patients with severe hemodynamic compromise or cardiogenic shock who fail to respond promptly to the above measures should be considered for intraaortic balloon counterpulsation, which can stabilize the patient and allow time for the right ventricle to recover (1).

Clinical Course and Prognosis

Right ventricular infarction has been associated with an increased incidence of advanced A-V nodal block, atrial fibrillation (due to simultaneous atrial infarction or increased RA pressure), and ventricular tachycardia and fibrillation. Tricuspid regurgitation due to papillary muscle dysfunction or rupture may occur, and ventricular septal and free wall rupture have also been reported (1). Severe hemodynamic decompensation progressing to cardiogenic shock occurs in up to 15% of cases (1). Rarely, the right atrial pressure may exceed the left atrial pressure in the presence of a patent foramen ovale, thus producing a right-to-left shunt with systemic arterial oxygen desaturation (16). This complication should be suspected if severe hypoxemia unresponsive to supplemental oxygen is present. Volume loading is contraindicated in this situation, since further increases in right atrial pressure will only serve to increase the magnitude of the shunt.

Despite these problems, prognosis in right ventricular infarction is generally more favorable than in left ventricular MI, even in patients with cardiogenic shock. This is most likely due to an early recovery of systolic function (9), which may begin within 24-72 hours after the onset of infarction (2). The long-term prognosis following right ventricular infarction is largely dependent on the extent of left ventricular dysfunction (2). Thus, in patients with inferior MI, the presence or absence of RV involvement does not influence late survival or functional status (17). For these reasons, maximal supportive therapy is justified in the early management of these patients.

REFERENCES

1. Kulbertus HE, Rigo P, Legrand V. Right ventricular infarction: Pathophysiology, diagnosis, clinical course, and treatment. Mod Concepts Cardiovasc Dis 1985;54:1-5.

2. Dell'Italia LJ. Right ventricular infarction. J Intensive Care Med 1986;1:246-256.

3. Dell'Italia LJ, Starling MR, O'Rourke RA. Physical examination for exclusion of hemodynamically important right ventricular infarction. Ann Intern Med 1983;99:608-611.

4. Cintron GB, Hernandez F, Linares E, Aranda JM. Bedside recognition, incidence and clinical course of right ventricular infarction. Am J Cardiol 1981;47:224-227.

5. Baigrie RS, Haq A, Morgan CD, Rakowski H, Drobac M, McLaughlin P. The spectrum of right ventricular involvement in inferior wall myocardial infarction: A clinical, hemodynamic, and noninvasive study. J Am Coll Cardiol 1983;1:1396-1404.

6. Cohn J, Guiha N, Broder M, Limas C. Right ventricular infarction: Clinical and hemodynamic features. Am J Cardiol 1974;33:209-214.

7. Chou TC, vander Bel-Kahn J, Allen J, Brockmeier L, Fowler NO. Electrocardiographic diagnosis of right ventricular infarction. Am J Med 1981;70:1175-1180.

8. Morgera T, Alberti E, Silvestri F, Pandullo C, della Mea MT, Camerini F. Right precordial ST and QRS changes in the diagnosis of right ventricular infarction. Am Heart J 1984;108:13-18.

9. Klein HO, Tordjman T, Ninio R, et al. The early recognition of right ventricular infarction. Diagnostic accuracy of the electrocardiographic V4R lead. Circulation 1983;67:558-565.

10. Marmor A, Geltman EM, Biello DR, Sobel BE, Siegel BA, Roberts R. Functional response of the right ventricle to myocardial infarction: Dependence on the site of left ventricular infarction. Circulation 1981;64:1005-1011.

11. Lopez-Sendon J, Coma-Canella I, Gamallo C. Sensitivity and specificity of hemodynamic criteria in the diagnosis of acute right ventricular infarction. Circulation 1981;64:515-525.

12. Lorell B, Leinbach RC, Pohost GM, et al. Right ventricular infarction: Clinical diagnosis and differentiation from cardiac tamponade and pericardial constriction. Am J Cardiol 1979; 43:465-471.

13. Dell'Italia LJ, Starling MR, Blumhardt R, Lasher JC, O'Rourke RA. Comparative effects of volume loading, dobutamine, and nitroprusside in patients with predominant right ventricular infarction. Circulation 1985;72:1327-1335.

14. Topol EJ, Goldschlager N, Ports TA, et al. Hemodynamic benefit of atrial pacing in right ventricular myocardial infarction. Ann Intern Med 1982;96:594-597.

15. Love JC, Haffajee CI, Gore JM, Alpert JS. Reversibility of hypotension and shock by atrial or atrioventricular sequential pacing in patients with right ventricular infarction. Am Heart J 1984;108:5-13.

16. Bansal RC, Marsa RJ, Holland D, Beehler C, Gold PM. Severe hypoxemia due to shunting through a patent foramen ovale: A correctable complication of right ventricular infarction. J Am Coll Cardiol 1985;5:188-192.

17. Haines DE, Beller GA, Watson DD, et al. A prospective, scintigraphic, angiographic, and functional evaluation of patients after inferior myocardial infarction with and without right ventricular dysfunction. J Am Coll Cardiol 1985;6:995-1003.

Chapter 20

Mechanical Complications

Mechanical complications of acute MI include ventricular septal perforation, papillary muscle dysfunction or rupture, free wall rupture, and left ventricular aneurysm and pseudoaneurysm. Although the occurrence of any of these complications is life-threatening, with prompt diagnosis and management, a catastrophic outcome may be averted in many cases. Careful cardiac examination should be performed daily throughout the hospital stay and any time there are new symptoms or a change in hemodynamic status. A systolic murmur that is either new or of increasing intensity, particularly in association with hemodynamic deterioration, suggests a ventricular septal perforation or mitral regurgitation due to papillary muscle dysfunction or rupture. Pulmonary artery catheterization in conjunction with echocardiography will confirm the diagnosis in most cases. Chest pain followed by sudden hemodynamic collapse suggests free wall rupture with acute pericardial tamponade. Emergency pericardiocentesis and surgical repair of the perforation offer the only hope for survival. Left ventricular aneursym should be suspected in patients with large anterior MIs, especially when complicated by CHF. Pseudoaneurysm occurs when a free wall rupture is locally contained by adherent pericardium and fibrous tissue resulting in an intrapericardial hematoma. The hemodynamic effect of pseudoaneurysm depends on its size and location. Differentiation from true aneurysm may be difficult, but the distinction is important because a pseudoaneurysm may rupture, leading to rapid cardiovascular collapse. The following sections discuss these problems in more detail.

Ventricular Septal Defect (VSD)

Acute VSD occurs in 2-4% of patients with acute transmural MI, typically 3-5 days after initial presentation (1). Older patients are at increased risk for VSD, and the majority of patients have severe multivessel coronary artery disease (2,3). The incidence of septal perforation is similar in anterior and inferior MI (2-6).

Clinical findings consist of a new, harsh, holosystolic murmur, often associated with a thrill, best heard along the lower left sternal border. Depending on the magnitude of the left-to-right shunt and pre-existing right and left ventricular function, the hemodynamic consequences of acute VSD may range from minimal to mild CHF, cardiogenic shock, and death.

Pulmonary artery catheterization is the procedure of choice to confirm the diagnosis of VSD, estimate the magnitude of the shunt, and guide subsequent therapy. A "step-up" in oxygen saturation in excess of 10% in crossing from the right atrium to the right ventricle is diagnostic. Note that in the presence of a VSD, both the thermodilation and Fick methods of calculating cardiac output will overestimate the true left-sided output (Chapter 18). Echocardiography, especially using the color flow doppler technique, may be helpful in confirming the diagnosis and localizing the defect. First-pass radionuclide angiography may be useful in estimating the degree of left-to-right shunting.

Acute management of VSD is dictated by the hemodynamic status. Stable patients can be treated with afterload reduction and continued close observation. Mild to moderate congestive heart failure should be treated with diuretics and vasodilators. More severe heart failure and shock mandate inotropic therapy, an intravenous vasodilator such as nitroprusside, intra-aortic balloon counterpulsation, and consideration for early operative intervention.

Virtually all acquired VSDs require surgical repair, as the mortality with medical management is 90% (1). In the past, medical stabilization for several weeks prior to VSD repair was recommended; more recently, earlier intervention has been advocated (7). Overall surgical mortality is about 50%. Patients with inferior MI have higher mortality than those with anterior MI; significant right ventricular dysfunction is also associated with poor surgical outcome (8). Long-term prognosis following successful VSD repair is good, with left ventricular ejection fraction being the most important prognostic variable (8).

Papillary Muscle Dysfunction and Rupture

Papillary muscle dysfunction (PMD) occurs when ischemia or infarction of an intact papillary muscle prevents normal mitral valve motion and leads to mitral regurgitation. Papillary muscle rupture (PMR) occurs when there is partial or complete transection of one of the heads, usually producing severe mitral insufficiency. In both PMD and PMR, the posteromedial papillary muscle is most frequently involved. Rarely, right ventricular papillary muscle dysfunction will result in clinically significant tricuspid regurgitation.

Clinical findings in PMD include a musical mid-to-late systolic murmur best heard at the lower left sternal border or apex, occasionally associated with a thrill. Mitral regurgitation may be mild, with minimal hemodynamic consequence, or more severe, with significant congestive heart failure which may progress to severe pulmonary edema. The diagnosis can usually be made from the physical findings but occasionally the murmur will be unimpressive. Less frequently, it may be difficult to distinguish PMD from PMR or VSD. PA catheterization does not show an oxygen saturation "step-up" with PMD or PMR, but will often reveal a significant v-wave in the PAOP tracing (Chapter 18). Note, however, that a v-wave may also be seen with a VSD, or may be absent despite severe mitral regurgitation. Echocardiography with doppler will demonstrate mitral regurgitation with an intact mitral valve apparatus.

The treatment of PMD depends on the severity of mitral regurgitation. In mild cases, no specific therapy is required, although afterload reduction may be desirable to prevent deterioration. In more severe cases, diuretics, inotropic therapy, intravenous vasodilators, or even intra-aortic balloon counterpulsation may be required to treat congestive heart failure and stabilize hemodynamics. If PMD is intermittent, suggesting recurrent ischemia, coronary angiography followed by transluminal angioplasty or bypass surgery may be indicated. Finally, moderate or severe papillary muscle dysfunction may lead to chronic mitral regurgitation requiring mitral valve repair or replacement.

Partial or complete rupture of a papillary muscle causes acute mitral regurgitation which is generally more severe than with simple papillary muscle dysfunction. This complication occurs in about 1% of patients with acute MI (1), usually following occlusion of the right coronary or left circumflex artery. In contrast to acute VSD, papillary muscle rupture may occur following a relatively small MI and in the absence of diffuse coronary atherosclerosis (4,9,10).

Total PMR usually results in overwhelming mitral regurgitation, rapid hemodynamic deterioration, and death. More often, there is partial rupture of the papillary muscle, presenting a clinical and hemodynamic picture similar to severe PMD. There is usually sudden worsening of congestive heart failure, often associated with a fall in blood pressure and a new systolic murmur. Pulmonary artery catheterization reveals low cardiac output with an elevated PAOP and a prominent v-wave, although absence of the latter does not exclude the diagnosis. Echocardiography will usually demonstrate the ruptured papillary muscle and flail mitral valve leaflet (11).

Since PMR often leads to rapid hemodynamic deterioration, prompt surgical intervention is usually indicated (12). Inotropic agents, vasodilators, and intra-aortic balloon counterpulsation may help stabilize the patient pre-operatively. Fewer than 10% of patients with PMR will survive without surgical intervention (1). Operative mortality is 40-90% (1,12); patients with preserved ventricular function, limited coronary disease, and less extensive rupture have the best prognosis (12).

Free Wall Rupture

Free wall rupture occurs in up to 10% of patients with transmural MI (1), although in recent years the incidence may be declining (13). It is the third leading cause of death in MI patients (after pump failure and arrhythmias). Rupture usually occurs within the first 10 days following MI, but may occur up to several weeks after the initial event (1,13). Predisposing factors include advanced age, female sex, hypertension on admission, and absence of a prior history of MI or angina (13).

Impending myocardial rupture is often presaged by persistent or recurrent chest pain unresponsive to conventional treatment in association with ST segment elevation or depression (13-15). When rupture occurs, there is usually rapid progression to cardiac tamponade, electromechanical dissociation, and death unless prompt recognition is followed by emergency treatment. In some cases, cardiac rupture may follow a subacute course (16), and in others, the rupture may be walled off by adherent pericardium, producing a pseudoaneurysm (see next section).

Management of free wall rupture begins with maintaining a high index of suspicion in patients at increased risk, and treating hypertension actively in the early post-MI period (13). When rupture is associated with rapid hemodynamic deterioration, immediate pericardiocentesis followed by emergency surgical repair provides the only hope for survival (17). Patients with subacute rupture may be stabilized with fluids, inotropic agents, and intra-aortic balloon counterpulsation, but urgent surgical intervention, with or without cardiac catheterization, is still necessary if the patient is to survive (16,18).

Left Ventricular Aneurysm and Pseudoaneurysm

In the early healing phase of acute MI, hemodynamic stresses within the heart may lead to expansion and thinning of the infarcted myocardium (19,20). As the healing process continues and the involved area becomes fibrotic, a discrete outpouching or aneurysm of the left ventricle may occur. Depending on the size of the aneurysm, various hemodynamic consequences may ensue, including congestive heart failure, angina due to an increased workload placed on adjacent viable myocardial tissue, and progressive dilatation of non-infarcted muscle with further decline in myocardial function. In addition, aneurysms are often the site of mural thrombus formation which can lead to systemic embolization, and aneurysms may provide the substrate for recurrent ventricular tachyarrhythmias.

Aneurysms occur in 10-15% of patients with acute MI (21), and are more frequent in large anterior infarcts involving the apex than in inferior or posterior MIs. Patients with total occlusion of the left anterior descending artery and poor collateral circulation are at increased risk of developing an aneurysm relative to those with either a patent vessel or good collateral blood flow (22).

Because aneurysm formation occurs during the healing phase of acute MI, pathologically discrete true aneurysms are not apparent until several weeks after the initial event. However, functional aneurysms producing similar hemodynamic stresses may be diagnosed within the first 48 hours after infarction (23).

Aneurysms should be suspected in patients with large anterior MIs, particularly when complicated by congestive heart failure. Electro-cardiographic findings suggestive of an aneurysm include persistent precordial ST segment elevation in association with low limb lead voltage, left atrial enlargement or atrial fibrillation, ventricular arrhythmias, and an upright QRS in lead AVR due to marked left or right axis deviation (Goldberger's sign). The diagnosis can be confirmed by echocardiography, radionuclide angiography, or contrast ventriculography.

Surgical repair of a left ventricular aneurysm is indicated for persistent congestive heart failure or angina pectoris, refractory life-threatening ventricular arrhythmias, or recurrent systemic embolization despite anticoagulation. Recently, it has been suggested that the angiotensin converting enzyme inhibitor captopril may be effective in preventing progressive ventricular dilatation and in improving hemodynamics and exercise tolerance in patients with anterior MI at risk for aneurysm formation (24).

The non-operative prognosis of patients with large, hemo-dynamically significant left ventricular aneurysms is poor, with only about 10% surviving 5 years (21). Survival and quality of life are improved with surgical intervention; patients with preserved ventricular function in the non-aneurysmal segments and favorable coronary anatomy have the best prognosis (25).

Left ventricular pseudoaneurysm (also called false aneurysm) occurs when a free wall rupture is contained within adherent peri-cardium. The resulting intrapericardial hematoma communicates with the left ventricle via a narrow channel and, depending on its size, may produce a similar hemodynamic picture to a true aneurysm. Rarely, embolization of thrombus contained within the false aneurysm may occur.

Differentiation of false aneurysm from true aneurysm may be difficult, but rests on identifying the narrow neck using non-invasive techniques or contrast ventriculography. If a pseudoaneurysm is sus-pected, surgical repair is indicated, since rupture tends to occur and the prognosis following correction of the defect is favorable (26,27).

REFERENCES

1. Labovitz AJ, Miller LW, Kennedy HL. Mechanical complications of acute myocardial infarction. Cardiovasc Rev Rep 1984;5:948-961.

2. Radford MJ, Johnson RA, Daggett WM, et al. Ventricular septal rupture: A review of clinical and physiologic features and an analysis of survival. Circulation 1981;64:545-553.

3. Edwards BS, Edwards WD, Edwards JE. Ventricular septal rupture complicating acute myocardial infarction: Identification of single and complex types in 53 autopsied hearts. Am J Cardiol 1984;54:1201-1205.

4. Vlodaver Z, Edwards JE. Rupture of ventricular septum or papillary muscle complicating myocardial infarction. Circulation 1977;55:815-822.

5. Feneley MP, Chang VP, O'Rourke MF. Myocardial rupture after acute myocardial infarction. Ten year review. Br Heart J 1983; 49:550-556.

6. Mann JM, Roberts WC. Acquired ventricular septal defect during acute myocardial infarction: Analysis of 38 unoperated necropsy patients and comparison with 50 unoperated necropsy patients without rupture. Am J Cardiol 1988;62:8-19.

7. Miyamoto AT, Lee ME, Kass RM, et al. Post-myocardial infarction ventricular septal defect. Improved outlook. J Thorac Cardiovasc Surg 1983;86:41-46.

8. Jones MT, Schofield PM, Dark JF, et al. Surgical repair of acquired ventricular septal defect. Determinants of early and late outcome. J Thorac Cardiovasc Surg 1987;93:680-686.

9. Nishimura RA, Schaff HV, Shub C, Gersh BJ, Edwards WD, Tajik AJ. Papillary muscle rupture complicating acute myocardial infarction: Analysis of 17 patients. Am J Cardiol 1983; 51:373-377.

10. Barbour DJ, Roberts WC. Rupture of a left ventricular papillary muscle during acute myocardial infarction. Analysis of 22 necropsy patients. J Am Coll Cardiol 1986;8:558-565.

11. Come PC, Riley MF, Weintraub R, Morgan JP, Nakao S. Echocardiographic detection of complete and partial papillary muscle rupture during acute myocardial infarction. Am J Cardiol 1985;56:787-789.

12. Clements SD, Story WE, Hurst JW, Craver JM, Jones EL. Ruptured papillary muscle, a complication of myocardial infarction: Clinical presentation, diagnosis, and treatment. Clin Cardiol 1985;8:93-103.

13. Nakano T, Konishi T, Takezawa H. Potential prevention of myocardial rupture resulting from acute myocardial infarction. Clin Cardiol 1985;8:199-204.

14. Friedman HS, Kuhn LA, Katz AM. Clinical and electrocardiographic features of cardiac rupture following acute myocardial infarction. Am J Med 1971;50:709-720.

15. Herlitz J, Samuelsson SO, Richter A, Hjalmarson A. Prediction of rupture in acute myocardial infarction. Clin Cardiol 1988; 11:63-69.

16. Coma-Canella I, Lopez-Sendon J, Gonzalez LN, Ferrufino O. Subacute left ventricular free wall rupture following acute myocardial infarction: Bedside hemodynamics, differential diagnosis, and treatment. Am Heart J 1983;106:278-284.

17. McMullan MH, Kilgore TL, Dear HD, Hindman SH. Sudden blowout rupture of the myocardium after infarction: Urgent management. J Thorac Cardiovasc Surg 1985;89:259-263.

18. Pifarre R, Sullivan HJ, Grieco J, et al. Management of left ventricular rupture complicating myocardial infarction. J Thorac Cardiovasc Surg 1983;86:441-443.

19. Hutchins GM, Bulkley BH. Infarct expansion versus extension: Two different complications of acute myocardial infarction. Am J Cardiol 1978;41:1127-1132.

20. Eaton LW, Weiss JL, Bulkley BH, Garrison JB, Weisfeldt ML. Regional cardiac dilatation after acute myocardial infarction. N Engl J Med 1979;300:57-62.

21. Cohn LH. Surgical management of acute and chronic cardiac mechanical complications due to myocardial infarction. Am Heart J 1981;102:1049-1060.

22. Forman MB, Collins HW, Kopelman HA, et al. Determinants of left ventricular aneurysm formation after anterior myocardial infarction: A clinical and angiographic study. J Am Coll Cardiol 1986;8:1256-1262.

23. Meizlish JL, Berger HJ, Plankey M, Errico D, Levy W, Zaret BL. Functional left ventricular aneurysm formation after acute anterior transmural myocardial infarction. N Engl J Med 1984;311:1001-1006.

24. Pfeffer MA, Lamas GA, Vaughan DE, Parisi AF, Braunwald E. Effect of captopril on progressive ventricular dilatation after anterior myocardial infarction. N Engl J Med 1988;319:80-86.

25. Brawley RK, Magovern GJ, Gott VL, Donahoo JS, Gardner TJ, Watkins L. Left ventricular aneurysmectomy. Factors influencing postoperative results. J Thorac Cardiovasc Surg 1983;85:712-717.

26. Vlodaver Z, Coe JI, Edwards JE. True and false left ventricular aneurysms. Propensity for the latter to rupture. Circulation 1975;51:567-572.

27. Shabbo FP, Dymond DS, Rees GM, Hill IM. Surgical treatment of false aneurysm of the left ventricle after myocardial infarction. Thorax 1983;38:25-30.

Chapter 21

Other Complications: Thromboembolism, Recurrent Ischemia, and Pericarditis

Thromboembolic Phenomena

Left ventricular mural thrombi can be detected echocardio-graphically in about one-third of patients with transmural anterior myocardial infarctions but are rare with infarcts in other locations (1). Clinically apparent embolic events, most commonly stroke, occur in approximately 10-20% of patients with mural thrombus, usually within the first three months after infarction (1). Patients with a protruding or freely mobile thrombus visualized on a two-dimensional echocardiogram are at increased risk for embolic events (2).

Low dose anticoagulation does not appear to inhibit mural thrombus formation, but several small series suggest that full heparinization initiated early in the course of transmural anterior infarction reduces the incidence of mural thrombus (3,4) and subsequent embolization (5). Based on these findings, we recommend full-dose heparin unless contraindicated in patients with large anterior MIs, particularly when complicated by CHF or atrial fibrillation. Subsequent treatment with coumadin for at least 3 months has been recommended (1,5), but the risk-benefit ratio of this strategy remains to be defined. Similarly, the effect of thrombolytic therapy on the incidence and natural history of mural thrombi is unclear (6,7).

Patients with acute MI are at risk for developing deep vein thrombosis (DVT) and pulmonary emboli (PE), particularly when CHF or prolonged immobilization is present. Full systemic anticoagulation and low dose subcutaneous heparin have both been shown to reduce the incidence of deep vein thrombosis in acute MI patients (8,9). Heparin 5000 units subcutaneously every 12 hours is routinely started on admission to our CCU and continued until the patient is ambulatory. Early mobilization and prophylactic anticoagulation have now rendered DVT and PE uncommon complications of acute MI.

Recurrent Ischemia and Infarction

Ischemic chest pain more than 48 hours after the initial infarct occurs in 15-25% of patients (10-13), and signifies additional myo-cardium at risk, either in the infarct zone or in a separate vascular distribution (10). Enzymatically confirmed infarct extension occurs in 7-17% of patients (12-15), and is clinically silent in 25-35%

of cases (11,15). Patients with non-Q-wave MI, prior angina, recurrent prolonged chest pain, or successful reperfusion with a thrombolytic agent are at increased risk for reinfarction (12-14,16).

Recurrent ischemia early after MI is associated with a poor prognosis unless specific therapy is instituted. In the largest series to date, hospital mortality was 30% among patients with documented reinfarction compared to 7% in patients without reinfarction (12). In another study, mortality after a mean of 6 months was 56% in 70 patients with early post-infarction angina (10).

In view of the adverse outcome associated with recurrent ischemia, an aggressive approach to management is justified. Patients at high risk for reinfarction (i.e. those with non-Q-wave MI or successful reperfusion) may be considered candidates for early catheterization before ischemia recurs. Diltiazem 240-360 mg/day may also be beneficial in these patients (17; Chapter 23). Anginal pain should be managed with nitrates, beta blockers, calcium antagonists and analgesics as described in Chapter 4. Aspirin should be continued; full heparinization may also be beneficial. If prolonged chest pain is associated with ECG evidence of reinfarction, thrombolytic therapy should be considered. If these measures are ineffective or if there is significant hemodynamic compromise, urgent catheterization with subsequent angioplasty or bypass surgery is indicated. Most patients with recurrent ischemia, particularly if reinfarction is ruled out, should undergo coronary angiography and revascularization (if appropriate) prior to hospital discharge (18).

Pericardial Disease

Pericardial effusion can be detected echocardiographically in one-fourth of patients with acute MI; effusions are more common with anterior infarcts and in the presence of congestive heart failure (19). Unless caused by myocardial rupture, MI-associated pericardial effusions tend to run a benign course, rarely progress to cardiac tamponade, and require no specific treatment. In most cases, anticoagulation need not be discontinued.

Transmural MI is often associated with low-grade pericardial inflammation, but clinical pericarditis is detected in only 6-10% of cases (20,21). A transient pericardial friction rub, usually during the first 4 days after infarction, is the most common finding. Pleuritic chest pain, fever, tachycardia, atrial or ventricular arrhythmias, and an elevated erythrocyte sedimentation rate (ESR) may occur, but diagnostic ECG changes are rare (21). Infarct-associated pericarditis is usually self-limited and does not require treatment in the absence of significant chest pain or fever. If necessary, aspirin 650 mg q4-6° for 1-3 days is usually sufficient. Other non-steroidal anti-inflammatory agents and corticosteroids are best avoided because they may retard infarct healing, promote sodium and fluid retention, or exacerbate ischemia (22-24). In patients refractory to or intolerant of aspirin, a short course of prednisone 20-40 mg/day can be used.

Dressler's post-myocardial infarction syndrome was first described in 1956 (25) as a rare complication of acute MI, occurring in less than 5% of patients. It is similar to the post-pericardiotomy syndrome which occurs following cardiac surgery. Both are associated with the presence of anti-myocardial antibodies (26,27) although a cause-effect relationship has not been established. The syndrome begins 1-12 weeks (usually 2-8 weeks) after MI or open heart surgery; typical features include pericarditis, pleuritis, fever, leukocytosis, an elevated ESR, and a tendency to develop a relapsing or protracted course (25). As with post-MI pericarditis, symptomatic therapy is warranted, beginning with a trial of aspirin 650 mg every 4 hours. Unlike early postinfarction pericarditis, significant pericardial bleeding and tamponade may occur in Dressler's syndrome; anticoagulation, if used, should be monitored closely. Treatment may be required for several weeks, and in more severe cases, moderate to high doses of corticosteroids may be necessary. Relapses may occur for several years and should be managed similarly.

REFERENCES

1. Meltzer RS, Visser CA, Fuster V. Intracardiac thrombi and systemic embolization. Ann Intern Med 1986;104:689-698.

2. Visser CA, Kan G, Meltzer RS, et al. Embolic potential of left ventricular thrombus after myocardial infarction: A two-dimensional echocardiographic study of 119 patients. J Am Coll Cardiol 1985;5:1276-1280.

3. Gueret P, DuBourg O, Ferrier A, Farcot JC, Rigaud M, Bourdarias JP. Effects of full-dose heparin anticoagulation on the development of left ventricular thrombosis in acute transmural myocardial infarction. J Am Coll Cardiol 1986;8:419-426.

4. Nordrehaug JE, Johannessen KA, von der Lippe G. Usefulness of high-dose anticoagulants in preventing left ventricular thrombus in acute myocardial infarction. Am J Cardiol 1985;55:1491-1493.

5. Weinreich DJ, Burke JF, Pauletto FJ. Left ventricular mural thrombi complicating acute myocardial infarction. Ann Intern Med 1984;100:789-794.

6. Eigler N, Maurer G, Shah PK. Effect of early systemic thrombolytic therapy on left ventricular mural thrombus formation in acute anterior myocardial infarction. Am J Cardiol 1984;54:261-263.

7. Sharma B, Carvalho A, Wyeth R, Franciosa JA. Left ventricular thrombi diagnosed by echocardiography in patients with acute myocardial infarction treated with intracoronary streptokinase followed by intravenous heparin. Am J Cardiol 1985;56:422–425.

8. Wray R, Maurer B, Shillingford J. Prophylactic anticoagulant therapy in the prevention of calf–vein thrombosis after myocardial infarction. N Engl J Med 1973;288:815–817.

9. Warlow C, Beattie AG, Terry G, Ogston D, Kenmure ACF, Douglas AS. A double blind trial of low doses of subcutaneous heparin in the prevention of deep–vein thrombosis after myocardial infarction. Lancet 1973;II:934–936.

10. Schuster EH, Bulkley BH. Early post–infarction angina. Ischemia at a distance and ischemia in the infarct zone. N Engl J Med 1981;305:1101–1105.

11. Buda AJ, MacDonald IL, Dubbin JD, Orr SA, Strauss HD. Myocardial infarct extension: Prevalence, clinical significance, and problems in diagnosis. Am Heart J 1983;105:744–749.

12. Muller JE, Rude RE, Braunwald E, et al. Myocardial infarct extension: Occurrence, outcome, and risk factors in the multi-center investigation of limitation of infarct size. Ann Intern Med 1988;108:1–6.

13. Bosch X, Theroux P, Waters DD, Pelletier GB, Roy D. Early post–infarction ischemia: Clinical, angiographic, and prognostic significance. Circulation 1987;75:988–995.

14. Marmor A, Sobel BE, Roberts R. Factors presaging early recurrent myocardial infarction ("extension"). Am J Cardiol 1981;48:603–610.

15. Baker JT, Bramlet DA, Lester RM, Harrison DG, Roe CR, Cobb FR. Myocardial infarct extension: Incidence and relationship to survival. Circulation 1982;65:918–923.

16. Gruppo Italiano per lo Studio della Streptochinasi nell'Infarto Miocardico (GISSI). Effectiveness of intravenous thrombolytic treatment in acute myocardial infarction. Lancet 1986;I:397–402.

17. Gibson RS, Boden WE, Theroux P, et al. Diltiazem and reinfarction in patients with non–Q–wave myocardial infarction. Results of a double–blind, randomized, multicenter trial. N Engl J Med 1986; 315:423–429.

18. Epstein SE, Palmeri ST, Patterson RE. Evaluation of patients after acute myocardial infarction. Indications for cardiac catheterization and surgical intervention. N Engl J Med 1982; 307:1487–1492.

19. Pierard LA, Albert A, Henrard L, et al. Incidence and significance of pericardial effusion in acute myocardial infarction as determined by two-dimensional echocardiography. J Am Coll Cardiol 1986;8:517-520.

20. Lichstein E, Liu HM, Gupta P. Pericarditis complicating acute myocardial infarction: Incidence of complications and significance of electrocardiogram on admission. Am Heart J 1974; 87:246-252.

21. Krainin FM, Flessas AP, Spodick DH. Infarction-associated pericarditis. Rarity of diagnostic electrocardiogram. N Engl J Med 1984;311:1211-1214.

22. Silverman HS, Pfeifer MP. Relation between use of anti-inflammatory agents and left ventricular free wall rupture during acute myocardial infarction. Am J Cardiol 1987;59:363-364.

23. Cannon PJ. Prostaglandins in congestive heart failure and the effects of non-steroidal anti-inflammatory drugs. Am J Med 1986; 81(Suppl 2B):123-132.

24. Friedman PL, Brown EJ, Gunther S, et al. Coronary vasoconstrictor effect of indomethacin in patients with coronary artery disease. N Engl J Med 1981;305:1171-1175.

25. Dressler W. A post-myocardial-infarction syndrome. JAMA 1956; 160:1379-1383.

26. van der Geld H. Anti-heart antibodies in the post-pericardiotomy and the post-myocardial-infarction syndromes. Lancet 1964; II:617-621.

27. McCabe JC, Ebert PA, Engle MA, Zabriskie JB. Circulating heart-reactive antibodies in the post-pericardiotomy syndrome. J Surg Res 1973;14:158-164.

Chapter 22

Prognosis in Myocardial Infarction

Improved public awareness of the symptoms of acute MI and increased availability of emergency medical services have reduced pre-hospital mortality from 30% to about 10-15%. In-hospital mortality has similarly declined since the advent of CCUs in the 1960s, primarily as a result of prompt recognition and treatment of rhythm disturbances. More recently, interventional therapy with thrombolytic agents, beta blockers, and acute angioplasty, and aggressive management of high risk patients (e.g., those with recurrent ischemia or non-Q-wave infarcts), have led to further declines in hospital mortality. One-year mortality among hospital survivors is 5-10%; mortality declines to 2-4% per year subsequently (1-3). A number of variables have important impact on hospital and long-term prognosis. These factors allow stratification of acute MI patients into risk categories, thus permitting a more rational selection of post-MI diagnostic tests and therapeutic strategies (3).

Hospital Phase

Simple clinical parameters (Table 22.1) assessed early in the hospital course have long been known to correlate closely with hospital mortality, and based on these parameters several indices for evaluating short-term prognosis have been developed (4-6). The most important prognostic factor is the presence and severity of congestive heart failure on physical examination or chest x-ray. In 1967, Killip (5) reported that acute MI patients without CHF had a hospital mortality of 6%. In contrast, mortality in patients with mild to moderate CHF was 17%, in those with frank pulmonary edema it was 38%, and in cardiogenic shock, 81%. Currently, mortality in each of these subgroups is lower, but the relative risk between groups has not changed (7).

Infarct size and location, assessed electrocardiographically and by serum enzymes, also have important prognostic implications. Larger infarcts carry a worse prognosis, and anterior MIs have a less favorable outcome than inferior MIs, even after adjusting for infarct size (8-10). Mortality is lower in patients with non-Q-wave rather than Q-wave infarcts, although the former have a higher re-infarction rate (11). Additional ECG findings associated with adverse outcome include bundle branch block, second and third degree atrioventricular block (esp. in the setting of anterior MI), atrial fibrillation,

Table 22.1
Factors Influencing Short-Term Prognosis after Acute MI

A. Demographics
   1. Age
   2. Sex
   3. Prior angina or infarction

B. Physical examination
   1. Heart rate
   2. Systolic blood pressure
   3. S_3 or S_4 gallop rhythm
   4. Pulmonary congestion

C. Electrocardiogram
   1. Rate
   2. Rhythm disturbances
   3. Conduction abnormalities
   4. Infarct type, size, and location

D. Chest x-ray
   1. Heart size
   2. Congestive heart failure

E. Hospital course and treatment
   1. Recurrent ischemia or infarction
   2. Thrombolytic therapy
   3. Intravenous beta blockade

frequent ventricular premature beats and more advanced grades of ventricular ectopic activity. Persistent sinus tachycardia usually occurs in the setting of large anterior MI complicated by CHF, but has been shown to correlate independently with an increased risk of major complications (12).

Advanced age is associated with higher mortality, presumably due to the presence of co-existing illness, more advanced coronary atherosclerosis, and diminished cardiovascular reserve (Chapter 32). Women have a higher mortality than men, but this difference disappears after correction for age and concordant risk factors (13). Systolic blood pressure on admission to the CCU correlates inversely with mortality (6), and the presence of diabetes is associated with a poorer prognosis. Other traditional coronary risk factors do not have a major impact on short-term outcome.

As discussed in Chapter 21, recurrent ischemia and reinfarction are associated with increased mortality. In addition, prior angina or MI usually indicate more extensive coronary disease and ventricular dysfunction and therefore correlate with an increased risk of major complications and death. Finally, recent studies have demonstrated that at least two pharmacologic interventions, intravenous beta blockade (14) and thrombolytic therapy (15), can favorably influence short-term prognosis when initiated within the first 6 hours of the onset of infarction (see Chapters 12-13).

Post-Hospital Phase

Many of the factors affecting short-term prognosis are also important following discharge. For example, a young patient with an inferior MI uncomplicated by CHF, arrhythmias, hypotension, or recurrent chest pain and without prior cardiac disease has an expected 1-year mortality of less than 3%. By contrast, an elderly patient with a large anterior infarction, previous inferior MI, severe congestive heart failure, atrial fibrillation, and bundle branch block has less than a 40% chance of surviving 1 year from discharge.

Residual left ventricular function, extent of viable but jeopardized myocardium, and severity of ventricular arrhythmias are the most important variables affecting long-term prognosis. Left ventricular function is the single most important factor, and there is an inverse curvilinear relationship between radionuclide ejection fraction and 1-year mortality (Fig. 22.1). Patients with additional

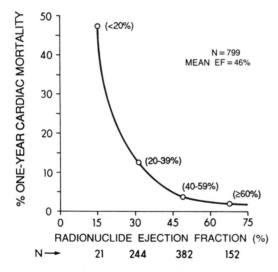

Figure 22.1 Relationship between radionuclide left ventricular ejection fraction and 1-year survival. Reprinted with permission from The Multicenter Postinfarction Research Group. Risk stratification and survival after myocardial infarction. N Engl J Med 1983;309:333.

myocardium at risk, as indicated by recurrent angina (16; Chapter 21), a positive stress test (17,18), or coronary angiography (19), also have increased mortality during follow-up. The presence of ventricular ectopic activity correlates with ventricular dysfunction but imparts independent prognostic information. Specifically, ≥ 3 VPCs/hour and salvos of 3 or more consecutive VPCs on a pre-discharge 24-hour Holter monitor have each been associated with a twofold increase in 2-year mortality (20), an effect independent of ejection fraction. Furthermore, ventricular arrhythmias may be an even more powerful predictor of mortality than ejection fraction in patients surviving more than 6 months after infarction (20). Finally, patients with sustained ventricular tachycardia occurring more than 48 hours after MI have a particularly poor prognosis, and are at high risk for sudden cardiac death (21).

Other factors which adversely affect prognosis following hospital discharge include anterior MI (8-10), poor exercise tolerance or inability to exercise (17), diabetes (22), continued smoking (23), black race (24,25), low education level (26), and social isolation or stress (27).

Risk Stratification

The ability to assess short and long-term prognosis based on clinical factors and non-invasive test results permits stratification of patients into various risk categories prior to hospital discharge (28-31). Patients at moderate to high risk for subsequent cardiac events who may benefit from more aggressive treatment strategies (e.g. early cardiac catheterization, revascularization, and anti-arrhythmic therapy) are thus identified (29,31). Similarly, low risk patients unlikely to benefit from these strategies are also identified (31). Finally, based on clinical data and the results of non-invasive tests, the physician is able to design an individualized program of physical activity, cardiac rehabilitation, and risk factor modification.

REFERENCES

1. Gomez-Martin O, Folsom AR, Kottke TE, et al. Improvement in long-term survival among patients hospitalized with acute myocardial infarction, 1970 to 1980. N Engl J Med 1987; 316:1353-1359.

2. Gruppo Italiano per lo Studio della Streptochinasi nell'Infarto Miocardico (GISSI). Long-term effects of intravenous thrombolysis in acute myocardial infarction: Final report of the GISSI study. Lancet 1987;II:871-874.

3. The Multicenter Postinfarction Research Group. Risk stratification and survival after myocardial infarction. N Engl J Med 1983;309:331-336.

4. Peel AAF, Semple T, Wang I, Lancaster WM, Doll JLG. A coronary prognostic index for grading the severity of infarction. Br Heart J 1962;24:745-760.

5. Killip T, Kimball JT. Treatment of myocardial infarction in a coronary care unit. A two year experience with 250 patients. Am J Cardiol 1967;20:457-464.

6. Norris RM, Brandt PWT, Caughey DE, Lee AJ, Scott PJ. A new coronary prognostic index. Lancet 1969;I:274-278.

7. Forrester JS, Diamond G, Chatterjee K, Swan HJC. Medical therapy of acute myocardial infarction by application of hemodynamic subsets. N Engl J Med 1976;295:1356-1362 and 1404-1413.

8. Thanavaro S, Kleiger RE, Province MA, et al. Effect on infarct location on the in-hospital prognosis of patients with first transmural myocardial infarction. Circulation 1982;66:742-747.

9. Hands ME, Lloyd BL, Robinson JS, deKlerk N, Thompson PL. Prognostic significance of electrocardiographic site of infarction after correction for enzymatic size of infarction. Circulation 1986;73:885-891.

10. Stone PH, Raabe DS, Jaffe AS, et al. Prognostic significance of location and type of myocardial infarction: Independent adverse outcome associated with anterior location. J Am Coll Cardiol 1988;11:453-463.

11. Roberts R. Recognition, pathogenesis, and management of non-Q-wave infarction. Mod Concept Cardiovasc Dis 1987;56:17-21.

12. Crimm A, Severance HW, Coffey K, McKinnis R, Wagner GS, Califf RM. Prognostic significance of isolated sinus tachycardia during first three days of acute myocardial infarction. Am J Med 1984;76:983-988.

13. Robinson K, Conroy RM, Mulcahy R, Hickey N. Risk factors and in-hospital course of first episode of myocardial infarction or acute coronary insufficiency in women. J Am Coll Cardiol 1988;11:932-936.

14. ISIS-1 (First International Study of Infarct Survival) Collaborative Group. Randomized trial of intravenous atenolol among 16,027 cases of suspected acute myocardial infarction: ISIS-1. Lancet 1986;II:57-66.

15. Gruppo Italiano per lo Studio della Streptochinasi nell'Infarto Miocardico (GISSI). Effectiveness of intravenous thrombolytic treatment in acute myocardial infarction. Lancet 1986;I:397-402.

16. Schuster BH, Bulkley BH. Early post-infarction angina. Ischemia at a distance and ischemia in the infarct zone. N Engl J Med 1981;305:1101-1105.

17. Krone RJ, Gillespie JA, Weld FM, Miller JP, Moss AJ, and the Multicenter Postinfarction Research Group. Low level exercise testing after myocardial infarction: Usefulness in enhancing clinical risk stratification. Circulation 1985;71:80-89.

18. Fioretti P, Brower RW, Simoons ML, et al. Prediction of mortality during the first year after myocardial infarction from clinical variables and stress test at hospital discharge. Am J Cardiol 1985;55:1313-1318.

19. Sanz G, Castaner A, Betriu A, et al. Determinants of prognosis in survivors of myocardial infarction. A prospective clinical angiographic study. N Engl J Med 1982;306:1065-1070.

20. Bigger JT, Fleiss JL, Kleiger R, Miller JP, Rolnitzky LM, and the Multicenter Postinfarction Research Group. The relationships among ventricular arrhythmias, left ventricular dysfunction, and mortality in the two years after myocardial infarction. Circulation 1984;69:250-258.

21. Marchlinski FE, Waxman HL, Buxton AE, Josephson ME. Sustained ventricular tachyarrhythmias during the early postinfarction period: Electrophysiologic findings and prognosis for survival. J Am Coll Cardiol 1983;2:240-250.

22. Smith JW, Marcus FI, Serokman R, with the Multicenter Postinfarction Research Group. Prognosis of patients with diabetes mellitus after acute myocardial infarction. Am J Cardiol 1984;54:718-721.

23. Aberg A, Bergstrand R, Johansson S et. al. Cessation of smoking after myocardial infarction. Effects on mortality after 10 years. Br Heart J 1983;49:416-422.

24. Tofler GH, Stone PH, Muller JE, et al. Effects of gender and race on prognosis after myocardial infarction: Adverse prognosis for women, particularly black women. J Am Coll Cardiol 1987; 9:473-482.

25. Castaner A, Simmons BE, Mar M, Cooper R. Myocardial infarction among black patients: Poor prognosis after hospital discharge. Ann Intern Med 1988;109:33-35.

26. Weinblatt E, Ruberman W, Goldberg JD, Frank CW, Shapiro S, Chaudhary BS. Relation of education to sudden death after myocardial infarction. N Engl J Med 1978;299:60-65.

27. Ruberman W, Weinblatt E, Goldberg JD, Chaudhary BS. Psychosocial influences on mortality after myocardial infarction. N Engl J Med 1984;311:552-559.

28. Cohn PF. The role of non-invasive cardiac testing after an uncomplicated myocardial infarction. N Engl J Med 1983;309:90-93.

29. Rapaport E, Remedios P. The high risk patient after recovery from myocardial infarction. J Am Coll Cardiol 1983;1:391-400.

30. DeBusk RF, Kraemer HC, Nash E. Stepwise risk stratification soon after myocardial infarction. Am J Cardiol 1983;52:1161-1166.

31. DeBusk RF, Blomqvist CG, Kouchoukos NT, et. al. Identification and treatment of low-risk patients after acute myocardial infarction and coronary artery bypass graft surgery. N Engl J Med 1986;314:161-166.

Chapter 23

Secondary Prevention of Recurrent Cardiac Events

The occurrence of acute myocardial infarction serves as a strong "risk factor" for subsequent cardiac events, since these patients have a substantially higher incidence of recurrent MI, revascularization procedures, and cardiac death than the general population. Secondary prevention refers to efforts designed to inhibit progression of coronary atherosclerosis and to reduce reinfarction rates and mortality following an index event such as an MI. Current strategies fall into three major categories: risk factor modification, pharmacotherapy, and invasive procedures.

Risk Factor Modification

Major risk factors (1) for the development of clinical coronary heart disease include age, male sex, serum cholesterol level, hypertension (both systolic and diastolic), cigarette smoking, glucose intolerance, and electrocardiographic left ventricular hypertrophy. Documented coronary heart disease in a first degree relative under age 50, obesity, physical inactivity, and certain psychosocial factors are also associated with increased risk. Several of these factors are modifiable, and the post-MI patient is an ideal candidate for intervention, since motivation is high and the potential yield is great (2).

Treatment of hypercholesterolemia in asymptomatic middle-aged men has been shown to reduce the incidence of major cardiac events (3,4), and the magnitude of benefit correlates directly with the degree to which cholesterol is lowered (3). In men with documented MI, nicotinic acid (niacin) reduced cardiac and total mortality as well as the incidence of non-fatal reinfarction during long-term follow-up (5). Thus, in high-risk patients, cholesterol reduction is associated with both primary and secondary prevention of cardiac events. The current recommendation (6) for post-MI patients is to treat a total serum cholesterol level in excess of 200 mg/dl (or low density lipoprotein level $\geq$ 130 mg/dl). Dietary therapy is used initially, and if this fails to lower cholesterol to a desirable range, drug therapy is added, with the bile acid sequestrants (cholestyramine, colestipol) and nicotinic acid being the agents of first choice (6).

Cessation of smoking after MI has been associated with up to 50% reduction in non-fatal reinfarction and cardiovascular death (7,8). Patients should be strongly encouraged to stop smoking; those unable

to quit may benefit from a formal smoking cessation program (2).
Treatment of persistent hypertension after MI is prudent because it is
associated with lower cardiovascular morbidity and mortality in
general, although no specific reduction in events after MI has been
documented (2). Normalization of blood pressure reduces afterload and
may diminish angina frequency by reducing myocardial oxygen demand.
Diabetes control and weight reduction to attain ideal body weight are
also desirable, but have not been proven to reduce cardiovascular
events.

Regular exercise has been associated with improved psychological
well-being and decreased mortality following myocardial infarction in
several randomized trials (2), and is recommended for patients who are
able to exercise without undue risk (see Chapter 24). The importance
of type A behavior in cardiac disease remains controversial, although
one study suggested a reduction in cardiac morbidity and mortality
when patients with type A behavior underwent counseling after MI (9).
Other psychosocial factors, such as depression, social isolation (10),
and low education level, have been associated with adverse outcome
after MI, but whether these effects can be altered with specific
interventions has not been determined (see Chapter 31).

Pharmacologic Treatment

In the early 1980s, three large, randomized, double-blind trials
(11-15) were published demonstrating conclusively that prophylactic
administration of beta adrenergic blocking agents after MI reduces
non-fatal reinfarction and total mortality (Table 23.1). Pooling the
results of these trials yields a 25% reduction in reinfarction and a
31% reduction in mortality. It is important to note that the doses of
beta blockers employed in these trials are moderately high, and that
smaller doses may not afford comparable protection. Also, although
the beneficial effects of beta blockers appear to be relatively
generic, a detailed review of all published trials (16) fails to
reveal a favorable effect among agents with intrinsic sympathomimetic
activity (ISA), and these drugs cannot be recommended for routine
post-MI prophylaxis.

Table 23.1
Secondary Prevention with Beta Blockers after MI

Agent	Dose	N	Follow-up	Non-fatal Reinfarction	Mortality
Timolol	10 mg BID	1884	17 mo	-32%	-36%
Metoprolol	100 mg BID	1395	3 mo	-34%	-36%
Propranolol	60-80 mg TID	3837	25 mo	-15%	-26%

The question of how long beta blockers should be continued has not been resolved, but is potentially important, since these agents may have unfavorable effects on serum lipids. Current data indicate that the beneficial effects of beta blockade persist for at least 3-6 years after MI (17,18). Another unresolved issue is whether all patients require treatment, since certain low-risk subgroups may have little to gain from such therapy (19). Despite these considerations, we recommend treating all patients with beta blockers following acute MI in the absence of contraindications, and continuing such therapy indefinitely in the absence of data suggesting it is safe to discontinue treatment. This policy is supported by a recent analysis of the cost-effectiveness of this treatment (20).

Diltiazem in doses of 360 mg/day has been shown to reduce early reinfarction but not mortality in patients with initial non-Q wave MI (21). Although the long-term effects of such therapy are not known, it would seem reasonable to continue diltiazem for at least several months after discharge in these patients. On the other hand, a large multicenter trial of long-term therapy with diltiazem 180-240 mg/day failed to demonstrate a reduction in mortality or non-fatal reinfarction during a 25 month followup period after acute MI (22). While patients with normal ventricular function and no congestive heart failure achieved a modest benefit with diltiazem, patients with pulmonary congestion or an ejection fraction less than 40% had increased mortality with this agent (22). Similarly, the calcium antagonists nifedipine and verapamil have not been shown to be effective in secondary prevention and cannot be recommended.

No prospective secondary prevention trials of long-acting nitrates have been conducted. Although one small, retrospective analysis suggested a beneficial effect of nitrates (23), in the absence of angina routine therapy with nitrates after MI is not justified. Similarly, although it is well established that complex ventricular arrhythmias are associated with adverse outcome, prophylactic anti-arrhythmic therapy has not been shown to improve long term survival (24). A large, multicenter trial (CAST: Cardiac Arrhythmia Suppression Trial) is now underway to assess the role of flecainide, encainide, and moricizine in post-MI patients at increased risk of arrhythmic death (25).

The use of long-term oral anticoagulation following acute MI remains controversial. A review of published trials failed to demonstrate consistent benefit, and treated patients were more prone to hemorrhagic complications (26). It is therefore recommended that long-term anticoagulation be reserved for those patients at high risk for venous or systemic thromboembolic events. This might include patients with severe left ventricular dysfunction, atrial fibrillation, mobile left ventricular mural thrombus, or prior embolization. The use of low-dose subcutaneous heparin (12,500 units/day) has recently been shown to reduce reinfarction and mortality after MI (27), but additional confirmation is needed before this strategy can be recommended for routine use. Data on secondary prevention with anti-platelet agents are conflicting (28,29). However, in view of the important role of platelets in atherosclerosis and thrombogenesis, the demonstrated benefit of aspirin in primary prevention of MI (30) and in unstable angina (Chapter 25), and the ease of administration and low cost, we recommend low-dose aspirin (1-5 grains/day) in all patients with documented coronary heart disease without contraindications.

Invasive Treatment Strategies

A full discussion of the role of cardiac catheterization, angioplasty, electrophysiologic testing, and cardiac surgery following myocardial infarction is beyond the scope of this manual. In general, none of these procedures can be recommended routinely, but each is of value in appropriately selected patients. The reader is referred to standard cardiology texts for further discussion of these issues.

Summary and Conclusions

Patients surviving acute myocardial infarction are at increased risk of recurrent cardiac events in subsequent years. Control of modifiable risk factors, including reduction of cholesterol, cessation of smoking, normalization of blood pressure, weight reduction in obese patients, and regular exercise is desirable. In the absence of contraindications, we routinely prescribe a non-ISA beta blocker and one aspirin a day (325 mg). Other interventions should be based on identification of patients at risk of specific complications, as indicated by the hospital course and the results of selected non-invasive diagnostic tests (Chapter 22).

REFERENCES

1. Kannel WB, McGee D, Gordon T. A general cardiovascular risk profile: The Framingham Study. Am J Cardiol 1976;38:46-51.

2. Siegel D, Grady D, Browner WS, Hulley SB. Risk factor modification after myocardial infarction. Ann Intern Med 1988; 109:213-218.

3. Lipid Research Clinics Program. The Lipid Research Clinics Coronary Primary Prevention Trial results. JAMA 1984;251:351-364 & 365-374.

4. Frick MH, Elo O, Haapa K, et al. Helsinki Heart Study: Primary prevention trial with gemfibrozil in middle-aged men with dyslipidemia. N Engl J Med 1987;317:1237-1245.

5. Canner PL, Berge KG, Wenger NK, et al. Fifteen year mortality in Coronary Drug Project patients: Long term benefit with niacin. J Am Coll Cardiol 1986;8:1245-1255.

6.   Report of the National Cholesterol Education Program Expert Panel on detection, evaluation, and treatment of high blood cholesterol in adults. Arch Intern Med 1988;148:36-69.

7.   Wilhelmsson C, Vedin JA, Elmfeldt D, Tibblin G, Wilhelmsen L. Smoking and myocardial infarction. Lancet 1975;I:415-420.

8.   Aberg A, Bergstrand R, Johansson S, et al. Cessation of smoking after myocardial infarction. Effects on mortality after 10 years. Br Heart J 1983;49:416-422.

9.   Friedman M, Thoresen CE, Gill JJ, et al. Alteration of type A behavior and its effect on cardiac recurrences in post myocardial infarction patients: Summary results of the recurrent coronary prevention project. Am Heart J 1986;112:653-665.

10. Ruberman W, Weinblatt E, Goldberg JD, Chaudhary BS. Psychosocial influences on mortality after myocardial infarction. N Engl J Med 1984;311:552-559.

11. The Norwegian Multicenter Study Group. Timolol induced reduction in mortality and reinfarction in patients surviving acute myocardial infarction. N Engl J Med 1981;304:801-807.

12. Hjalmarson A, Elmfeldt D, Herlitz J, et al. Effect on mortality of metoprolol in acute myocardial infarction. Lancet 1981; II:823-827.

13. Hjalmarson A, Herlitz J, Holmberg S, et al. The Goteborg Metoprolol Trial: Effects on mortality and morbidity in acute myocardial infarction. Circulation 1983;67(Suppl I):I-26-32.

14. Beta Blocker Heart Attack Trial Research Group. A randomized trial of propranolol in patients with acute myocardial infarction. I. Mortality results. JAMA 1982;247:1707-1714.

15. Beta Blocker Heart Attack Trial Research Group. A randomized trial of propranolol in patients with acute myocardial infarction. II. Morbidity results. JAMA 1983;250:2814-2819.

16. Yusuf S, Peto R, Collins R, Sleight P. Beta blockade during and after myocardial infarction: An overview of the randomized trials. Prog Cardiovasc Dis 1985;27:335-371.

17. Olsson G, Rehnqvist N, Sjogren A, Erhardt L, Lundman T. Long term treatment with metoprolol after myocardial infarction: Effect on 3-year mortality and morbidity. J Am Coll Cardiol 1985;5:1428-1437.

18. Pedersen TR for the Norwegian Multicenter Study Group. Six year follow-up of the Norwegian Multicenter Study on timolol after acute myocardial infarction. N Engl J Med 1985;313:1055-1058.

19. Ahumada GG. Identification of patients who do not require beta antagonists after myocardial infarction. Am J Med 1984; 76:900-904.

20. Goldman L, Sia STB, Cook EF, Rutherford JD, Weinstein MC. Cost and effectiveness of routine therapy with long term beta-adrenergic antagonists after acute myocardial infarction. N Engl J Med 1988;319:152-157.

21. Gibson RS, Boden WE, Theroux P, et al. Diltiazem and reinfarction in patients with non-Q-wave myocardial infarction. Results of a double-blind, randomized, multicenter trial. N Engl J Med 1986;315:423-429.

22. The Multicenter Diltiazem Postinfarction Trial Research Group. The effect of diltiazem on mortality and reinfarction after myocardial infarction. N Engl J Med 1988;319:385-392.

23. Rapaport E. Influence of long-acting nitrate therapy on the risk of reinfarction, sudden death, and total mortality in survivors of acute myocardial infarction. Am Heart J 1985;110:276-280.

24. Gottlieb SH, Achuff SC, Mellits ED, et al. Prophylactic antiarrhythmic therapy of high risk survivors of myocardial infarction: lower mortality at one month but not at one year. Circulation 1987;75:792-799.

25. The Cardiac Arrhythmia Pilot Study (CAPS) Investigators. Effects of encainide, flecainide, imipramine, and moricizine on ventricular arrhythmias during the year after myocardial infarction: The CAPS. Am J Cardiol 1988;61:501-509.

26. Goldberg RJ, Gore JM, Dalen JE, Alpert JS. Long-term anti-coagulant therapy after acute myocardial infarction. Am Heart J 1985;109:616-622.

27. Serneri GGN, Rovelli F, Gensini GF, et al. Effectiveness of low-dose heparin in prevention of myocardial reinfarction. Lancet 1987;I:937-942.

28. Aspirin Myocardial Infarction Study Research Group. A randomized controlled trial of aspirin in persons recovered from myocardial infarction. JAMA 1980;243:661-669.

29. Klimt CT, Knatterud GL, Stamler J, Meier P. Persantine-Aspirin Reinfarction Study. Part II. Secondary coronary prevention with persantine and aspirin. J Am Coll Cardiol 1986;7:251-269.

30. The Steering Committee of the Physician's Health Study Research Group. Preliminary report: Findings from the aspirin component of the ongoing Physician's Health Study. N Engl J Med 1988; 318:262-264.

Chapter 24

Cardiac Rehabilitation after Myocardial Infarction

Allen D. Soffer, M.D.

The rehabilitation process following myocardial infarction begins almost immediately after the acute event and consists of 3 phases: a gradual increase in activity while in the hospital, early post-discharge convalescence, and long-term rehabilitation. While cardiac rehabilitation programs must be tailored to meet individual patient requirements, their goals are generally uniform: to return the patient to the pre-MI state of physical and psychological health and to provide educational information designed to address issues of secondary prevention. Although decreased cardiac morbidity and mortality have not been conclusively demonstrated (1), rehabilitation programs have been shown to be safe (2,3) and to result in improved exercise performance (2,4,5), psychological well-being (1), and quality of life (1). This chapter will focus on the in-hospital phase of cardiac rehabilitation.

Complications of prolonged bed rest include orthostatic hypotension, thromboembolic events, atelectasis, pneumonia, physical deconditioning, and psychological stress, conditions which may be particularly hazardous in patients having sustained recent myocardial damage. Despite initial fears, early mobilization has been shown to be safe (6,7) and indeed beneficial (7) in patients with uncomplicated acute myocardial infarction, and should be encouraged in patients without evidence of ongoing ischemia, significant arrhythmias, or congestive heart failure.

Bed rest during the first 24-48 hours following admission should be accompanied by active assisted range of motion exercises. Patients should sit in a chair several times daily by the second or third day, and progress to limited ambulation by the third or fourth day post-MI. Physical activity is increased progressively in a structured fashion, with modifications in the program made on an individual basis as necessitated by symptoms or hemodynamic abnormalities. Hospital discharge is usually possible in uncomplicated MIs by day 7-10; discharge instructions should include specific recommendations concerning physical, sexual, and vocational activities. At our institution, the following 10-step rehabilitation program is used.

In-Hospital Cardiac Rehabilitation Program Post-Myocardial Infarction

(patients normally progress one step per day)

Step 1

Supine:
a. active assisted range of motion exercises (5 repetitions)
    1. shoulder flexion/extension
    2. shoulder abduction/adduction
    3. elbow flexion/extension
    4. hip and knee flexion/extension
    5. hip abduction/adduction
    6. hip internal/external rotation
b. active ankle pumps (5 repetitions)
c. deep breathing

Step 2

Supine:
a. active range of motion exercises (5 repetitions)
    1. perform exercises 1-6 above without assistance; upper
       extremity exercises may be performed bilaterally
b. active ankle pumps (5 repetitions)
c. deep breathing

Step 3

Sitting:
a. active range of motion exercises (5 repetitions, may be
   performed bilaterally)
    1. shoulder flexion/extension
    2. shoulder abduction/adduction
    3. elbow flexion/extension
    4. hip flexion/extension (marching in place)
b. active ankle pumps (perform throughout the day, 10 reps/hr)
c. deep breathing

Step 4

Warm Up:

Standing:
a. active range of motion exercises, as in step 3

Exercise:
a. ambulate 50-100 feet

Cool Down:

Sitting:
a. marching in place for at least 3 minutes, sitting in chair with back supported, lifting feet completely off of floor

Throughout the Day:
a. active ankle pumps
b. deep breathing

Step 5

Warm Up:
a. active range of motion exercises, 5 repetitions, as in step 4
b. lateral trunk bending with hands on hips

Exercise:
a. ambulate 100-200 feet, or double the distance performed the previous day

Cool Down:

Sitting:
a. march in place at least 3 minutes, as above

Throughout the Day:
a. active ankle pumps
b. deep breathing

Step 6

Warm Up:

Standing:
a. active range of motion as in step 5, increase to 5 - 10 repetitions

Exercise:
a. ambulate 200-400 feet, or double the distance of the previous day

Cool Down:

Sitting:
a. march in place at least 3 minutes

Throughout the Day:
a. active ankle pumps
b. deep breathing

Step 7

Warm Up:

Standing:
a. active range of motion as in step 6 with 1-pound cuff weight on each upper extremity, 5 - 10 repetitions

Exercise:
a. ambulate 400-800 feet (approximately 5 minutes), or double the distance of the previous day
b. stair climbing, up and down 1 flight

Cool Down:

Sitting/Standing:
a. march in place at least 3 minutes

Throughout the Day:
a. active ankle pumps
b. deep breathing

Step 8

Warm Up:

Standing:
a. active range of motion as in step 7; 10 repetitions

Exercise:
a. ambulate up to 10 minutes
b. stair climbing, up and down 1 flight

Cool Down:

Sitting/Standing:
a. march in place at least 3 minutes

Throughout the Day:
a. active ankle pumps
b. deep breathing

Steps 9 and 10

Warm Up:

Standing:
a. active range of motion as in step 8; 10 - 15 repetitions

Exercise:
a. ambulate 10-15 minutes
b. stair climbing, up and down 1 flight

Cool Down:

Sitting/Standing:
a. march in place at least 3 minutes

Throughout the Day:
a. active ankle pumps
b. deep breathing

REFERENCES

1. Oldridge NB, Jones NL. Preventive use of exercise rehabilitation after myocardial infarction. Acta Med Scand 1986;711(Suppl): 123-129.

2. Squires RW, Lavie CJ, Brandt TR, Gau GT, Bailey KR. Cardiac rehabilitation in patients with severe ischemic left ventricular dysfunction. Mayo Clin Proc 1987;62:997-1002.

3. Van Camp SP, Peterson RA. Cardiovascular complications of out-patient cardiac rehabilitation programs. JAMA 1986;256:1160-1163.

4. Hoffmann A, Lengyel M, Majer K. The effect of training on the physical working capacity of myocardial infarction patients with left ventricular dysfunction. Europ Heart J 1987;8(Suppl G):43-49.

5. Hertanu JS, Davis L, Focseneanu M, Lahman L. Cardiac rehabilitation exercise program: Outcome assessment. Arch Phys Med Rehabil 1986;67:431-435.

6. Hayes MJ, Morris GK, Hampton JR. Comparison of mobilization after two and nine days in uncomplicated myocardial infarction. Br Med J 1974;3:10-13.

7. Bloch A, Maeder J, Haissly J, Felix J, Blackburn H. Early mobilization after myocardial infarction: A controlled study. Am J Cardiol 1974;34:152-157.

Chapter 25

Unstable Angina and Variant Angina

Unstable Angina

Unstable angina is a frequent cause for admission to the CCU and encompasses several clinical syndromes:

1) Worsening of a previously stable angina pattern, manifested by increased frequency, intensity, or duration of pain, or angina that occurs with minimal exertion or at rest, or by pain that responds less readily to standard therapy;

2) New onset angina occurring with minimal exertion or at rest;

3) Angina occurring within the first few weeks after acute MI.

Unstable angina may or may not be associated with ischemic changes on ECG; cardiac enzymes are normal.

Pathophysiology

At cardiac catheterization, unstable angina patients are usually found to have one or more severely narrowed coronary arteries (1,2). The lesions are of comparable severity to those seen in chronic stable angina, although involvement of the left main coronary artery is somewhat more frequent. Recently, it has been suggested that platelet activation may play an important role in unstable angina (3), and coronary angioscopic studies have revealed a high incidence of ruptured atherosclerotic plaque and non-occlusive thrombi in patients with unstable angina (4). These findings indicate that progression from stable to unstable angina may be caused by plaque rupture, resulting in platelet activation and thrombus formation. If sustained total coronary occlusion ensues, the result is acute MI (5). It is likely that alterations in coronary vasomotor tone also contribute to the unstable pattern. The pathogenesis of unstable angina and acute MI is thus similar, resulting in a spectrum of acute coronary syndromes.

Treatment

On presentation, patients with unstable angina frequently cannot be readily distinguished from those with acute MI. Such patients should

be admitted to the CCU and placed on standard protocol. Optimal
initial medical therapy consists of nitrates, a beta blocker and/or
calcium antagonist, and aspirin.

Many patients will respond to bed rest and institution of anti-
anginal therapy. Intravenous nitroglycerin is superior to other
nitrate preparations (6), and should be administered to patients with
severe symptoms, marked ischemic ECG changes, or recurrent pain after
admission. Intravenous nitroglycerin should be tapered to relieve
symptoms or to reduce mean arterial pressure by 7-10 mm Hg. Usual
doses are 10-200 mcg/min; occasionally higher doses are required.
Most centers combine nitrates with a beta blocker or calcium
antagonist; both classes of agents are effective in reducing symptoms,
either alone or in combination (7-9). Nifedipine in the absence of
beta blockade may exacerbate ischemia in acute MI (Chapter 11) and
unstable angina patients (10), and is not recommended as a single
agent. Intravenous metoprolol (Chapter 13) or verapamil may be useful
in patients with recurrent or refractory symptoms.

Two large trials have demonstrated that aspirin 325-1300 mg/day
reduces infarction and mortality by 50% in patients with unstable
angina (11,12), thus providing additional support for the role of
platelets in this syndrome. The higher aspirin dose resulted in more
side effects without additional benefit (12); we therefore prescribe
aspirin 325 mg/day, beginning on admission to the unit, in all
patients with suspected unstable angina. Full-dose heparin also
limits progression to myocardial infarction in unstable angina
patients (13-15). We recommend heparinization of patients with
recurrent severe symptoms unresponsive to conventional therapy
(including aspirin). Thrombolytic therapy may also be effective in
unstable angina, but is associated with a higher incidence of bleeding
complications than aspirin or heparin (16); this strategy may be useful in selected patients, but is not recommended routinely at present.

The principal goal of medical therapy is stabilization of the
patient and prevention of progression to acute myocardial infarction.
The above measures will be effective in over 90% of cases. Because
unstable angina patients are at increased risk for myocardial
infarction and have a significant incidence of left main coronary
stenosis, we recommend elective cardiac catheterization in most
patients who are suitable candidates for angioplasty (PTCA) or bypass
surgery. Gradual ambulation followed by a stress test to determine
the need for catheterization is an acceptable alternative. Patients
who cannot be stabilized warrant more aggressive intervention.
Intra-aortic balloon counterpulsation (Chapter 37) is often effective,
but does not obviate the need for urgent cardiac catheterizaton.
Depending on the results of coronary angiography, angioplasty (17,18)
or coronary bypass surgery (19) may be advisable.

Prognosis

One-year mortality in patients hospitalized with unstable angina is 5-15% (20,21). Non-fatal infarctions occur in an additional 10-15% of patients (20,21). The long-term prognosis is thus similar to that of hospital survivors with documented myocardial infarction (22). Patients with recurrent chest pain and ECG changes (20,21), evidence for silent myocardial ischemia (23,24), or a positive stress test (25) are at increased risk for adverse outcome.

Two large studies failed to show a favorable effect of early surgery on either infarction rate or mortality in unstable angina patients (26,27). In the subgroup of patients with depressed left ventricular function (ejection fraction 30-49%), 2-year survival was higher with surgery (27). Patients with left main coronary disease or severe 3-vessel disease with involvement of the proximal left anterior descending artery are also likely to benefit from surgical treatment. In addition, patients undergoing surgery have less angina than those treated medically (26,28). PTCA has also been associated with symptomatic improvement during short-term follow-up (16), although restenosis occurs in up to 30% of cases. The effects of PTCA on infarction and mortality have not been established.

Variant (Prinzmetal's) Angina

Prinzmetal's angina (29), also called variant or vasospastic angina, is a dramatic syndrome of typical ischemic chest pain and ST segment elevation which is due to focal coronary artery spasm (30). Episodes occur predominantly at rest, often during the early morning hours. In two-thirds of cases, spasm occurs at or near the site of fixed coronary obstruction, while in the remaining one-third there is little or no significant coronary narrowing (31,32). The diagnosis is confirmed by typical symptoms and ECG changes which resolve with standard therapy (see below) or, if necessary, by provocative testing with ergonovine (33). Although lesser alterations in coronary vasomotor tone may play an important role in other acute coronary ischemic syndromes, classic vasospastic angina is a relatively infrequent cause for admission to the CCU.

In the acute phase, vasospastic angina usually responds to nitrates and calcium antagonists (34). For long-term management, the calcium blockers are superior to nitrates (34) and are the treatment of choice. Beta blockers and large doses of aspirin are best avoided, as these agents may exacerbate the syndrome in some patients. In patients with fixed coronary disease, PTCA may be effective in controlling symptoms (35). Coronary bypass surgery has also been performed successfully, even in the absence of obstructive coronary disease (36).

The natural history of vasospastic angina is variable. Although over 50% of patients eventually undergo spontaneous remission (37), during the active phase 10-20% of patients develop acute MI, usually within 1-3 months of initial presentation (38-40). In addition, attacks may be complicated by life-threatening arrhythmias, including ventricular tachycardia, fibrillation, and high-degree A-V block, and sudden cardiac death has been reported in up to one-sixth of patients during long-term followup (41).

The long-term prognosis of patients with variant angina has not been well characterized. Clinical characteristics on presentation are of little value in predicting outcome (39). Among medically treated patients, those free of significant coronary disease tend to have a more favorable course. Patients with fixed coronary disease and variant angina appear to have a worse prognosis than patients with typical angina, and patients with multivessel disease tend to do better with surgery than with medical therapy (40). Patients treated with calcium antagonists also have an improved outcome (42).

In summary, vasospastic angina is an uncommon syndrome of ischemic chest pain and ST-segment elevation which simulates acute MI or unstable angina. Treatment consists initially of nitrates and calcium antagonists. Most patients should undergo cardiac catheterization, and consideration should be given to PTCA or CABG when the anatomy is appropriate. Patients with documented vasospasm should be followed closely because they are at high risk of MI and death within the first several months of presentation.

REFERENCES

1. Alison HW, Russell RO, Mantle JA, Kouchoukos NT, Moraski RE, Rackley CE. Coronary anatomy and arteriography in patients with unstable angina pectoris. Am J Cardiol 1978;41:204-209.

2. Victor MF, Likoff MJ, Mintz GS, Likoff W. Unstable angina pectoris of new onset: A prospective clinical and arteriographic study of 75 patients. Am J Cardiol 1981;47:228-232.

3. Fitzgerald DJ, Roy L, Catella F, Fitzgerald GA. Platelet activation in unstable coronary disease. N Engl J Med 1986; 315:983-989.

4. Sherman CT, Litvack F, Grundfest W, et al. Coronary angioscopy in patients with unstable angina pectoris. N Engl J Med 1986; 315:913-919.

5. Fuster V, Chesebro JH. Mechanisms of unstable angina. N Engl J Med 1986;315:1023-1025.

6. Kaplan K, Davison R, Parker M, Przybylek J, Teagarden JR, Lesch M. Intravenous nitroglycerin for the treatment of angina at rest unresponsive to standard nitrate therapy. Am J Cardiol 1983;51:694-698.

7. Theroux P, Taeymans Y, Morissette D, Bosch X, Pelletier GB, Waters DD. A randomized study comparing propranolol and diltiazem in the treatment of unstable angina. J Am Coll Cardiol 1985;5:717-722.

8. Muller JE, Turi ZG, Pearle DL, et al. Nifedipine and conventional therapy for unstable angina pectoris: A randomized, double-blind comparison. Circulation 1984;69:728-739.

9. Gottlieb SO, Weisfeldt ML, Ouyang P, et al. Effect of the addition of propranolol to therapy with nifedipine for unstable angina pectoris: A randomized, double-blind, placebo-controlled trial. Circulation 1986;73:331-337.

10. Report of the Holland Interuniversity Nifedipine/Metoprolol Trial (HINT) Research Group. Early treatment of unstable angina in the coronary care unit: A randomized, double-blind, placebo controlled comparison of recurrent ischemia in patients treated with nifedipine or metoprolol or both. Br Heart J 1986;56:400-413.

11. Lewis HD, Davis JW, Archibald DG, et al. Protective effects of aspirin against acute myocardial infarction and death in men with unstable angina. N Engl J Med 1983;309:396-403.

12. Cairns JA, Gent M, Singer J, et al. Aspirin, sulfinpyrazone, or both in unstable angina. N Engl J Med 1985;313:1369-1375.

13. Telford AM, Wilson C. Trial of heparin versus atenolol in prevention of myocardial infarction in intermediate coronary syndrome. Lancet 1981;I:1225-1228.

14. Oliva PB. Unstable rest angina with ST-segment depression. Ann Intern Med 1984;100:424-440.

15. Theroux P, Ouimet H, McCans J, et al. Aspirin, heparin, or both to treat acute unstable angina. N Engl J Med 1988;319:1105-1111.

16. Gold HK, Johns JA, Leinbach RC, et al. A randomized, blinded, placebo-controlled trial of recombinant human tissue-type plasminogen activator in patients with unstable angina pectoris. Circulation 1987;75:1192-1199.

17. deFeyter PJ, Serruys PW, van den Brand M, et al. Emergency coronary angioplasty in refractory unstable angina. N Engl J Med 1985;313:342-346.

18. Quigley PJ, Erwin J, Maurer BJ, Walsh MJ, Gearty GF. Percutaneous transluminal coronary angioplasty in unstable angina: Comparison with stable angina. Br Heart J 1986;55:227-230.

19. McCormick JR, Schick EC, McCabe CH, Kronmal RA, Ryan TJ. Determinants of operative mortality and long term survival in patients with unstable angina. The CASS experience. J Thorac Cardiovasc Surg 1985;89:683-688.

20. Gazes PC, Mobley EM, Faris HM, Duncan RC, Humphries GB. Preinfarctional (unstable) angina: A prospective study. Ten year follow-up. Circulation 1973;48:331-337.

21. Mulcahy R, Awadhi AHA, deBuitleor M, Tobin G, Johnson H, Contoy R. Natural history and prognosis of unstable angina. Am Heart J 1985;109:753-758.

22. Schroeder JS, Lamb IH, Hu M. Do patients in whom myocardial infarction has been ruled out have a better prognosis after hospitalization than those surviving infarction? N Engl J Med 1980;303:1-5.

23. Swahn E, Areskog M, Berglund U, Walfridsson H, Wallentin L. Predictive importance of clinical findings and a predischarge exercise test in patients with suspected unstable coronary artery disease. Am J Cardiol 1987;59:208-214.

24. Gottlieb SO, Weisfeldt ML, Ouyang P, Mellits ED, Gerstenblith G. Silent ischemia as a marker for early unfavorable outcomes in patients with unstable angina. N Engl J Med 1986;314:1214-1219.

25. Gottlieb SO, Weisfeldt ML, Ouyang P, Mellits ED, Gerstenblith G. Silent ischemia predicts infarction and death during two year follow-up of unstable angina. J Am Coll Cardiol 1987;10:756-760.

26. National Cooperative Unstable Angina Study Group. Unstable angina pectoris: National Cooperative Study Group to compare surgical and medical therapy. Am J Cardiol 1978;42:839-848.

27. Luchi RJ, Scott SM, Deupree RH, et al. Comparison of medical and surgical treatment for unstable angina pectoris. Results of a Veterans Administration Cooperative Study. N Engl J Med 1987; 316:977-984.

28. Rahimtoola SH, Nunley D, Grunkemeier G, Tepley J, Lambert L, Starr A. Ten-year survival after coronary bypass surgery for unstable angina. N Engl J Med 1983;308:676-681.

29. Prinzmetal M, Kennamer R, Merliss R, et al. Angina pectoris. I. A variant form of angina pectoris. Am J Med 1959;27:375-388.

30. Oliva PB, Potts DE, Pluss RG. Coronary arterial spasm in Prinzmetal angina. Documentation by coronary arteriography. N Engl J Med 1973;288:745-751.

31. Selzer A, Langston M, Ruggeroli C, Cohn K. Clinical syndrome of variant angina with normal coronary arteriogram. N Engl J Med 1976;295:1343-1347.

32. Bott-Silverman C, Heupler FA, Yiannikas J. Variant angina: Comparison of patients with and without fixed severe coronary artery disease. Am J Cardiol 1984;54:1173-1175.

33. Health and Public Policy Committee, American College of Physicians. Performance of ergonovine provocative testing for coronary artery spasm. Ann Intern Med 1984;100:151-152.

34. Ginsburg R, Lamb IH, Schroeder JS, Hu M, Harrison DC. Randomized double-blind comparison of nifedipine and isosorbide dinitrate therapy in variant angina pectoris due to coronary artery spasm. Am Heart J 1982;103:44-48.

35. Corcos T, David PR, Bourassa MG, et al. Percutaneous transluminal coronary angioplasty for the treatment of variant angina. J Am Coll Cardiol 1985;5:1046-1054.

36. Sussman EJ, Goldberg S, Poll DS, et al. Surgical therapy of variant angina associated with nonobstructive coronary disease. Ann Intern Med 1981;94:771-774.

37. Waters DD, Bouchard A, Theroux P. Spontaneous remission is a frequent outcome of variant angina. J Am Coll Cardiol 1983; 2:195-199.

38. Waters DD, Miller DD, Szlachcic J, et al. Factors influencing the long term prognosis of treated patients with variant angina. Circulation 1983;68:258-265.

39. Waters DD, Szlachcic J, Miller DD, Theroux P. Clinical characteristics of patients with variant angina complicated by myocardial infarction or death within one month. Am J Cardiol 1982;49:658-664.

40. Mark DB, Califf RM, Morris KG, et al. Clinical characteristics and long term survival of patients with variant angina. Circulation 1984;69:880-888.

41. Miller DD, Waters DD, Szlachcic J, Theroux P. Clinical characteristics associated with sudden death in patients with variant angina. Circulation 1982;66:588-592.

42. Yasue H, Takizawa A, Nagao M, et al. Long term prognosis for patients with variant angina and influential factors. Circulation 1988;78:1-9.

Chapter 26

Pericardial Disease
Allen D. Soffer, M.D.

Pericardial disease is generally manifest clinically by either acute pericarditis, pericardial effusion, or constrictive pericarditis.

Acute Pericarditis

The conditions that may lead to inflammation of the pericardium are numerous and diverse (Table 26.1), but the resultant clinical syndrome of acute pericarditis is generally of similar presentation, regardless of its etiology. Acute pericarditis is characterized by chest pain, a pericardial friction rub, electrocardiographic changes, and non-specific laboratory findings.

Clinical Presentation

While the chest pain associated with pericarditis may be mistaken for that caused by myocardial ischemia, it is usually characterized by several distinguishing features. Pericardial pain is often sharp, pleuritic, and positional. It may be exacerbated by deep inspiration, coughing, and recumbency, and diminished by sitting upright and leaning forward. It is typically substernal or left precordial in location, may radiate to the neck, shoulders, or back, and often persists for hours or days.

The pericardial friction rub has been called the pathognomonic physical finding of acute pericarditis (1). It is classically comprised of 3 separate components, occurring in mid-systole, mid-diastole, and late-diastole, though at times only one or two of the components may be discernable. Exercise is useful in bringing out all 3 components. Pericardial rubs can best be heard with the diaphragm of the stethoscope applied firmly to the chest wall, with the patient sitting upright and leaning forward. The most common location is between the lower left sternal border and apex (2), but rubs may be heard anywhere over the precordium. Pericardial rubs are typically scratchy, but are also characterized by their changing quality, varying intensity, and transient nature.

The ECG manifestations of pericarditis must be distinguished from those caused by ischemia. Four distinct ECG stages evolve in 50% of patients with acute pericarditis (3). ECG changes may be noted within hours or days after the onset of chest pain and consist of the

Table 26.1
Etiology of Pericarditis

Idiopathic
Viral
Post myocardial infarction
  Acute
  Dressler's syndrome
Cancer
  Primary
  Metastatic
    Lung
    Breast
    Lymphoma
    Leukemia
Collagen vascular disorders
  Systemic lupus erythematosus
  Rheumatoid arthritis
  Mixed connective tissue disease
  Progressive systemic sclerosis
  Polyarteritis nodosa
Drug-induced
  Procainamide
  Hydralazine
  Isoniazid
  Phenytoin
Trauma
  Closed chest
  Surgical (post-pericardiotomy syndrome)
  Procedure-related
Infectious (non-viral)
  Bacterial
  Fungal
  Tuberculosis
  Parasitic
  Rickettsial
Radiation
Uremia
Hypothyroidism
Aortic dissection
Sarcoidosis
Amyloidosis
Inflammatory bowel disease
Pancreatitis

sequential appearance of diffuse ST-segment elevation with or without
PR-segment depression (stage I), normalization of the ECG (stage II),
T-wave inversion with or without PR-segment depression (stage III),
and normalization of the ECG (stage IV). The ST-segment elevation
seen in pericarditis is distinguished from that of acute MI by its
concave upward appearance, diffuse nature, and absence of reciprocal

changes. (Exception: ST-depression may be seen in leads AVR and V1.) In addition, the T-wave changes associated with acute MI may occur simultaneously with ST-segment elevation, whereas in pericarditis T-wave changes occur only after the ST-segment has returned to baseline. PR-segment depression (or elevation in AVR) should be carefully sought, as it is present in 80% of patients with acute pericarditis and it is helpful in confirming the diagnosis (4).

Non-specific signs and laboratory findings often associated with acute pericarditis include fever, sinus tachycardia, leukocytosis, and elevation of the erythrocyte sedimentation rate. Occasionally cardiac isoenzymes may be modestly elevated (5).

General Management

Management of patients with acute pericarditis consists of an evaluation for etiology, control of symptoms, and observation for complications. Most patients should be hospitalized until it has been established that pericarditis is not caused by an acute myocardial infarction, non-viral infection, or other treatable disorder, and that it is not associated with a hemodynamically significant pericardial effusion. Bedrest is usually recommended until chest pain and fever subside. Pericardial chest pain typically responds to conventional nonsteroidal anti-inflammatory agents (aspirin 650 mg q 3-4 hr or indomethacin 25-100 mg q 4-6 hr), but prednisone (40-80 mg/day in divided doses, tapered and discontinued as quickly as possible) may be required in refractory cases. Anticoagulant therapy is usually contraindicated in acute pericarditis.

Pericardial Effusion

Pericardial effusions can complicate pericarditis of any etiology or may occur without clinical evidence of pericardial inflammation. Excessive amounts of pericardial fluid may compromise hemodynamics if increased pericardial pressure results in cardiac tamponade.

Diagnostic Evaluation

Pericardial effusions should be suspected in patients with underlying conditions which predispose to pericarditis. While significant fluid accumulation in the pericardial space may lead to enlargement of the cardiac silhouette on chest x-ray or result in a decrease in ECG voltage and heart sound intensity, such findings are neither sensitive nor specific, and indeed the most important aspect of evaluating suspected pericardial effusions is maintaining a high index of suspicion. Non-invasive evaluation should include an echocardiogram, which has become the diagnostic test of choice because it can be readily performed at bedside, it allows an assessment of effusion size and hemodynamic significance, and it provides useful information about other cardiac structures. Computed tomography (6) and magnetic resonance imaging (7) may provide additional information in selected cases. Invasive techniques include cardiac catheterization, which is occasionally needed to determine the effusion's hemodynamic significance, and pericardiocentesis, which can be diagnostic as well as therapeutic. Flexible fiberoptic pericardioscopy may also be of value if available (8).

Once a pericardial effusion is suspected or identified, an assessment of its hemodynamic significance must be made. This can be accomplished by careful clinical evaluation aided by ancillary studies such as echocardiography and cardiac catheterization.

Pericardial Tamponade

Cardiac tamponade is a life-threatening complication of pericardial effusion which occurs when the pressure exerted by a tense pericardial sac impairs ventricular diastolic filling to the point that stroke volume falls to dangerously low levels. The rise in intrapericardial pressure is dependent not only on the amount of pericardial fluid, but on the rapidity of its accumulation. Thus, as little as 200 cc of fluid may cause tamponade if it accumulates rapidly, as in cases of trauma, while 1000 cc or more of gradually accumulating fluid may be of little hemodynamic consequence due to the ability of the pericardium to stretch and adapt.

Clinical Evaluation

Patients with cardiac tamponade classically present with hypotension, jugular venous distention, distant or inaudible heart sounds and, in advanced cases, signs of inadequate systemic perfusion. However, in the early stages and in patients with slowly developing tamponade, many of these findings may be absent. The most common physical finding in patients with tamponade is jugular venous distention (9). Tachypnea, tachycardia, and pulsus paradoxus are frequently noted. Only one-third of patients have a systolic blood pressure less than 100 mm Hg. Neck vein examination should include an attempt to define jugular venous waveforms, as tamponade is characterized by a prominent x descent and absent y descent (see Chapter 18). A careful examination for pulsus paradoxus (inspiratory decline in systolic blood pressure of greater than 10 mm Hg) should also be performed; in severe cases, complete disappearance of systolic blood pressure with inspiration may be detected (total paradox).

ECG findings typical of pericarditis may or may not be seen in cardiac tamponade. Tachycardia and decreased voltage are the most frequent abnormalities. Electrical alternans (most commonly of the QRS complex; occasionally involving the P and T waves) is not specific for cardiac tamponade, but in the presence of a pericardial effusion and appropriate clinical circumstances, it is highly suggestive.

Echocardiographic findings indicative of tamponade include swinging of the heart within the pericardial space and right atrial and ventricular diastolic collapse (10).

Cardiac catheterization is not necessary in cases of tamponade with typical clinical and echocardiographic features, but can be extremely useful in more subtle cases. Catheterization of the right side of the heart will show an elevated right atrial pressure with a prominent x and absent y descent. Equalization of the diastolic pressures in the right atrium, right ventricle, pulmonary artery, and pulmonary occlusive position may be present, but is not essential to the diagnosis of tamponade.

Treatment

Treatment of cardiac tamponade includes volume expansion while immediate preparations are made for pericardial fluid drainage. Therapeutic options include percutaneous pericardiocentesis, subxiphoid pericardiotomy (pericardial "window"), and pericardiectomy. Patients with severe cardiac tamponade require emergency pericardiocentesis. When possible, this is best performed using fluoroscopy or echocardiography, but in life-threatening situations, the procedure must be performed at the bedside (1).

Technique of Emergency Bedside Pericardiocentesis

Using sterile technique and local anesthesia, the skin is incised with a scalpel 0.5 cm below and to the left of the xiphoid process. An 8-inch large bore needle attached to a syringe is inserted under the skin and slowly advanced toward the right or left shoulder while aspirating continuously. Once the pericardial membrane is pierced and pericardial fluid appears, the needle should be held in position while 50-100 cc of fluid are removed. The removal of even small amounts of pericardial fluid may be associated with dramatic clinical improvement, after which the needle may be withdrawn. If the etiology of the effusion is in question, fluid should be sent for appropriate chemistries, cultures, and cytologic studies. After the patient has been stabilized, a more definitive procedure may be required.

Constrictive Pericarditis

The healing process of pericarditis may result in obliteration of the pericardial space by granulation and scar tissue with resultant fusion and thickening of parietal and visceral pericardium. Such pericardium loses its normal elastic properties, encasing the heart and restricting diastolic filling of its chambers. Constrictive pericarditis may occur following tuberculous, uremic, collagen vascular, neoplastic, radiation, or traumatic pericarditis. The most common etiology today is idiopathic, possibly as a sequela of prior subclinical viral pericarditis (11). Although constrictive pericarditis is uncommon, its recognition is important because complete resection of the pericardium is often curative.

Clinical Presentation

Patients typically present with symptoms of fatigue and dyspnea and clinical evidence of right-sided congestive heart failure. Jugular venous distention is common, and careful inspection reveals a prominent x and y descent (as opposed to the absent y descent in cardiac tamponade). Kussmaul's sign (paradoxic inspiratory expansion of the jugular veins) is often present and should be carefully sought. On auscultation, a diastolic pericardial knock may be heard. Hepatomegaly and other signs of hepatic congestion are frequently present. Pericardial calcification may be seen on chest x-ray. ECG findings may include low QRS voltage and non-specific T-wave abnormalities. Documentation of a thickened pericardium by echocardiography (12), computed tomography (13), or magnetic resonance imaging (14) is helpful when accompanied by appropriate clinical characteristics. Cardiac catheterization typically shows elevated right atrial, right ventricular diastolic, and pulmonary artery occlusive pressures, and the right atrial tracing reveals prominent x and y descents. The right and left ventricular diastolic pressure waveforms show an early diastolic dip followed by a rapid rise and plateau. The latter finding, referred to as the "square-root" sign, is not usually seen in cardiac tamponade.

At times it may be impossible to distinguish constrictive pericarditis from restrictive cardiomyopathy, since the two disorders share many clinical and hemodynamic features. In such cases, endomyocardial biopsy or thoracotomy may be necessary.

Treatment

Satisfactory medical treatment of constrictive pericarditis does not exist, but surgical resection of the thickened, fibrotic pericardium may be curative. Frequently, the initial hemodynamic benefit is modest, but patients may show progressive improvement over the ensuing months.

REFERENCES

1. Lorell BH, Braunwald E. Pericardial disease. In: Braunwald E, ed. Heart disease: A textbook of cardiovascular medicine, 3rd ed. W.B. Saunders Co, Philadelphia, 1988:1484-1534.

2. Shabetai R. The pericardium and its diseases. In: Hurst JW, ed. The heart, 6th ed. McGraw Hill Book Co, New York, 1985:1249-1275.

3. Spodick DH. Electrocardiographic changes in acute pericarditis. Am J Cardiol 1974;33:470-474.

4. Spodick DH. Diagnostic electrocardiographic sequences in acute pericarditis: Significance of PR segment and PR vector changes. Circulation 1973;48:575-580.

5. Marmor A, Grenadir E, Keidar A, Edward S, Palant A. The MB fraction of creatine phosphokinase: An indicator of myocardial involvement in acute pericarditis. Arch Intern Med 1979; 139:819-820.

6. Isner JM, Carter BL, Bankoff MS, Konstam MA, Salem DN. Computed tomography in the diagnosis of pericardial heart disease. Ann Intern Med 1982;97:473-479.

7. Sechtem U, Tscholakoff D, Higgins CB. MRI of the abnormal pericardium. Am J Roentgenol 1986;147:245-252.

8. Kondos GT, Rich S, Levitsky S. Flexible fiberoptic pericardioscopy for the diagnosis of pericardial disease. J Am Coll Cardiol 1986;7:432-434.

9. Guberman BA, Fowler NO, Engel PJ, Gueron M, Allen JM. Cardiac tamponade in medical patients. Circulation 1981;64:633-640.

10. Singh S, Wann LS, Schuchard GH, et al. Right ventricular and right atrial collapse in patients with cardiac tamponade. A combined echocardiographic and hemodynamic study. Circulation 1984;70:966-971.

11. Blake S, Bonar S, O'Neill H, et al. Aetiology of chronic constrictive pericarditis. Br Heart J 1983;50:273-276.

12. Schnittger I, Bowden RE, Abrams J, Popp RL. Echocardiography: Pericardial thickening and constrictive pericarditis. Am J Cardiol 1978;42:388-395.

13. Moncada R, Baker M, Salinas M, et al. Diagnostic role of computed tomography in pericardial heart disease: Congenital defects, thickening, neoplasms, and effusions. Am Heart J 1982;103:263-282.

14. Soulen RL, Stark DD, Higgins CB. Magnetic resonance imaging of constrictive pericardial disease. Am J Cardiol 1985;55:480-484.

Chapter 27

Congestive Heart Failure and Pulmonary Edema

Congestive heart failure (CHF) is not a diagnosis per se, but rather represents the "final common pathway" resulting from a variety of primary cardiac disturbances (Table 27.1). It is one of the most common indications for hospitalization, and at our institution accounts for about 15% of CCU admissions, being second only to chest pain. The management of CHF associated with acute ischemic heart disease was discussed in Chapter 17. The present chapter deals with other causes of CHF and the management of severe or refractory CHF in the CCU.

Table 27.1
Common Causes of Congestive Heart Failure in the CCU

Ischemic heart disease
    Acute ischemia, with or without MI
    Ischemic cardiomyopathy
Valvular heart disease
    Aortic stenosis or insufficiency
    Mitral stenosis or insufficiency
    Tricuspid insufficiency
    Infective endocarditis
Hypertensive heart disease
Cardiomyopathy
    Dilated (congestive) cardiomyopathy
    Hypertrophic cardiomyopathy
    Infiltrative cardiomyopathy (e.g. amyloid)
Arrhythmias
    Atrial fibrillation or flutter
    Other supraventricular tachycardias
    Ventricular tachycardia
    Severe bradycardia
Miscellaneous
    Acute ventricular septal defect
    Myocarditis

Diagnosis and Etiology

The diagnosis of CHF is straightforward in patients with typical symptoms (dyspnea, orthopnea, paroxysmal nocturnal dyspnea, easy fatigability, ankle swelling), physical findings (inspiratory rales, elevated jugular venous pressure, displaced apical impulse, S_3 gallop, pitting edema), and chest x-rays (cardiomegaly, pulmonary vascular congestion, alveolar infiltrates, pleural effusions). Occasionally, the presence of chronic lung disease, atelectasis, pulmonary embolism, pericardial disease, non-cardiogenic pulmonary edema (adult respiratory distress syndrome), or other acute pulmonary disorder makes the diagnosis more difficult.

Once the presence of CHF is confirmed, a careful assessment should be performed in order to determine its etiology and mechanism, since proper management ultimately depends on treatment of the primary cardiac disorder (Table 27.1). In addition, a number of other factors may play a role in precipitating or exacerbating heart failure (Table 27.2), and these factors should be carefully searched for in patients with worsening heart failure of uncertain cause. Not uncommonly, multiple etiologies or other factors contribute to the development of CHF. It is therefore important to perform a careful history and physical examination on all patients presenting with heart failure so that potentially treatable or reversible causes are not overlooked.

Table 27.2
Factors Contributing to the Development of CHF

Excess sodium intake
Excess fluid administration
Failure to take prescribed medications
Drugs
    Beta blockers
    Calcium antagonists
    Anti-arrhythmic agents
    Non-steroidal anti-inflammatory agents
    Steroids
    Alcohol
    Cocaine
Associated medical conditions
    Hyperthyroidism
    Hypothyroidism
    Anemia
    Infections
    Renal insufficiency
    Pulmonary embolism
    Chronic lung disease

Management

Mild to moderate heart failure usually responds to bed rest, supplemental oxygen, dietary sodium restriction, and a diuretic. Furosemide 20-40 mg intravenously results in venodilation and a prompt diuresis in most patients with preserved renal function. Patients with more severe heart failure or renal impairment may require a higher dose. Bumetamide (Bumex) is often used as an alternative to furosemide because of its increased potency (1 mg bumetamide = 40 mg furosemide) but it is substantially more expensive. Patients with severe CHF who do not respond well to furosemide or bumetamide may benefit from the addition of metolazone 5-10 mg p.o., spironolactone 25-50 mg p.o. TID-QID, or chlorothiazide 250-500 mg intravenously.

In the acute setting, digoxin is used primarily to control the ventricular rate in patients with supraventricular tachyarrhythmias, particularly atrial fibrillation or flutter. In addition, its modest inotropic effect may benefit some patients with severe CHF due to systolic (contractile) dysfunction. The usual loading dose is 1 mg in divided doses over 24 hours (see Chapter 38). Digoxin is not indicated in patients with sinus rhythm and normal left ventricular systolic function (e.g. hypertrophic cardiomyopathy), and the use of digitalis in chronic congestive heart failure remains controversial (1). The use of other inotropic agents is discussed below.

Vasodilators are playing an increasingly important role in the management of CHF as a result of recent studies showing favorable effects of these agents on symptoms, exercise tolerance, and mortality in chronic heart failure (2-4). In the acute phase, vasodilators alter the loading characteristics of the left ventricle, thus reducing left ventricular work while improving hemodynamics. Sublingual nitroglycerin produces a prompt reduction in preload, thereby improving dyspnea even in patients without active ischemia. Oral and transcutaneous nitrates provide a more sustained effect. In patients with severe CHF, intravenous nitroglycerin or nitroprusside can be used (see below). Tolerance to the hemodynamic effects of nitrates may occur rapidly (5), but can be minimized by intermittent dosing (6). Several other vasodilators have beneficial short-term effects, but the angiotensin converting enzyme inhibitors captopril and enalapril have become the agents of choice for long-term management because of their sustained beneficial actions and proven value in reducing symptoms and mortality (2,4). Starting doses of captopril range from 6.25-25 mg TID and of enalapril from 2.5-5 mg once or twice daily, depending on blood pressure, renal function, and CHF severity. Isosorbide dinitrate (160 mg/day) in combination with hydralazine (300 mg/day) has also been shown to improve ventricular function and decrease mortality (3).

The above measures will be appropriate in most patients with heart failure, but three situations warrant special consideration. Severe decompensated CHF due to critical aortic stenosis is associated with a poor prognosis without early surgical intervention. Furthermore, overzealous diuresis can compromise cardiac output by reducing preload, and the use of vasodilators can lead to severe hypotension if cardiac output across the severely narrowed valve cannot be increased. Thus, these treatment modalities must be used cautiously if critical aortic stenosis is suspected. In patients with hypertrophic cardiomyopathy and outflow tract obstruction, diuretics, vasodilators, and inotropic agents can all increase the severity of obstruction, further decreasing cardiac output and leading to hypotension. Medical therapy of these patients is directed at ensuring adequate ventricular filling by controlling heart rate and optimizing diastolic relaxation with a beta blocker and/or calcium antagonist. Diltiazem may be the preferred calcium antagonist in this setting because nifedipine can cause excessive vasodilatation and hypotension whereas verapamil has been associated with hemodynamic deterioration in some patients. Atrial fibrillation with loss of the atrial contribution to ventricular filling (atrial "kick") can lead to sudden hemodynamic deterioration in these patients and should be managed aggressively, often with prompt cardioversion. Finally, CHF due to diastolic dysfunction with preserved systolic function may be seen in elderly patients and in chronic hypertensives. These patients are also best managed with beta blockers or calcium antagonists (8).

Acute Pulmonary Edema

The term acute pulmonary edema refers to the sudden development of severe congestive heart failure. Symptoms include extreme dyspnea, air hunger, a sense of suffocation, cough, expectoration of frothy sputum (often pink or blood-tinged), diaphoresis, and marked anxiety. Patients are tachypneic, tachycardic, and in obvious respiratory distress. The skin is pale and clammy and may be cyanotic. Diffuse inspiratory crackles are present; wheezing may also be heard. Cardiac auscultation may be difficult, but frequently reveals an S_3 or summation gallop.

Treatment consists of placing the patient in an upright position and administering oxygen by nasal cannula, face mask, or, if indicated, endotracheal intubation and mechanical ventilation (Chapter 9). Morphine sulfate 5-10 mg intravenously over 5-15 minutes reduces preload and decreases anxiety. Intravenous furosemide 40-100 mg should also be given. Nitroglycerin sublingually or transcutaneously is a useful adjunct in the acute phase, and intravenous aminophylline may be helpful if there is associated bronchospasm. Rotating tourniquets decrease preload by reducing venous return and may be particularly helpful if there is a delay in establishing intravenous access. Phlebotomy is also effective acutely but rarely required. Following stabilization of the patient with these measures, the cause of pulmonary edema should be investigated. Subsequent therapy should be based on the results of this evaluation and on the clinical course.

Refractory Chronic Congestive Heart Failure

In many patients, the natural history of chronic congestive heart failure is one of progressive deterioration until compensation can no longer be maintained with the standard measures described above. Such patients may be admitted to the CCU for more intensive therapy. In all cases, it is imperative to rule out potentially treatable causes of heart failure, including active ischemia, left ventricular aneurysm, valvular disease, uncontrolled hypertension, hypertrophic cardiomyopathy, myocarditis, endocarditis, and drug effects.

Assuming treatable causes have been excluded, patients with refractory CHF are best managed using a pulmonary artery catheter to guide therapy (Chapter 18). Baseline hemodynamic data usually reveal a cardiac index < 2.2 L/min/M^2, pulmonary artery occlusive pressure > 18 mm Hg, and mixed venous oxygen saturation < 50%. (Note: If these findings are not present, the diagnosis of "refractory" CHF should be reassessed.) Initiation of intravenous inotropic and/or vasodilator therapy will often produce salutory hemodynamic effects. Dobutamine 5-10 mcg/kg/min is used most frequently in the absence of severe hypotension or shock. Additional benefit may be obtained in some patients at doses up to 20 mcg/kg/min but higher doses do not usually result in further improvement. Tolerance to dobutamine has been reported during prolonged infusions (9), but this has not been a major problem in this author's experience. Amrinone, a phospho-diesterase inhibitor with inotropic and vasodilatory properties, produces hemodynamic changes comparable to those seen with dobutamine (10). Amrinone is initiated with a loading dose of 0.75 mg/kg given as an intravenous bolus over 3-5 minutes followed by a continuous infusion at 5-10 mcg/kg/min. The loading dose may be repeated after 15-30 minutes if desired. The principal disadvantage of amrinone is that its relatively long half-life (4-6 hours) makes titration difficult, and if adverse reactions occur, they may persist for several hours. Dopamine is less effective than dobutamine in improving hemodynamics (11), but it is useful when severe hypotension precludes the use of dobutamine or amrinone. Inotropic doses of dopamine range from 4-10 mcg/kg/min. At lower doses, the drug has important renal and mesenteric vasodilating effects, and at higher doses vasoconstrictor effects predominate without further increases in cardiac output. In severely decompensated patients, combination therapy with dobutamine and dopamine (12) or dobutamine and amrinone (13) may be superior to a single agent.

Intravenous nitroglycerin or nitroprusside often results in further hemodynamic improvement when added to an inotropic agent. Both drugs are usually titrated until the desired effect is achieved or until hypotension limits further increases in dosage. Both agents may decrease arterial oxygen saturation as a result of intrapulmonic shunting. Other vasodilators, including converting enzyme inhibitors, hydralazine, and prazosin, also exert a prompt, beneficial effect on hemodynamics.

If the patient responds to the above interventions, an attempt should be made to wean the patient off intravenous therapy while maintaining therapeutic doses of digoxin, diuretics, and oral vasodilators. Levodopa 1.5-2.0 g/day in divided doses has also been used in some patients (14), and newer oral inotropic agents such as enoximone (15) may soon be available. In patients who fail to improve with aggressive management but who are candidates for corrective cardiac surgery or heart transplantation, invasive measures such as intra-aortic balloon counterpulsation or a left ventricular assist device should be considered.

Unfortunately, although patients with refractory heart failure may experience temporary hemodynamic improvement, the prognosis remains poor unless the underlying disease process is amenable to specific therapy or the patient is eligible for transplantation. Of available medical options, only vasodilator therapy has been shown to significantly improve survival and quality of life (2-4).

REFERENCES

1. Parmley WW, Smith TW, Pitt B. Should digoxin be the drug of first choice after diuretics in chronic congestive heart failure? J Am Coll Cardiol 1988;12:265-273.

2. Captopril Multicenter Research Group. A placebo-controlled trial of captopril in refractory chronic congestive heart failure. J Am Coll Cardiol 1983;2:755-763.

3. Cohn JN, Archibald DG, Ziesche S, et al. Effect of vasodilator therapy on mortality in chronic congestive heart failure. Results of a Veteran's Administration cooperative study. N Engl J Med 1986;314:1547-1552.

4. The CONSENSUS Trial Study Group. Effects of enalapril on mortality in severe congestive heart failure. Results of the Cooperative North Scandinavian Enalapril Survival Study (CONSENSUS). N Engl J Med 1987;316:1429-1435.

5. Jordan RA, Seth L, Casebolt P, Hayes MJ, Wilen MM, Franciosa J. Rapidly developing tolerance to transdermal nitroglycerin in congestive heart failure. Ann Intern Med 1986;104:295-298.

6. Packer M, Lee WH, Kessler PD, Gottlieb SS, Medina N, Yushak M. Prevention and reversal of nitrate tolerance in patients with congestive heart failure. N Engl J Med 1987;317:799-804.

7. Epstein SE, Rosing DR. Verapamil: Its potential for causing serious complications in patients with hypertrophic cardiomyopathy. Circulation 1981;64:437-441.

8. Topol EJ, Traill TA, Fortuin NJ. Hypertensive hypertrophic cardiomyopathy of the elderly. N Engl J Med 1985;312:277-283.

9. Unverferth DV, Blanford M, Kates RE, Leier CV. Tolerance to dobutamine after a 72 hour continuous infusion. Am J Med 1980; 69:262-266.

10. Klein N, Siskind S, Frishman W, Sonnenblick E, LeJemtel T. Hemodynamic comparison of intravenous amrinone and dobutamine in patients with chronic congestive heart failure. Am J Cardiol 1981;48:170-175.

11. Leier CV, Heban PT, Huss P, Bush CA, Lewis RP. Comparative systemic and regional hemodynamic effects of dopamine and dobutamine in cardiogenic shock. Circulation 1978;58:466-475.

12. Richard C, Ricome JL, Rimailho A, Bottineau G, Auzepy P. Combined hemodynamic effects of dopamine and dobutamine in cardiogenic shock. Circulation 1983;67:620-626.

13. Gage J, Rutman H, Lucido D, LeJemtel TH. Additive effects of dobutamine and amrinone on myocardial contractility and ventricular performance in patients with severe heart failure. Circulation 1986;74:367-373.

14. Rajfer FI, Anton AH, Rossen JD, Goldberg LI. Beneficial hemodynamic effects of oral levodopa in heart failure. Relation to the generation of dopamine. N Engl J Med 1984;310:1357-1362.

15. Maskin CS, Weber KT, Janicki JS. Long term oral enoximone therapy in chronic cardiac failure. Am J Cardiol 1987;60:63C-67C.

Chapter 28

Hypertensive Emergencies and Urgencies

Hypertensive emergencies are defined as those conditions requiring reduction of blood pressure within 1 hour to minimize the risk of progressive end-organ damage, while hypertensive urgencies are those situations in which severe hypertension should be treated within several hours despite the absence of acute end-organ dysfunction (1). Specific examples of hypertensive emergencies and urgencies are listed in Table 28.1. Note that it is the immediate threat of major complications which defines hypertensive emergencies and urgencies, rather than the severity of blood pressure elevation itself. Thus, a patient with a chronically elevated blood pressure of 240/140 mm Hg certainly requires treatment, but in the absence of acute complications, rapid reduction of blood pressure is not justified and could be harmful (see below).

Management

Since hypertensive emergencies are often associated with cardiovascular complications (acute pulmonary edema, myocardial infarction or unstable angina, or less frequently, aortic dissection), these patients may be admitted to the coronary care unit for management. The patient should be placed at bed rest in a quiet room, and reduction of blood pressure should be initiated promptly. In general, hypertensive emergencies are treated with parenteral agents, whereas rapidly acting oral agents are usually appropriate for hypertensive urgencies. Several classes of drugs are now available (Table 28.2), and selection of an agent should be based on the clinical circumstances. Thus, nitroprusside and nitroglycerin (in conjunction with a diuretic) are appropriate intravenous agents if congestive heart failure is present, and captopril is a suitable oral agent (3). In the presence of acute MI or unstable angina, intravenous nitroglycerin, alone or in combination with a beta blocker, would be a rational choice, and if aortic dissection is suspected, nitroprusside is often used in conjunction with a beta blocker (Chapter 30). Other agents include diazoxide (4,5), labetalol (6), hydralazine, minoxodil (7), clonidine (8,9), and nifedipine (10,11). Methyldopa, trimethaphan camsylate, and phentolamine are used less frequently.

Table 28.1
Hypertensive Emergencies and Urgencies*

Hypertensive emergencies
    Hypertensive encephalopathy
    Intracranial hemorrhage
    Acute left ventricular failure
    Acute myocardial infarction
    Unstable angina
    Aortic dissection
    Eclampsia or severe hypertension during pregnancy
    Head trauma
    Extensive burns
    Rapidly progressing renal insufficiency
    Severe post-operative bleeding

Hypertensive urgencies
    Perioperative hypertension
    Papilledema without other immediate complications
    Antihypertensive drug withdrawal syndrome
    Pheochromocytoma
    Diastolic blood pressure ≥ 130 mm Hg not
       known to be chronic

*Adapted from Ferguson RK, Vlasses PH. Hypertensive emergencies and urgencies. JAMA 1986;255:1608. Copyright 1986, American Medical Association. Used with permission.

In patients with immediately life-threatening complications of severe hypertension, nitroprusside is often the agent of first choice. This is because its rapid efficacy and ease of titration minimize the risk of complications associated with overly rapid blood pressure reduction (2). Use of an intra-arterial pressure line to guide therapy is often desirable but not mandatory. Complications may arise if the fall in blood pressure exceeds the central nervous system's autoregularity capacity for maintaining cerebral perfusion, thus producing symptoms or signs of cerebral ischemia. Similarly, myocardial ischemia may be aggravated if coronary perfusion pressure is compromised, and a prolonged reduction in renal perfusion may cause a deterioration in renal function (2). To prevent these complications, a reasonable goal of therapy is to reduce the mean arterial pressure by 20 mm Hg during the first 1-4 hours, with normalization of blood pressure over the next 1-3 days.

Table 28.2
Treatment of Hypertensive Emergencies and Urgencies*

Agent	Dose	Onset, min	Adverse reactions
Nitroprusside	0.5-10 mcg/kg/min IV	<1	Nausea, vomiting, thiocyanate toxicity
Nitroglycerin	5-100 mcg/kg/min IV	2-5	Headache, tachycardia, vomiting
Diazoxide	50-150 mg IV boluses or 15-30 mg/min IV infusion	1-2	Hypotension, tachycardia, angina, hyperglycemia
Hydralazine	5-20 mg IV, 10-40 mg IM	10-30	Tachycardia, headache, vomiting, angina
Labetalol	20-80 mg IV bolus q10 min 2 mg/min IV infusion	5-10	Bronchoconstriction, heart block, CHF, orthostatic hypotension
Trimethaphan	1-4 mg/min IV	1-5	Ileus, orthostatic hypotension, blurred vision
Methyldopa	250-500 mg IV infusion	30-60	Drowsiness
Phentolamine	5-15 mg IV	1-2	Tachycardia, orthostatic hypotension
Captopril	25 mg po, repeat prn	<60	Renal dysfunction
Clonidine	0.1-0.2 mg po q1° prn	30-60	Sedation, rebound hypertension
Minoxodil	2.5-5 mg po	15-30	Tachycardia, hypotension, fluid retention
Nifedipine	10 mg po or SL, repeat prn	10-30	Tachycardia, angina, headache, flushing

*Adapted from The 1988 report of the Joint National Committee on detection, evaluation, and treatment of high blood pressure. Arch Intern Med 1988;148;1032. Copyright 1988, American Medical Association. Used with permission.

REFERENCES

1. 1988 Joint National Committee. The 1988 report of the Joint National Committee on detection, evaluation, and treatment of high blood pressure. Arch Intern Med 1988;148:1023-1038.

2. Ferguson RK, Vlasses PH. Hypertension emergencies and urgencies. JAMA 1986;255:1607-1613.

3. Case DB, Atlas SA, Sullivan PA, Laragh JH. Acute and chronic treatment of severe and malignant hypertension with the oral angiotensin converting enzyme inhibitor captopril. Circulation 1981;64:765-771.

4. Ram C, Kaplan NM. Individual titration of diazoxide dosage in the treatment of severe hypertension. Am J Cardiol 1979;43:627-630.

5. Garrett BN, Kaplan NM. Efficacy of slow infusion of diazoxide in the treatment of severe hypertension without organ hypoperfusion. Am Heart J 1982;103:390-394.

6. Cressman MD, Vidt DG, Gifford RW, Moore WS, Wilson DJ. Intravenous labetalol in the management of severe hypertension and hypertensive emergencies. Am Heart J 1984;107:980-985.

7. Wood BC, Sharma JN, Crouch T. Oral minoxidil in the treatment of hypertensive crisis. JAMA 1979;241:163.

8. Anderson RJ, Hart GR, Crumpler CP, Reed WG, Matthews CA. Oral clonidine loading in hypertensive urgencies. JAMA 1981; 246:848-850.

9. Houston MC. Treatment of hypertensive emergencies and urgencies with oral clonidine loading and titration. Arch Intern Med 1986; 146:586-589.

10. Bertel O, Conen D, Radu EW, Muller J, Lang C, Dubach UC. Nifedipine in hypertensive emergencies. Br Med J 1983;286:19-21.

11. Given BD, Lee TH, Stone PH, Dzau VJ. Nifedipine in severely hypertensive patients with congestive heart failure and preserved ventricular systolic function. Arch Intern Med 1985;145:281-285.

Percutaneous Transluminal Coronary Angioplasty

Patricia L. Cole, M.D.

Widespread availability of percutaneous transluminal coronary angioplasty (PTCA) coupled with recent advances in technology have made this technique a preferred treatment for a large subgroup of patients with coronary artery disease. In 1986 alone, over 110,000 PTCAs were performed in the United States. In many institutions, arterial sheaths are left in place for 12-24 hours after angioplasty, and patients are admitted to the CCU or intermediate care unit for routine observation and monitoring. Care of the post-PTCA patient has thus become an important part of the CCU rotation for the house officer.

PTCA involves the use of a balloon-tipped catheter to dilate focal stenoses in coronary arteries. The catheter usually has a double lumen: the central lumen is for hemodynamic measurements and angiography; the outer lumen is used to inflate the balloon. The coronary artery is cannulated using a preformed guiding catheter that is introduced into the arterial system via the femoral or brachial artery. An 8 or 9 French arterial sheath is used to maintain access to the artery. Under certain circumstances (most notably when angioplasty of the right coronary artery is planned) a 5 or 6 French temporary pacing wire is placed transvenously into the right ventricle.

The histologic mechanism of PTCA involves dislodgement of any clot present at the stenotic site, endothelial desquamation, and rupture of the intimal plaque. Atheromatous material becomes compressed against the arterial wall, and presumably small fragments of plaque and endothelial remnants are released into the circulation. Although distal embolization cannot usually be identified angiographically, it may account for some episodes of persistent pain which occur after PTCA despite continued vessel patency. Intimal plaque rupture results in exposure of the vascular subendothelium, causing platelet activation and adherence. This may lead to early closure of the vessel (0-48 hrs), and is the reason for routine anticoagulation with aspirin or heparin following PTCA.

In most respects, the management of the post-PTCA patient involves routine CCU care. However, it is important to make the distinction between residual post-PTCA chest discomfort and chest pain that represents acute ischemia due to vessel closure. The latter usually has a typical anginal quality and may worsen over several minutes to hours. It is often associated with ECG changes in an anatomic pattern consistent with the involved vessel. Suspected vessel closure warrants prompt treatment with IV nitroglycerin and a calcium antagonist. Symptoms caused by local coronary spasm usually resolve with medical therapy; persistent pain may necessitate re-catheterization to assess vessel patency. In contrast, "benign" post-PTCA pain is usually less intense, eases over several hours and is not associated with ECG changes or hemodynamic instability.

Patients admitted to the CCU with an arterial sheath in place should be fully anticoagulated with heparin to keep the PTT at 2.0-2.5 times control. During the evening following PTCA, the patient with a femoral sheath should remain supine, with the head of the bed elevated no more than 30 degrees to prevent buckling of the sheath and catheter. Persistent oozing of blood around the sheath may respond to reducing the heparin rate and applying a more effective pressure bandage. An enlarging hematoma may represent vessel perforation or a crack in the wall of the arterial sheath. If the hematoma continues to expand despite application of pressure for 20 minutes, heparin should be stopped and the arterial sheath removed. Evidence for arterial insufficiency is another indication for removal of the sheath. Pain, loss of distal pulses, pallor, and poor capillary refill suggest arterial insufficiency and warrant prompt attention.

If the patient remains stable and free of arterial complications for 12-24 hours, heparin is discontinued for 2-4 hours to allow the sheath to be removed. Firm pressure should be maintained over the arterial puncture site for at least 20-30 minutes until adequate hemostasis has been achieved. A pressure dressing and sandbag (if desired) should be used to reduce the risk of bleeding. Subsequent resumption of anticoagulation with heparin or coumadin varies with the clinical situation and local preferences, but antiplatelet agents are usually initiated prior to the procedure and continued for at least several months thereafter.

Once the sheath has been pulled and hemostasis achieved, the patient can be transferred to a general medical floor if continued hospitalization is necessary. Patients should be given instructions to avoid heavy lifting or exertion for a period of 1-2 weeks after the angioplasty to allow the access artery to heal.

Long-term post-PTCA care involves risk factor modification (cessation of smoking, control of blood pressure and cholesterol levels), and routine administration of aspirin and dipyridamole for at least 3-6 months. In some centers, thallium stress testing is performed to assess vessel patency, but the value of this procedure in the absence of recurrent symptoms has not been established.

FURTHER READING

1. Baim DS, Faxon DP. Coronary angioplasty. In: Grossman W, ed. Cardiac catheterization and angiography, 3rd ed. Lea & Febiger, Philadelphia, 1986:473-492.

2. Chokshi SK, Meyers S, Abi-Mansour P. Percutaneous transluminal coronary angioplasty: Ten years experience. Prog Cardiovasc Dis 1987;30:147-210.

3. Jang GD, ed. Angioplasty. McGraw-Hill Book Co, New York, 1986.

Chapter 30

Dissection of the Aorta

Edward C. Miller, M.D.

Although a variety of conditions may affect the thoracic or abdominal aorta in adults, only acute aortic dissection will be discussed in this chapter, in part because it is the most common disease of the aorta resulting in admission to the CCU, and in part because it may mimic other life-threatening intrathoracic events, including acute myocardial infarction.

The normal aorta consists of a thin intima, a muscular and elastic media, and a fibrous adventitia. Aortic dissection is thought to occur when an intimal tear allows dissection and expansion of a hematoma into the media. Such tears usually occur at the site of prior disease or injury; common predisposing factors include hypertension (70-90% of cases), atherosclerosis, collagen diseases, degenerative processes such as cystic medial necrosis, and trauma (both accidental and surgical). Dissections most commonly originate within a few centimeters of the aortic valve or just distal to the left subclavian artery, but can occur anywhere along the aorta. Propagation of the dissecting hematoma usually proceeds distally, but can extend proximally or in both directions. The pulsatile sheer force produced by ventricular systole is the principal factor contributing to progression of the dissection.

Classification

Aortic dissections are classified by age and location. Patients presenting within 2 weeks of onset are considered to have acute dissections; those more than 2 weeks old are termed chronic. This distinction derives from the fact that the mortality of untreated dissection is 65-80% within 2 weeks, while the prognosis is substantially better after 2 weeks.

DeBakey defined three types of dissections based on location. Type I involves both the ascending and descending aorta, Type II is limited to the ascending aorta, and Type III is confined to the descending aorta. Type III is subdivided into subtypes A (above the diaphragm) and B (extending below the diaphragm). Involvement of the ascending aorta (Types I and II) is associated with a worse prognosis, which has led to the simplified classification scheme proposed by Daily et al. In this system, Type A is any dissection involving the ascending aorta; all others are classified as Type B.

Clinical Presentation

The cardinal manifestation of acute aortic dissection is severe chest pain, which is present in 90% of cases. Pain is maximal at onset and frequently described as ripping or tearing in quality. Anterior or posterior location of the pain often correlates with involvement of the ascending or descending aorta respectively, and migration of the pain may localize the course of extension. Neurologic deficits are the second most common symptom, but are often evanescent. Stroke, paraparesis or paraplegia, ischemic peripheral neuropathy, or altered mental status ranging from mild confusion to syncope or obtundation may occur. Symptoms due to limb or visceral ischemia are less common.

On physical examination, hypertension is often present proximal to the dissection, while pulses may be diminished or asymmetric in distal vessels due to compromised blood flow. Hypertension may be exacerbated by renin release from a hypoperfused kidney or by reflex sympathetic stimulation. Hypotension and shock are more common in Type A dissections and may be due to aortic rupture into one of the cardiac chambers or the pericardial sac, aortic insufficiency, or acute MI. Free rupture of the aorta usually results in rapid hemodynamic deterioration and death.

Acute aortic insufficiency occurs in two-thirds of Type A dissections and is the most common cause of congestive heart failure. Acute MI complicates 1-2% of dissections, and may be due to involvement of the coronary ostia (most commonly the right coronary artery) or underlying atherosclerosis. Signs and symptoms caused by displacement, compression, ischemia, or infarction of other mediastinal structures or visceral organs may also occur.

Diagnosis

Acute aortic dissection should be considered in any patient with typical chest pain, particularly if there is a history of longstanding hypertension. Because the symptoms may simulate acute MI, the importance of performing a detailed physical examination, including a careful assessment of peripheral pulses, in all patients admitted to the CCU with acute chest pain cannot be overemphasized.

Routine blood tests are usually not helpful, and cardiac enzymes must be interpreted cautiously, since ischemia of the limbs, brain, and other viscera may produce confusing enzyme patterns with or without associated myocardial infarction. The ECG may demonstrate left ventricular hypertrophy or evidence for myocardial ischemia. The chest x-ray reveals an abnormality in the aortic size or shape in 90% of cases, with mediastinal widening being the most common finding. The aortic contour should be inspected carefully, since a separation of 1 cm or more between intimal calcification and adventitial outline strongly suggests dissection.

Definitive diagnosis rests on demonstrating an intimal tear or false lumen with contrast angiography. Computed tomography with contrast is a useful screening test and has a sensitivity of 90%. Digital subtraction angiography, magnetic resonance imaging, and echocardiography (especially esophageal echo) have also been used, but in most cases catheterization will still be required to define the extent of dissection and to evaluate the coronary arteries and aortic valve.

Management

Aortic dissection carries a 20-25% mortality in the first 6 hours; thus, prompt diagnosis and treatment is imperative. Medical therapy is aimed at stabilizing the patient and preventing extension of the dissection, and consists of lowering the blood pressure and reducing myocardial contractility, thus decreasing the sheer force at the site of the intimal tear. Unless contraindicated, intravenous beta blockade with propranolol, metoprolol, or esmolol should be instituted promptly to lower heart rate to 50-70/min. Esmolol as a continuous infusion may be particularly useful in this setting, as it allows titration to the desired heart rate and blood pressure. In patients who cannot tolerate beta blockers, verapamil can be used to reduce contractility, but this agent is less effective in lowering heart rate.

Systolic blood pressure should be maintained within a narrow range (usually 100-120 mm Hg) without compromising organ perfusion; this is best accomplished using an arterial line for continuous blood pressure monitoring. Intravenous nitroprusside has become the standard agent in our institution because it can be easily titrated to maintain the desired blood pressure. However, nitroprusside increases the force of ejection in the absence of effective beta blockade. For this reason, intravenous trimethaphan and labetalol have been used as alternative agents.

Surgical consultation is advised in all cases where there is a high index of suspicion for aortic dissection. Surgical repair is indicated in patients with acute type A dissections, acute type B dissections that cannot be stabilized with medical therapy, all dissections associated with Marfan's syndrome, and chronic dissections with recurrent symptoms. Stable type B dissections and most chronic type A dissections can be managed medically, as can some stable dissections involving the aortic arch, since the latter carry a higher surgical morbidity and mortality. Patients with acute aortic insufficiency and congestive heart failure or pericardial tamponade require emergency surgical intervention.

Prognosis

Untreated acute aortic dissection is associated with a 20-25% mortality within 6 hours and 65-80% mortality at 2 weeks. Type A dissections carry a worse prognosis, especially when associated with aortic insufficiency, myocardial infarction, or pericardial tamponade. Surgical mortality has fallen from 25% to less than 10% in acute type A dissections, and from 36% to 13% in acute type B dissections which have failed to respond to medical therapy. Nonoperative mortality in stable acute type B dissections is 10-20%. The long-term prognosis in hospital survivors is relatively good; up to 60% 10-year survival has been reported. Factors adversely affecting long-term outlook include aneurysm formation, recurrent dissection, chronic aortic insufficiency, stroke, renal insufficiency, and MI.

Long-term follow-up care should include a beta blocker (if tolerated) in all patients, strict blood pressure control, and periodic chest x-rays (3-6 month intervals). High risk patients (e.g., Marfan's syndrome) may also benefit from more aggressive screening, such as annual or semi-annual computed tomographic scanning.

FURTHER READING

1. Amparo EG, Higgins CB, Hricak H, et al. Aortic dissection: Magnetic resonance imaging. Radiology 1985;155:399-406.

2. Daily PO, Trueblood W, Stinson EB, et al. Management of acute aortic dissections. Ann Thorac Surg 1970;10:237-247.

3. DeBakey ME, Henly WS, Cooley DA, et al. Surgical management of dissecting aneurysms of the aorta. J Thorac Cardiovasc Surg 1965; 49:130-149.

4. DeBakey ME, McCollum CH, Crawford ES, et al. Dissection and dissecting aneurysms of the aorta: Twenty-year follow-up of five hundred twenty-seven patients treated surgically. Surgery 1982; 92:1118-1134.

5. DeSanctis RW, Doroghazi RM, Austen WG, Buckley MJ. Aortic dissection. N Engl J Med 1987;317:1060-1067.

6. Doroghazi RM, Slater EE, DeSanctis RW, et al. Long-term survival of patients with treated aortic dissection. J Am Coll Cardiol 1984;3:1026-1034.

7. Earnest F, Muhm JR, Sheedy PF. Roentgenographic findings in thoracic aortic dissection. Mayo Clin Proc 1979;54:43-50.

8. Goldman AP, Kotler MN, Scanlon MH, et al. The complimentary role of magnetic resonance imaging, doppler echocardiography, and computed tomography in the diagnosis of dissecting thoracic aneurysms. Am Heart J 1986;111:970-981.

9. Greenwood WR, Robinson MD. Painless dissection of the thoracic aorta. Am J Emerg Med 1986;4:330-333.

10. Guthaner DR, Miller DC. Digital subtraction angiography of aortic dissection. AJR 1983;141:157-161.

11. Gutierrez FR, Gowda S, Ludbrook PA, McKnight RC. Cineangiography in the diagnosis and evaluation of aortic dissection. Radiology 1980;135:759-761.

12. Haverich A, Miller DC, Scott WC, et al. Acute and chronic aortic dissections: Determinants of long-term outcome for operative survivors. Circulation 1985;72(Suppl II):II-24-34.

13. Kouchoukos NT, Marshall WG, Wedige-Stecher TA. Eleven-year experience with composite graft replacement of the ascending aorta and aortic valve. J Thorac Cardiovasc Surg 1986;92:691-705.

14. Larson EW, Edwards WD. Risk factors for aortic dissection: A necropsy study of 161 cases. Am J Cardiol 1984;53:849-855.

15. Mathew T, Nanda NC. Two-dimensional and doppler echocardiographic evaluation of aortic aneurysm and dissection. Am J Cardiol 1984;54:379-385.

16. Miller DC, Mitchell RS, Oyer PE, et al. Independent determinants of operative mortality for patients with aortic dissections. Circulation 1984;70(Suppl I):I-153-164.

17. Murdoch JL, Walker BA, Halpern BL, et al. Life expectancy and causes of death in the Marfan's syndrome. N Engl J Med 1972; 286:804-808.

18. Murphy DA, Craver JM, Jones EL, et al. Recognition and management of ascending aortic dissection complicating cardiac surgical operations. J Thorac Cardiovasc Surg 1983;85:247-256.

19. Singh H, Fitzgerald E, Ruttley MS. Computed tomography: The investigation of choice for aortic dissection? Br Heart J 1986; 56:171-175.

20. Slater EE, DeSanctis RW. The clinical recognition of dissecting aortic aneurysm. Am J Med 1976;60:625-633.

21. Wheat MW, Palmer RF, Seelman RC. Treatment of dissecting aneurysms of the aorta without surgery. J Thorac Cardiovasc Surg 1965;50:364-373.

22. Wilson SK, Hutchins GM. Aortic dissecting aneurysms: Causative factors in 204 cases. Arch Pathol Lab Med 1982;106:175-180.

Chapter 31

Psychosocial Aspects of Coronary Care

Robert M. Carney, Ph.D.

Admission to the coronary care unit is a highly stressful experience for patients and their families, and may engender acute and long-term emotional responses which can have an important impact on the hospital course, early convalescence, and late functional and cardiovascular prognosis.

Anxiety

Almost all patients experience some degree of anxiety during hospitalization for a suspected acute cardiac event. This anxiety arises from fears and uncertainties about the future as patients face issues related to their own mortality and to possible major changes in lifestyle. Denial is the patient's principal means of combating anxiety and, when exercised appropriately, serves an important adaptive function. Excessive denial, however, may interfere with the physician-patient relationship and cause the patient to reject indicated diagnostic and therapeutic interventions. These patients are also unlikely to make modifications in lifestyle or to comply with other medical instructions after discharge and, as a result, may be at increased risk for rehospitalization.

There are several ways of reducing anxiety in cardiac patients. First, the CCU environment itself offers some measure of reassurance because of the constant surveillance provided by the cardiac monitor and the prompt availability of trained nurses and physicians. In fact, anxiety levels peak just prior to the patient's discharge from the CCU, despite the fact that this transfer generally implies improvement and stabilization of the patient's condition. The physician and CCU staff can provide considerable reassurance to the patient and family through empathic explanations about the CCU environment, the patient's diagnosis and expected hospital course, and the anticipated long-term outlook. Anxiety will be substantially reduced if the physician maintains a confident, optimistic attitude (without presenting false hope) which conveys to the patient the feeling that he is "in good hands" and that the long-term outlook is not as bleak as he might otherwise have thought.

Because patient anxiety is often underestimated due to associated denial, many hospitals routinely prescribe anxiolytics to all patients admitted to the CCU. On the other hand, since such therapy has not been shown to influence prognosis and may be associated with undesirable side effects, we continue to use these agents on an "as needed" basis. Benzodiazepines (e.g., diazepam 2-10 mg, oxazepam 10-30 mg, or alprazolam 0.25-1 mg 3-4 times/day) have become the drugs of choice for anxiety.

Depression

In the days following myocardial infarction, when patients are trying to come to grips with their illness, they may feel a sense of sadness and loss, thinking that their normal, "care-free" existence has come to an end. Concerns about mortality and quality of life may contribute to a sense of demoralization, which is further fueled by easy fatigability and diminished exercise tolerance due to in-hospital deconditioning and, in patients with large infarctions, the MI itself. These feelings often abate spontaneously within 2-3 months as activities return to normal or new limitations are accepted. However, in 15-30% of post-MI patients, feelings of diminished self-worth and hopelessness may escalate into a major depressive episode. Early signs may be detected in the CCU, and include a prior history of depression, excessive moodiness, ill-humor, and marked sleep disturbances, particularly when these behaviors represent a change from the patient's baseline.

Non-pharmacologic treatment of depressive symptomatology is similar to that for anxiety, with which it frequently coexists. Continued reassurance, emphasizing favorable prognostic aspects, is important, and early initiation of cardiac rehabilitation, if possible, may help overcome feelings of helplessness. In patients with severe mood disturbances, early psychiatric consultation is advised.

Psychosis

Acute, unexplained delirium ("ICU psychosis") is uncommon in the CCU. If symptoms fail to resolve after discontinuation of potentially offending medications (e.g., lidocaine) and correction of metabolic disorders (including hypoxemia), haloperidol 0.5-10 mg is usually effective.

Prognostic Implications

It is thought that psychosocial factors play an important role in determining whether the post-MI patient will return to work and continue to pursue an active and productive lifestyle. In addition, several studies have demonstrated that the presence of depression is associated with increased morbidity and mortality during the year after infarction, an effect which is independent of illness severity. Related variables, such as social isolation and a high degree of life stress, are also associated with increased mortality after MI. Finally, chronic anxiety about one's cardiac status may in some cases lead to psychological cardiac invalidism. Thus, proper early recognition and management of the emotional response to cardiac illness is important not only to relieve psychic stress, but to diminish increased cardiovascular morbidity and mortality and to reduce the adverse social outcomes associated with these commonly occurring psychiatric disorders in the post myocardial infarction patient.

FURTHER READING

1. Blumenthal JA, Burg M, Barefoot J, Williams R, Haney T, Zimet G. Social support, type A behavior, and coronary artery disease. Psychosom Med 1987;49:331-340.

2. Blumenthal JA, Williams RS, Wallace AG, Williams RB, Needles TL. Physiological and psychological variables predict compliance to prescribed exercise therapy in patients recovering from myocardial infartion. Psychosom Med 1982;44:519-527.

3. Carney RM, Rich MW, teVelde A, Saini J, Clark K, Jaffe AS. Major depressive disorder in coronary artery disease. Am J Cardiol 1987;60:1273-1275.

4. Cassem NH, Hackett TP. Psychiatric consultation in a coronary care unit. Ann Intern Med 1971;75:9-14.

5. Cay EL, Vetter N, Philip AE, Dugard P. Psychological status during recovery from an acute heart attack. J Psychosom Res 1972;16:425-435.

6. Falgar P, Appels A. Psychological risk factors over the life course of myocardial infarction patients. Adv Cardiol 1982; 29:132-139.

7. Hackett PP, Cassem NH. The psychologic reactions in patients in the pre and post hospital phase of myocardial infarction. Postgrad Med 1975;57:43.

8. Levine J, Warrenburg S, Kerns G, et al. The role of denial in recovery from coronary heart disease. Psychosom Med 1987; 49:109-117.

9. Mayou R, Foster A, Williamson B. Psychosocial adjustment in patients one year after myocardial infarction. J Psychosom Res 1978;22:447-453.

10. Philip AE, Cay EL, Stuckey AN. Short-term fluctuations in anxiety in in-patients with myocardial infarction. J Psychosom Res 1979;23:277-280.

11. Reich P, DeSilva RA, Lown B, Murawski BJ. Acute psychological disturbances preceding life-threatening ventricular arrhythmias. JAMA 1981;246:232-235.

12. Ruberman W, Weinblatt E, Goldberg JD, Chaudhary BS. Psychosocial influences on mortality after myocardial infarction. N Engl J Med 1984;311:552-559.

13. Stern JJ, Pascale L, Ackerman A. Life adjustment post myocardial infarction: Determining predictive variables. Arch Intern Med 1977;137:1680-1685.

14. Stern TA, Caplan RA, Cassem NH. Use of benzodiazepines in a coronary care unit. Psychosomatics 1987;28:19-23.

Chapter 32

The Geriatric Patient in the Coronary Care Unit

The number of elderly patients with coronary heart disease is increasing steadily. As a result, a greater number of elderly patients are being admitted to the CCU. Important age-related changes in the cardiovascular system include a decreased responsiveness to beta adrenergic and other autonomic stimuli, and an increased "stiffness" or decreased compliance of the left ventricle and arterial tree. These changes compromise the ability of the elderly heart to respond to stress. In addition, there are age-related declines in pulmonary, renal, hepatic, and cerebrovascular function, and there is an increased prevalence of coexisting illness. It is thus not surprising that the clinical presentation, hospital course, and prognosis in elderly patients with acute myocardial infarction are often different from those in younger patients.

Pathology

Although in general the location of coronary atherosclerosis in elderly patients does not differ from that of younger patients, the elderly tend to have more diffuse disease and an increased incidence of significant multivessel and left main coronary stenoses. The lesions also tend to be more calcified, a factor which may be important in determining angioplasty success rates. Finally, as a result of the relatively slow progression of coronary atherosclerosis, collateral vessels are frequently more extensive in older patients.

As in younger patients, acute myocardial infarction in the elderly is most frequently due to acute thrombotic coronary occlusion at the site of a pre-existing atherosclerotic plaque. However, due to the presence of diffuse atherosclerosis and diminished coronary reserve, myocardial infarction in elderly patients may occur in the absence of acute thrombus when there is a sustained imbalance between oxygen supply and demand due to hypoxemia, hypotension, uncontrolled hypertension, valvular lesions (e.g., severe aortic stenosis), or stress related to other acute illness. Such infarcts are frequently associated with only modest enzyme elevations and the absence of pathological Q waves. The presence of a more extensive collateral circulation may also contribute to the increased incidence of non-Q-wave MIs in elderly patients.

202

Clinical Presentation

Symptoms

The initial presentation of acute MI is more variable in older patients, with typical ischemic chest pain occurring in only 19-64% (1-5). Furthermore, the likelihood of "classic" symptoms decreases with increasing age, from 76.0% in patients less than 70 years old to 37.5% in patients 85 years or older (5). By contrast, neurological symptoms, including syncope, confusion, dizziness, weakness, and stroke, occur with increased frequency in elderly patients and may be the initial complaint in up to 36% of patients over age 65 (1). Dyspnea without chest pain is the presenting complaint in about 20% of acute MI patients and does not appear to vary significantly with age.

Signs

Physical findings of congestive heart failure, including pulmonary rales, an S_3 gallop, jugular venous distention, and peripheral edema, are more frequent in elderly patients with acute MI. An S_4 gallop and a systolic murmur of aortic or mitral origin are also commonly heard. The presence of neurological findings such as confusion or stroke may preclude an accurate history and may mislead the physician into suspecting a non-cardiac event. A variety of supraventricular and ventricular arrhythmias and conduction disturbances are seen in elderly patients admitted to the CCU, but these are also seen in healthy elderly patients and thus should not be considered specific for an acute ischemic episode.

Laboratory

Typical ECG changes of transmural myocardial infarction are seen in only about one-half of elderly patients with acute MI (4), reflecting the higher incidence of non-Q-wave infarcts in this age group. The lack of diagnostic ECG findings coupled with atypical symptomatology often leads to a delay in establishing a definitive diagnosis until serum enzyme levels can be obtained. Serum enzyme elevations have a similar pattern in old and young subjects; however, the peak levels may be lower in older patients, and in some patients with small infarctions, the total CK may not rise above the normal range.

Cardiomegaly, left ventricular prominence, and aortic, coronary, and valvular calcifications are common radiographic findings in elderly patients. Evidence for congestive heart failure may be seen in 40-60% of patients over 70 years of age with acute MI.

Complications

Table 32.1 summarizes the relative incidence of various complications of acute MI in old versus younger patients (3,4,6-10). Congestive heart failure occurs 2-3 times more frequently in elderly

Table 32.1
Incidence of Acute MI Complications by Age

	Elderly (%)	Young (%)
Conduction disturbances	12-35	21
Atrial flutter or fibrillation	14-25	8
Ventricular fibrillation	4-9	6-18
Congestive heart failure	44-61	16-30
Shock	26-30	15
Pericarditis	5-12	8-13
Death	23	8

patients, and cardiogenic shock occurs twice as often. Atrial arrhythmias are also more common in older patients, but ventricular fibrillation appears to occur less frequently.

Mortality data in Table 32.1 are taken from the control group of the recently reported Italian streptokinase trial (10). The mortality rate for patients over 65 was threefold higher than for patients under 65. Furthermore, the hospital mortality for patients 66-75 years of age was 18.1%, while for patients over 75 years of age, it was 33.1%. Although these data apply principally to transmural MIs (elderly patients with non-Q-wave infarcts may have a more favorable prognosis), it is clear that acute MI in the elderly is associated with a substantially higher mortality than in younger patients.

In addition to the above complications, rupture of the left ventricular free wall, septum, or papillary muscle occurs with increased frequency in elderly patients (11,12). Women without prior angina or infarction who are hypertensive on admission to the CCU appear to be at particularly high risk (12).

Management

In general, the management of acute MI in elderly patients is similar to that in younger patients. However, elderly patients are at increased risk for adverse drug reactions and interactions. In addition, the greater hemodynamic impairment seen in elderly MI patients may lead to deterioration in the function of other organ systems, most notably the central nervous system, kidneys, and lungs. Therefore, caution is advised in prescribing drugs, and close attention to noncardiac as well as cardiac function is essential.

Several specific situations warrant further comment. With regard to thrombolytic therapy, in the Italian streptokinase trial, benefit was limited to patients 65 years of age or less (10). In the ISIS-2 trial (13), mortality was significantly reduced in patients over 70 years of age receiving streptokinase, but the magnitude of benefit was less than in younger patients. In the large trial using TPA (14), patients over 75 years of age were excluded, but patients up to 75 years of age had a lower mortality with TPA. In these trials, the risk of hemorrhagic complications was not increased in elderly patients, although Lew et al (15) found that major hemmorhage occurred more frequently in patients over 75 years of age receiving streptokinase. Thus, thrombolytic therapy can be given safely in properly selected patients up to 75 years of age, but its ability to reduce mortality in patients over 75 has not yet been proven. In light of these data, caution is advised in using thrombolytic agents in patients over 75 years of age, particularly if hypertension, diabetes, or cerebrovascular disease is present. On the other hand, it is likely that subgroups of elderly patients will benefit from this treatment; therefore age alone should not be considered an absolute contraindication to thrombolytic therapy (see also Chapter 12).

As noted previously, elderly patients exhibit a decreased responsiveness to beta adrenergic stimulation. As a result, dopamine and dobutamine may be less effective inotropic agents in elderly patients (16). Digitalis glycosides, which are not reliant on beta adrenergic mechanisms, appear to maintain their inotropic effect with increasing age (17, 18). Beta blockers may also be less effective and may be associated with a higher incidence of side effects in patients over 75. Therefore, when intravenous beta blockers are used in elderly patients, a lower initial dose and careful monitoring during and after the infusion are warranted.

Ventricular arrhythmias are common in elderly patients with or without acute MI, but primary ventricular fibrillation appears to be a less frequent complication of myocardial infarction in older patients (Table 32.1). Furthermore, successful cardioversion is highly successful in the treatment of ventricular fibrillation in the elderly. By contrast, adverse reactions to lidocaine occur more frequently in older patients. Therefore, the risk-benefit ratio for "prophylactic" lidocaine in acute MI becomes unfavorable in elderly patients, and this treatment strategy should be used cautiously, if at all.

The increased incidence of congestive heart failure in elderly patients with acute MI is most likely due to decreased myocardial contractile reserve, increased diastolic "stiffness," altered loading conditions (especially increased afterload), and the presence of associated cardiac pathology such as valvular disease or prior myocardial infarction. Thus, congestive heart failure in these patients may be multifactorial, and treatment should be directed at the multiple underlying pathologies. Although diuretic therapy is usually appropriate, inotropic agents and vasodilators are not always indicated. Therefore, early assessment of ventricular function and of valvular lesions by echocardiography is often helpful. In addition, recent data indicate that elderly patients with acute mechanical complications, including septal perforation, papillary muscle rupture, or ventricular aneurysm, may derive substantial benefit from early surgical repair (19), so that these potentially treatable causes of congestive heart failure should not be overlooked.

Psychosocial factors should always be addressed in hospitalized patients, but are particularly important in elderly patients admitted to an intensive care unit. The sterile, "high-tech" environment, disruption of normal eating and sleep habits, and the use of myriad medications may lead to confusion, disorientation, or "sundowning" in elderly patients. Unnecessary drugs should be omitted, and nocturnal awakenings and excessive activity restrictions should be avoided. When feasible, liberal visitation privileges for close family members can help the elderly patient maintain orientation and a sense of identity. Spending additional time with the patient and family to discuss the clinical condition, management plans, and prognosis will help make the CCU course run as smoothly as possible.

Prognosis

As noted above, elderly patients with acute MI have an increased hospital mortality due to a higher rate of both cardiac and noncardiac complications. Following hospital discharge, older patients have an increased 2-year mortality rate which is independent of the severity of ventricular arrhythmias (20). In one study, age was also an independent predictor of reinfarction (21), but this finding has not been confirmed by others (22).

Ethical Issues

Occasionally, questions may arise as to the appropriateness of admitting an elderly patient to the CCU or of continuing aggressive supportive care. As technology improves and the number of elderly patients with coronary heart disease continues to rise, these issues will gain increased importance. Although specific decisions must be based on the wishes of the individual patient, family, and attending physician, as well as on local hospital and community policies, it should be noted that several studies have now shown that elderly patients are at least as likely as younger patients to derive benefit from admission to the CCU. This is not surprising, since high-risk patients, of which the elderly are a major subgroup, have the most to gain from intensive care. In a recent series of acute MI patients 75 years or older admitted to the CCU or a general ward, 28% of ward patients died suddenly, as compared with only 2.4% of CCU patients (9). Thus, age per se should not be an exclusion criteria for admission to the CCU.

REFERENCES

1. Pathy MS. Clinical presentation of myocardial infarction in the elderly. Br Heart J 1967;29:190-199.

2. Tinker GM. Clinical presentation of myocardial infarction in the elderly. Age Ageing 1981;10:237-240.

3. MacDonald JB, Baillie J, Williams BO, Ballantyne D. Coronary care in the elderly. Age Ageing 1983;12:17-20.

4. Applegate WB, Graves S, Collins T, Vander Zwaag R, Akins D. Acute myocardial infarction in elderly patients. South Med J 1984;77:1127-1129.

5. Bayer AJ, Chadha JS, Farag RR, Pathy MS. Changing presentation of myocardial infarction with increasing old age. J Am Geriatr Soc 1986;34:263-266.

6. Chaturvedi NC, Walsh MJ, Shivalingappa G, et al. Myocardial infarction in the elderly. Lancet 1972;I:280-282.

7. Williams BO, Begg TB, Semple T, McGuinness JB. The elderly in a coronary care unit. Br Med J 1976;II:451-453.

8. Latting CA, Silverman ME. Acute myocardial infarction in hospitalized patients over age 70. Am Heart J 1980;100:311-318.

9. Sagie A, Rotenberg Z, Weinberger I, Fuchs J, Agmon J. Acute transmural myocardial infarction in elderly patients hospitalized in the coronary care unit versus the general medical ward. J Am Geriatr Soc 1987;35:915-919.

10. Gruppo Italiano per lo Studio della Streptochinasi nell'Infarto Miocardico (GISSI). Effectiveness of intravenous thrombolytic treatment in acute myocardial infarction. Lancet 1986;I:397-402.

11. Zeman FD, Rodstein M. Cardiac rupture complicating myocardial infarction in the aged. Arch Intern Med 1960;105:431-443.

12. Nakano T, Konishi T, Takezawa H. Potential prevention of myocardial rupture resulting from acute myocardial infarction. Clin Cardiol 1985;8:199-204.

13. ISIS-2 (Second International Study of Infarct Survival) Collaborative Group. Randomised trial of intravenous strepto-kinase, oral aspirin, both, or neither among 17,187 cases of suspected acute myocardial infarction: ISIS-2. Lancet 1988; II:349-360.

14. Wilcox RG, von der Lippe G, Olsson CG, et al. Trial of tissue plasminogen activator for mortality reduction in acute myocardial infarction. Anglo-Scandinavian Study of Early Thrombolysis (ASSET). Lancet 1988;II:525-530.

15. Lew AS, Hanoch H, Cercek B, Shah PK, Ganz W. Mortality and morbidity rates of patients older and younger than 75 years with acute myocardial infarction treated with intravenous strepto-kinase. Am J Cardiol 1987;59:1-5.

16. Kyriakides ZS, Kelesides K, Melanidis J, Kardaras F, Caralis DG, Voridis F. Systolic functional response of normal older and younger adult left ventricles to dobutamine. Am J Cardiol 1986;58:816-819.

17. Cokkinos DV, Tsartsalis GD, Heimonas ET, Gardikas CD. Comparison of the inotropic action of digitalis and isoproterenol in younger and older individuals. Am Heart J 1980;100:802-806.

18. Ware JA, Snow E, Luchi JM, Luchi RJ. Effect of digoxin on ejection fraction in elderly patients with congestive heart failure. J Am Geriatr Soc 1984;32:631-635.

19. Weintraub RM, Wei JY, Thurer RL. Surgical repair of remediable postinfarction cardiogenic shock in the elderly. J Am Geriatr Soc 1986;34:389-392.

20. Moss AJ, DeCamilla J, Engstrom F, Hoffman W, Odoroff C, Davis H. The post-hospital phase of myocardial infarction. Identification of patients with increased mortality risk. Circulation 1974; 49:460-466.

21. Elveback LR, Connolly DC. Coronary heart disease in residents of Rochester, Minnesota. V. Prognosis of patients with coronary heart disease based on initial manifestation. Mayo Clin Proc 1985;60:305-311.

22. Marmor A, Geltman EM, Schechtman K, Sobel BE, Roberts R. Recurrent myocardial infarction: clinical predictors and prognostic implications. Circulation 1982;66:415-421.

FURTHER READING

1. Fowler NO. Acute myocardial infarction in the elderly. In: Messerli FH, ed. Cardiovascular disease in the elderly, 2nd ed. Martinus Nijhoff Publishing, Boston, 1988:187-196.

2. Gersh BJ. Clinical manifestations of coronary heart disease in the elderly. In: Wenger NK, Furberg CD, Pitt B, eds. Coronary heart disease in the elderly. Elsevier Science Publishing Inc, New York, 1986:276-302.

3. Harris R. Clinical geriatric cardiology. Management of the elderly patient, 2nd ed. J. B. Lippincott Co, Philadelphia, 1986:197-241.

Chapter 33

Cardioversion

Transthoracic direct current electrical shock is a safe and effective method for terminating most sustained supraventricular and ventricular tachyarrhythmias (1). Cardioversion refers to the delivery of an impulse synchronized with the QRS complex, whereas defibrillation refers to an asynchronously delivered impulse, usually of higher energy, which is used in emergencies to terminate ventricular flutter or fibrillation. This chapter will focus on cardioversion; defibrillation is discussed in Chapter 7.

Indications and Contraindications

Urgent electrical cardioversion is indicated for sustained tachyarrhythmias associated with significant hemodynamic compromise (hypotension, severe heart failure, persistent ischemia). Elective cardioversion is used to treat selected patients with hemodynamically stable, sustained tachyarrhythmias that do not revert spontaneously or with standard anti-arrhythmic therapy. Atrial fibrillation, atrial flutter, and ventricular tachycardia are the most common arrhythmias requiring either elective or urgent cardioversion.

Rhythms that do not normally respond to cardioversion include multifocal atrial tachycardia (MAT), longstanding atrial fibrillation with marked left atrial enlargement, and sinus tachycardia. Additional contraindications include severe electrolyte imbalance and digitalis intoxication, but digitalis concentrations in the therapeutic range should not be considered a contraindication to cardioversion (2,3). Finally, in patients with underlying sick sinus syndrome, cardioversion may result in severe bradycardia or asystole.

Technique

For elective cardioversion, informed consent is obtained and the patient is sedated with intravenous diazepam (Valium) 5-20 mg, midolazam (Versed) 2.5-10 mg, or methohexital (Brevital) 50-120 mg. These steps may be omitted in urgent situations or if the patient is obtunded. Supplemental oxygen is administered, and the patient is monitored continuously with ECG and pulse oximetry (if available). The electrode paddles are well lubricated with gel, and one paddle is placed anteriorly over the right upper sternal border while the other paddle is placed laterally over the left ventricular apex or posteriorly at the angle of the left scapula (4).

Once the patient has been adequately anesthetized and the monitor indicates that QRS complexes are being sensed appropriately, the electrodes are charged to the desired energy level and the impulse is delivered. We recommend an initial energy level of 50-100 joules for atrial fibrillation, and 20-50 joules for atrial flutter or ventricular tachycardia. If sinus rhythm is not restored, incremental shocks of 50, 100, and 200 joules may be given.

Following termination of the procedure, the vital signs, respiratory status, and rhythm should be monitored carefully until the patient's sensorium has returned to baseline. An additional period of monitoring may be desirable, particularly if anti-arrhythmic therapy is to be initiated.

Complications

In the absence of digitalis toxicity, severe electrolyte disturbances, or an asynchronously delivered shock, serious arrhythmias following cardioversion are uncommon. In addition, although transient ECG changes (5) and modest elevations of the total CK occur commonly after cardioversion, significant myocardial necrosis, as evidenced by a rise in the MB fraction, is rare, unless repeated high energy shocks are administered (6,7).

Other complications are usually minor, and are related either to the anesthesia or to skin irritation at the site of paddle placement. The latter can be minimized by liberal use of electrode gel.

Chronic Atrial Fibrillation

Questions frequently arise about the indications, timing, and role of anticoagulation in the cardioversion of stable atrial fibrillation. The risk of embolic events following cardioversion increases progressively with the duration of atrial fibrillation and with echocardiographic left atrial dimensions in excess of 4.0 cm. Patients with chronic mitral valve disease, especially rheumatic disease, or congestive heart failure are also at increased risk. The same factors also influence the likelihood of maintaining sinus rhythm after cardioversion. Thus, the risk-benefit ratio for cardioversion is unfavorable in patients with longstanding atrial fibrillation (> 1 year) or with a left atrial size greater than 5.5-6.0 cm. Patients with congestive heart failure due to severe left ventricular dysfunction or mitral valve disease are also unlikely to maintain sinus rhythm for prolonged periods of time, but cardioversion may nonetheless be justified if favorable hemodynamic effects are anticipated (8).

With regard to anticoagulation, patients with atrial fibrillation of more than 2-4 days duration should be anticoagulated with coumadin for 3-4 weeks prior to elective cardioversion, and anticoagulation should be continued for at least 4 weeks after restoration of sinus rhythm (9). Long-term anticoagulation is also indicated in patients with chronic atrial fibrillation in association with valvular heart disease or congestive (dilated) cardiomyopathy (9).

In addition to anticoagulation, we recommend a trial of anti-arrhythmic therapy (e.g. quinidine sulfate 300 mg q 6 hrs) for a period of 12-48 hours prior to attempting electrical cardioversion. Not only will some patients revert to sinus rhythm (obviating the need for countershock), but the likelihood of maintaining sinus rhythm after cardioversion may be enhanced. If cardioversion is successful, anti-arrhythmic therapy should be continued for at least several weeks.

REFERENCES

1. DeSilva RA, Graboys TB, Podrid PJ, Lown B. Cardioversion and defibrillation. Am Heart J 1980;100:881-895.

2. Ditchey RV, Karliner JS. Safety of electrical cardioversion in patients without digitalis toxicity. Ann Intern Med 1981; 95:676-679.

3. Mann DL, Maisel AS, Atwood E, Engler RL, LeWinter MM. Absence of cardioversion-induced ventricular arrhythmias in patients with therapeutic digoxin levels. J Am Coll Cardiol 1985;5:882-888.

4. Kerber RE, Jensen SJ, Grayzel J, Kennedy J, Hoyt R. Elective cardioversion: Influence of paddle-electrode location and size on success rates and energy requirements. N Engl J Med 1981; 305:658-662.

5. Eysmann SB, Marchlinski FE, Buxton AE, Josephson ME. Electro-cardiographic changes after cardioversion of ventricular arrhyth-mias. Circulation 1986;73:73-81.

6. Ehsani A, Ewy GA, Sobel BE. Effects of electrical countershock on serum creatine phosphokinase (CPK) isoenzymye activity. Am J Cardiol 1976;37:12-18.

7. Reiffel JA, Gambino SR, McCarthy DM, Leahey EB. Direct current cardioversion. Effect on creatine kinase, lactic dehydrogenase, and myocardial isoenzymes. JAMA 1978;239:122-124.

8. Mancini GB, Goldberger AL. Cardioversion of atrial fibrillation: Consideration of embolization, anticoagulation, prophylactic pacemaker, and long-term success. Am Heart J 1982;104:617-621.

9. Dunn M, Alexander J, deSilva R, Hildner F. Antithrombtic therapy in atrial fibrillation. Chest 1986;89(Suppl):68S-74S.

Chapter 34

Central Venous and Pulmonary Artery Catheterization

Patricia L. Cole, M.D.

Access to the central venous system for intravenous line placement and for placement of pulmonary artery catheters and temporary pacemakers is an important part of the management of critically ill patients since it often provides diagnostic information or permits therapeutic interventions that cannot be obtained or accomplished through other means.

There are numerous veins that can be used for central venous access, with a wide range of technical difficulty and safety. Use of the basilic vein in the arm is quite safe, but it can be difficult to maneuver a catheter through axillary and subclavian veins down into the superior vena cava. On the other hand, cannulation of the subclavian vein is technically easier, but is associated with a somewhat higher incidence of complications. Other sites include the internal and external jugular veins, the femoral vein, and the cephalic vein. Use of the cephalic vein is less desirable due to difficulty in advancing the catheter into the central venous system. The choice of access site varies with the clinical setting and local preferences. We use the right internal jugular approach in most elective situations because the technique is relatively straight-forward with an acceptable complication rate. This location also permits easy manipulation of pulmonary artery catheters and pacemakers.

Internal Jugular Vein

To minimize the risk of complications, one must be familiar with the normal anatomic landmarks before attempting central venous catheterization from the neck. It is also important to recognize that the vein will occasionally lie in an anomalous position relative to the usual landmarks. If the vein cannot be entered after several attempts, another site should be chosen for line insertion. Repeated attempts at the same location often lead to a higher incidence of complications.

There are three commonly used approaches for entry into the internal jugular vein: the "medial" (or "central") approach, the "posterior" approach, and the "low" (or "anterior") approach. The medial approach is generally felt to be the safest, and involves identification of the apex of the triangle formed by the two heads of the sternocleidomastoid muscle and the clavicle (Fig. 34.1). The internal jugular vein courses just under the posterior head of the sternocleidomastoid, and laterally and slightly anteriorly to the common carotid artery. When the medial approach is used, the operator should stand at the patient's head, which is turned away from the side of insertion. The carotid artery should be manually retracted medially (but without compressing it), and the exploring needle (see below) inserted at the apex of the triangle (approximately three fingerbreadths from the clavicle). The needle should be aimed at the ipsilateral nipple and inserted at a 30° angle to the frontal plane.

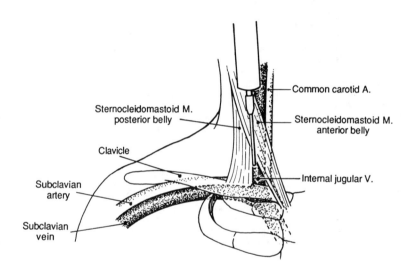

Common carotid A.

Sternocleidomastoid M.
posterior belly

Sternocleidomastoid M.
anterior belly

Clavicle

Internal jugular V.

Subclavian
artery

Subclavian
vein

__Figure 34.1__   Anatomic landmarks for right internal jugular central venous catheterization.

The "posterior" approach involves cannulation of the internal jugular from an orientation lateral to the posterior head of the sternocleidomastoid muscle. Since this approach generally directs the needle toward the common carotid artery, it carries a higher risk and is used infrequently. The "low" approach consists of entering the internal jugular vein at its junction with the subclavian vein. The needle is inserted at a 45° angle to the skin surface, bisecting the angle formed by the lateral margin of the posterior belly of the sternocleidomastoid muscle and the clavicle. The advantages of this approach are: 1) there is no need to identify a "distant" landmark (nipple), and 2) the "target" (internal jugular at the subclavian) is larger. The disadvantage is an increased risk of pneumothorax. At our institution, the medial approach is most often used because of its lower incidence of complications. The right internal jugular vein is preferred over the left for several reasons: 1) this approach avoids the large thoracic duct, which is on the left; 2) the dome of the right lung is lower; and 3) the catheter can be advanced directly into the right atrium.

Once the approach has been selected and the landmarks identified, the skin is cleansed with a betadine or alcohol solution, and a small skin wheal is made at the entry site using a 1% xylocaine solution. A 1.5-inch 22-gauge needle attached to a syringe containing xylocaine is used to anesthetize the deeper tissues and as an "exploring" needle for the initial venipuncture. Once the needle enters the vein, its orientation is carefully noted, and the needle is removed, keeping its path visually memorized. A large bore needle attached to a 10-20 cc syringe is then positioned in the same orientation. The needle is inserted under the skin and slowly advanced toward the vein while applying gentle negative pressure to the syringe. Entry into the vein is confirmed by free backflow of venous blood. The syringe is carefully removed, and a short guidewire is introduced into the vessel (Caution: Never force the guidewire). The needle is then withdrawn leaving the guidewire in place. (Note: While the needle hub is open to air, the patient should be instructed to avoid taking a deep breath in order to prevent drawing air into the vein through the open needle.)

Once the needle has been removed, a scalpel is used to enlarge the skin incision to facilitate passage of a vascular sheath and dilator over the guidewire. A sheath with a diaphragm is preferred to prevent back-bleeding around the catheter. The sheath and dilator are carefully advanced over the guidewire using caution not to release the wire. Gentle forward pressure and a slight twisting motion may be necessary to advance the sheath into the vein. The dilator should be locked or held securely inside the sheath so that it does not back out as the sheath is advanced into the vein. Once the sheath has been properly positioned, the guidewire and central dilator are removed and the sheath is sutured securely in place. If the sheath has a sidearm, the latter is flushed to remove any air bubbles. A central venous catheter, pulmonary artery catheter, or transvenous pacemaker can then be advanced through the lumen of the sheath if desired.

After placement of a central venous line from the neck, a chest x-ray should be obtained to assess its location and to evaluate for complications (e.g., pneumothorax, hemothorax). If an unsuccessful attempt to cannulate one of the internal jugular veins has resulted in hematoma formation, the opposite side of the neck should not be used, since development of bilateral hematomas may compromise the airway.

Subclavian Vein

Another commonly used approach to central venous access is the subclavian vein. Patients prefer this approach because it is generally more comfortable than when the internal jugular vein is used. In the very obese patient, this approach may be somewhat safer because there tends to be less distortion of the landmarks.

The subclavian artery and vein run roughly parallel to the clavicle in its proximal third (Fig. 34.2), and skin incision should be made approximately 1 cm below the clavicle in its middle third. The needle should be inserted under the clavicle parallel to the frontal plane, and directed toward the manubrium. It may be helpful to place the index finger of the free hand in the suprasternal notch, and use the thumb of the free hand to guide the needle under the clavicle. The needle is slowly advanced, aspirating on the attached syringe until free flowing venous blood is obtained as described previously. If pulsatile arterial blood appears in the syringe (indicating entry into the subclavian artery), the needle should be withdrawn and the patient should be carefully observed for possible development of a hemothorax.

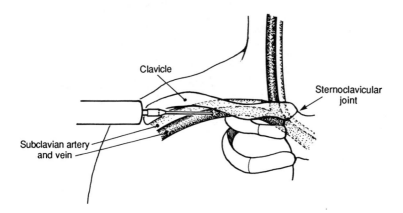

Clavicle

Sternoclavicular joint

Subclavian artery and vein

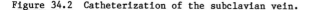

Figure 34.2 Catheterization of the subclavian vein.

Femoral Vein

Cannulation of the femoral vein is relatively easy, and is especially useful when quick access is needed to facilitate short-term management (e.g., during cardiac arrest when cardiopulmonary resuscitation makes jugular and subclavian access more difficult). Drawbacks of this approach include a higher risk of contamination or infection, need for the patient to remain supine, and in some cases, greater difficulty in positioning a pulmonary artery catheter, especially if fluoroscopy is not available.

The femoral vein lies just medial to the femoral artery, and skin puncture is usually made at or slightly below the femoral skin crease (Fig. 34.3). Entry into the vein above the inguinal ligament should be avoided, since bleeding above this level cannot be adequately controlled with external pressure. The needle is inserted at a 45° angle 1 cm medial to the femoral artery, and slowly advanced until venous blood appears in the syringe, as described previously. Aspiration of pulsatile arterial blood signifies entry into the femoral artery; withdraw the needle and apply pressure for 5-10 minutes.

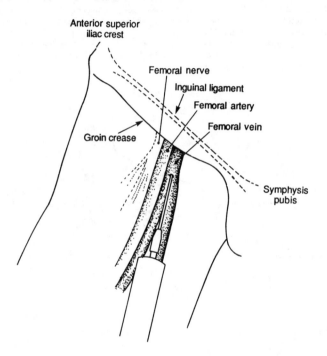

Figure 34.3   Catheterization of the right femoral vein.

Brachial Vein

The brachial approach is readily accessible and safe but has the drawback of requiring the arm to be immobilized on an armboard. In addition, maneuvering catheters into the heart may be difficult.

In the antecubital fossa, the median vein bifurcates into the median cephalic and median basilic branches. The cephalic vein travels up the lateral aspect of the arm and joins the axillary vein at a 90° angle; this makes catheter manipulation difficult. The basilic vein courses up the medial side of the arm and joins the brachial vein to become the axillary vein. When using the brachial approach, the basilic vein is preferable to the cephalic vein.

The basilic vein lies slightly lateral to and more superficial than the brachial artery. Entry should be just above the elbow crease, as the vein courses deep to the biceps muscle proximal to that point. Applying a tourniquet to the upper arm or lowering the arm below the level of the right atrium may facilitate the procedure by distending the vein. Venous cannulation can then be performed as described previously. Be sure to remove the tourniquet before attempting to advance a catheter.

Pulmonary Artery Catheterization

Once central venous access is established and a sheath is in place, a pulmonary artery (PA) catheter can be inserted for intracardiac pressure measurements. The basic PA or "Swan-Ganz" catheter is equipped with a triple lumen and a thermistor at the distal tip, which is used for measuring cardiac output. Air can be injected into one of the lumens to inflate a small balloon located near the distal end of the catheter. This permits the catheter to be easily advanced through the right heart chambers and into the pulmonary artery in a flow-directed fashion. The balloon is also inflated when measuring the pulmonary artery occlusive ("wedge") pressure. The other two lumens are used for pressure measurements and fluid administration; one lumen exits the catheter at the distal tip, the other exits 30 cm proximally (normally in the right atrium or vena cava). Several modifications of the basic catheter are also available, and include a fourth lumen with a proximal exit port used as an additional intravenous line, an exit port in the right ventricle, which permits introduction of a pacing electrode, and an oximeter, which allows continuous meaurement of mixed venous oxygen saturation.

Placement of the pulmonary artery catheter is performed through the venous access sheath under sterile conditions. The area should be cleaned with betadine and covered with a sterile drape. Use of a sterile gown and gloves by the primary operator is also advised. Before starting the procedure, the balloon should be inflated with 1 cc of air and submerged in sterile saline to ensure proper function and to check for leaks. The proximal and distal ports should be connected via sterile tubing to pressure transducers, and the lines flushed with sterile saline to remove air bubbles. With the balloon deflated, the catheter tip is introduced into the sheath and advanced until the tip has cleared the distal end of the sheath by several centimeters. The balloon is then inflated with 1 cc of air and the catheter is carefully advanced sequentially into the right atrium, the right ventricle, and out the right ventricular outflow tract into the pulmonary artery. Location of the catheter tip can be identified fluoroscopically or by recognition of the characteristic hemodynamic waveform in each chamber (see Fig. 18.1). With optimal placement of the catheter, a PA waveform is seen when the balloon is deflated and a PA occlusive pressure waveform appears when the balloon is inflated.

Several caveats with respect to the insertion of PA catheters are worth noting. If there is difficulty in advancing the catheter from one chamber to the next, have the patient take a deep breath. This is often helpful because it increases bloodflow through the right heart chambers. If there is a possibility of a left-to-right shunt, blood gases should be obtained as the catheter is passed through each chamber to evaluate for an oxygen "step-up." Occasionally, it may be difficult to tell whether the catheter is "wedged" without fluoroscopy. This can be checked by carefully aspirating blood from the distal port; blood obtained from the wedge position should be oxygenated (O_2 saturation > 85-90%). In patients with left bundle branch block, femoral insertion of a PA catheter may traumatize the right bundle, resulting in complete heart block; prophylactic pacemaker insertion should be considered. Finally, the balloon should never be left inflated in the occlusive position for prolonged periods of time, as pulmonary infarction or infection may occur.

Once the catheter has been properly positioned, its shaft should be securely sutured to the hub of the venous sheath and to the skin to prevent inadvertent dislodgement. Finally, a sterile dressing should be applied at the insertion site.

Care of Central Venous and Pulmonary Artery Catheters

Infection is the most common major complication occurring after successful insertion of a central venous catheter. Scrupulous attention to sterile technique during line placement is the most important factor in preventing infection, but the risk can be further reduced by daily inspection of the insertion site and periodic dressing changes. The occurrence of an unexplained fever should prompt further investigation for possible line infection and, if fever persists, all indwelling catheters should be removed or replaced. In the absence of signs of infection, neck lines should not be left in place for more than 5-7 days, and femoral lines should be routinely changed every 3-5 days. (Note: Use of silver nitrate impregnated subcutaneous catheter cuffs may permit catheters to be left in place for more prolonged periods of time in the absence of infection.

Complications

Serious complications resulting from central venous or pulmonary artery catheterization are infrequent when the procedure is performed electively by an experienced physician observing proper technique. Complication rates vary directly with the urgency of the clinical situation and inversely with the skill of the operator. Possible complications are listed in Table 34.1.

Table 34.1
Complications of Central Venous or Pulmonary Artery Catheterization

Major
  Sepsis, endocarditis
  Pneumonia
  Major bleeding (e.g. after thrombolytic therapy)
  Vascular perforation or dissection
  Myocardial perforation
  Ventricular tachycardia or fibrillation
  Complete heart block
  Pneumothorax, hemothorax
  Pulmonary embolus or infarction

Minor
  Local infection
  Minor bleeding
  Minor arrhythmias
  Transient conduction disturbances
  Phlebitis
  Vagal Reactions

FURTHER READING

1. Antman EM, Rutherford JD. Coronary care medicine. Martinus Nijhoff Publishing, Boston, 1986:259–274.

2. Kaye W. XII. Intravenous techniques; and XIII. Invasive monitoring techniques. In: McIntyre KM, Lewis AJ, eds. Textbook of advanced cardiac life support. American Heart Association, Dallas, 1981:XII-1-12 & XIII-1-32.

Chapter 35

Temporary Pacemaker Insertion
Patricia L. Cole, M.D.

There are numerous situations in the coronary care unit in which a temporary pacemaker is required for actual or potential symptomatic bradycardia or rate-related hypotension (Chapter 16). Except in emergencies, placement of a temporary pacing wire should be done under the supervision of a physician skilled in the technique, and the patient should remain in a carefully monitored setting for as long as the temporary wire remains in place.

Methods of Temporary Pacemaker Therapy

There are four basic techniques of temporary cardiac pacing: thump pacing, external transthoracic electrical pacing, percutaneous transthoracic pacing, and transvenous endocardial pacing. Although all four of these techniques are useful in the appropriate clinical setting, the transvenous approach is the one most commonly employed.

Thump Pacing

Thump pacing is an infrequently used technique for very short term pacing needs. A precordial thump, administered with a clenched fist held 8-12 inches above the patient, delivers approximately one joule of energy. This energy can traverse the chest wall and capture the ventricle. Repetitive "thumps" at 1-second intervals can serve as a temporary pacemaker until a more effective form of therapy can be initiated.

External Transthoracic Pacing

The first version of the external pacemaker was developed by Zoll in 1952. This technique utilizes external electrodes which deliver an electrical impulse through the chest wall resulting in electrical stimulation of the heart and myocardial capture. Although this can be an extremely effective measure in true emergencies, it is not the best solution to the problem of temporary pacing because of patient discomfort (due to skeletal muscle contractions), inability to effectively pace some patients, and electrical interference. Many emergency rooms and coronary care units now use the external pacemaker as a bridge until a transvenous wire can be placed.

Percutaneous Transthoracic Pacing

This technique involves direct placement of a pacing wire into the endocardium of the right ventricle by the transthoracic approach. A long pericardial needle with an alligator clip connecting the metal shaft of the needle to an exploring V-lead electrode is inserted under the xyphoid or in the lower left parasternal area and aimed toward the right shoulder, aspirating as the needle is advanced. Contact with the right ventricle is confirmed by the presence of an acute injury current on the V-lead. The needle is advanced until there is free flow of blood. A J-tip bipolar wire is then advanced through the needle lumen to the endocardial surface. The needle is removed, and the wire is connected to a pacing box with the distal electrode to the negative pole and the proximal electrode to the positive pole. Effective placement is confirmed by the presence of a paced rhythm on the electrocardiogram. Complications of the transthoracic approach are discussed later in this chapter, but include needle entry into other organs (lung, pleural space) and excessive bleeding (tamponade, coronary artery laceration). Because of the low efficacy and high complication rate, this approach is usually reserved for emergencies when other options are not available.

Transvenous Endocardial Pacing

In most situations, this is the method of choice for temporary cardiac pacing. The technique involves placement of an electrode wire into the right-sided cardiac chambers via the central venous system. Possible entry sites include the internal or external jugular, subclavian, antecubital or femoral veins (Chapter 34). The internal jugular vein is the preferred approach at our institution due to the ease of placement and slightly lower incidence of complications. The subclavian approach is also useful, but manipulation of the wire may be more difficult. The femoral approach usually requires fluoroscopy to ensure proper placement; patient mobility is also limited and this site may be more prone to infectious complications. The brachial approach also requires fluoroscopic guidance and has the disadvantage of easy dislodgement.

Technique of Transvenous Pacemaker Insertion

Equipment

The standard temporary pacing wire is bipolar (i.e. it has a positive and negative pole) and is designed to facilitate positioning in the right ventricular apex. A variety of wires of differing caliber and stiffness are available. Balloon-tipped wires that can be placed in a flow-directed fashion are also available. Balloon-tipped wires can be placed at bedside; other wires are usually placed under fluoroscopic guidance to minimize the risk of perforation. The main disadvantage of balloon-tipped wires is that they tend to become dislodged more easily.

Placement

When appropriate, informed consent should be obtained prior to pacemaker insertion. Cannulation of the central venous system is then performed as described in Chapter 34, and the pacemaker is introduced through the venous sheath.

If a flow-directed electrode is to be used, it can be positioned without fluoroscopic guidance using the distal pole as an exploring electrode. The wire is attached to a V-lead with an alligator clip, and the ECG pattern is monitored. When a right ventricular electrogram showing an injury current (ST segment shift) is obtained, the distal pole is connected to the impulse generator, and the pacing threshold is evaluated. When a non-balloon-tipped wire is used, it is maneuvered across the tricuspid valve under fluoroscopic guidance by applying torque to its shaft, and the tip is then positioned at the right ventricular apex. Placement of the electrode tip in the right ventricular outflow tract or coronary sinus should be avoided. Coronary sinus placement should be suspected if the catheter is directed posteriorly on a lateral chest x-ray. Finally, in positioning the electrode tip against the endocardium, avoid using pressure to advance the catheter, since excessive force can result in perforation of the thin-walled right ventricle. Ventricular perforation is more common with stiff catheters and in the setting of right ventricular infarction.

Atrial or atrioventricular (AV) sequential pacing may be performed by placing a specially shaped electrode in the right atrium in a manner similar to that described for placing a ventricular wire. AV sequential pacing requires a pacing box capable of dual stimulation.

Testing Pacemaker Function

After satisfactory placement of the wire has been accomplished, the pacemaker function should be tested. To evaluate the pacing threshold (i.e. the amount of current needed to produce ventricular capture), the output current (Fig. 35.1) is initially set at 0 mA, sensitivity is placed on full demand, and the rate is set at 10-20 beats/min higher than the intrinsic heart rate. Under electrocardiographic guidance, the output current is then slowly increased until capture is noted on the ECG (pacing spike followed by wide QRS). The output is set at a level approximately 2-3 times the threshold (or at 3 mA), and the rate is set at a level appropriate to maintain adequate blood pressure and cardiac output. The sensitivity is then adjusted so that native QRS complexes (but not T waves) are sensed and pacemaker function is appropriately inhibited.

If AV sequential pacing is desired, the generator output for each chamber is adjusted independently, and the AV delay (PR interval) is specified. The temporary AV sequential systems currently in use are unable to sense atrial activity (i.e., only the QRS is sensed). However, atrial output in close proximity to the ventricular sensing

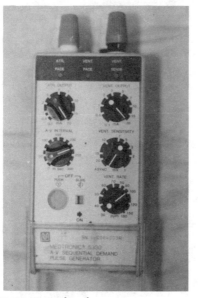

Figure 35.1 Temporary pacemaker box.

electrode may lead to "crosstalk." In this situation, the ventricular electrode senses atrial pacing, interprets it as a "QRS," and inhibits ventricular output. Reducing atrial output or repositioning the atrial lead will usually eliminate crosstalk.

After the electrode has been properly positioned and tested, it should be sutured to the skin near the entry site to prevent dislodgement. A chest x-ray should be obtained to check placement and assess for pneumothorax or other complications.

Maintenance of a temporary pacing system includes: 1) scrupulous attention to sterility, 2) daily examination of the entry site and application of a clean bandage, 3) daily evaluation of the pacing threshold (a threshold of more than 5 mA usually indicates a need for repositioning), and 4) continuous monitoring to ensure proper pacemaker function.

Complications

There are a number of complications that can occur during or after placement of a temporary pacemaker, but these can be kept to a minimum by proper technique. Local or systemic infections usually arise as a result of poor sterile technique during pacemaker insertion. Endocarditis of the tricuspid valve or right ventricular myocardium can also occur. The treatment for infectious complications is removal of the wire and appropriate antibiotics. Other complications related to insertion technique include: vessel laceration, pneumothorax, hemothorax, hematoma, and rarely, development of an AV fistula.

Right ventricular perforation occurs in 1-3% of pacemaker insertions and may result in the rapid development of cardiac tamponade. This complication should be suspected in any patient with unexplained hemodynamic deterioration within several hours of pacemaker insertion or repositioning. Treatment of pericardial tamponade is discussed in Chapter 26. Finally, phlebitis and thromboembolic complications can occur due to the presence of the foreign body in the venous circulation.

FURTHER READING

1. Antman EM, Rutherford JD. Coronary care medicine. Martinus Nijhoff Publishing, Boston, 1986:219-247.

2. Harthorne JW, McDermott J, Poulin F. Cardiac pacing. In: Johnson RA, Haber E, Austen WG, eds. The practice of cardiology. Little, Brown and Co, Boston, 1980:219-261.

3. Hauser RG, Vicari RM. Temporary pacing. Med Clin North Am 1986; 70:813-827.

4. Ludmer P, Goldschlager N. Cardiac pacing in the 1980's. N Engl J Med 1984;311:1671-1680.

5. Zipes DP, Duffin EG. Cardiac pacemakers. In: Braunwald E, ed. Heart disease: A textbook of cardiovascular medicine, 3rd ed. W.B. Saunders Co, Philadelphia, 1988:717-741.

Chapter 36

Arterial Lines

Patricia L. Cole, M.D.

Hemodynamic monitoring of critically ill patients in the CCU often requires placement of an arterial line. The radial, femoral, and brachial arteries are most commonly used.

Preliminary evaluation prior to insertion of a radial arterial line should include an Allen's test to ensure that ulnar blood flow to the hand is adequate. The arterial blood supply to one hand is occluded by compressing both the radial and ulnar arteries at the wrist. When the hand pales, pressure over the ulnar artery is released. If perfusion to the hand remains impaired, as indicated by persistent pallor, the radial artery of that hand should not be used for an arterial line. Normally, the brachial and femoral arteries are large enough that the presence of an arterial catheter does not compromise blood flow to the distal extremity.

Technique of Radial Artery Cannulation

After obtaining informed consent (if appropriate) and performing an Allen's test as described above, the hand and wrist are secured to an armboard in palm-up fashion, and a 1-2" diameter roll of gauze is inserted between the wrist and armboard to extend the hand at a 30-45° angle. This angle simplifies access to the radial artery. The wrist area is then thoroughly cleaned with betadine and alcohol. If desired, xylocaine 1-2% may be used to infiltrate the skin and subcutaneous tissues overlying the radial artery just proximal to the bones of the wrist. We recommend using a prepackaged peripheral arterial cannulation kit containing an arterial sheath, needle, and guidewire as a single unit. The radial artery is palpated with one hand while the other hand slowly advances the needle into the skin at a 45° angle. Free flow of pulsatile blood into the catheter hub signifies entry into the artery. The central wire is then carefully advanced (never forced) into the arterial lumen, and the needle is withdrawn. The catheter can then be advanced over the guidewire into the arterial lumen. The needle and wire are withdrawn, and the hub of the catheter is connected to an arterial pressure transducer.

If an arterial kit is not available, a short (3-4 cm), 18-20 gauge plastic cannula of the type used for intravenous lines is a suitable alternative. The needle and cannula are inserted, bevel up, at a 45° angle to the skin along the course of the radial artery. When blood appears in the hub, the needle and cannula are advanced through the artery. The needle is then removed, and the hub of the cannula is gently and slowly withdrawn until pulsatile blood flow is seen. The soft-tipped cannula is then carefully advanced into the radial artery up to the hub and connected to a pressure transducer. Although other methods are used, this technique decreases the likelihood of intimal dissection which can occur if the tip of the needle is left in the artery while the catheter is advanced over it.

Femoral and Brachial Arterial Lines

Insertion of a femoral arterial line is somewhat easier because the luminal diameter is larger. Femoral artery cannulation using an arterial kit is performed as described above. If an arterial kit is not available, a standard 7 or 8 French arterial sheath with a side arm or a long (10-20 cm) intravenous catheter can be used. The femoral artery is palpated, and an area 1-2 fingerbreadths distal to the femoral crease is prepped, draped, and anesthezied with 1-2% xylocaine. When using an arterial sheath, a 16-gauge percutaneous entry needle capable of accepting a guidewire (be sure needle and guidewire are compatible) is slowly advanced into the artery at a 30-45° angle. When free-flowing, pulsatile arterial blood is obtained, the guidewire is carefully advanced through the needle into the vessel lumen. (Caution: If passage of the guidewire is associated with undue resistance, the needle may need to be repositioned. Never force a guidewire into a vessel.) After the wire is in position, the needle is withdrawn, and the sheath with an arterial dilator locked into place is advanced over the wire. A gentle rotating and pushing motion may be necessary to advance the dilator into the artery. The dilator and wire are then removed, and the sidearm is attached to the pressure transducer. If a long intravenous catheter is used, the technique is similar except the catheter and stylet are passed into the artery through the needle lumen, and the stylet and needle are then withdrawn. Again, check in advance to be sure that the catheter passes easily through the needle.

Cannulation of the brachial artery is performed in a similar manner. The arm is immobilized on an armboard in the palm-up position. The brachial artery is palpated just medial and deep to the biceps muscle at the elbow crease. The needle is inserted at a 30-45° angle 1-2 fingerbreadths above the crease. When arterial blood appears, the catheter is advanced into the artery as previously described.

Care of Arterial Lines

Once an acceptable arterial pressure waveform has been obtained, the line should be securely sutured in place to prevent it from kinking or slipping out of the artery. Betadine ointment should be applied to the catheter entry site, which is then covered by a sterile dressing. The site should be inspected daily for signs of infection (more common with femoral lines), and the dressing should be changed regularly. The extremity distal to the insertion site should be checked frequently for evidence of ischemia or embolization, especially when the radial artery is used. As with other intravascular catheters, arterial lines should generally not be left in place for more than a few days, and indications for continued use should be reassessed daily. When the catheter is removed, pressure should be applied until adequate hemostasis is achieved (minimum 5-10 minutes).

FURTHER READING

1. Antman EM, Rutherford JD. Coronary care medicine. Martinus Nijhoff Publishing, Boston, 1986:259-274.

2. Kaye W. XIII. Invasive monitoring techniques. In: McIntyre KM, Lewis AJ, eds. Textbook of advanced cardiac life support. American Heart Association, Dallas, 1981:XIII-1-32.

Chapter 37

Intra-Aortic Balloon Pumps
Stanley I. Biel, M.D.

The intra-aortic balloon pump (IABP) consists of an elongated balloon attached to a driving unit via a catheter and vacuum tubing. The balloon is inserted into the descending thoracic aorta, usually through the femoral artery, and the balloon is rapidly inflated with CO_2 or helium gas during diastole, transiently increasing aortic volume and pressure. At the onset of systole, the balloon is rapidly deflated, creating a partial vacuum which reduces afterload and augments stroke volume. Inflation and deflation are triggered by the electrocardiogram, arterial pressure waveform, or an internal stimulator.

Beneficial hemodynamic effects of IABP counterpulsation include:

1. Decreased left ventricular afterload through a reduction in peak aortic systolic pressure of 10-15%

2. Decreased left ventricular end diastolic pressure and pulmonary artery occlusive pressure by 10-15%

3. Increased coronary perfusion pressure through augmentation of the diastolic aortic pressure by more than 70%

4. Decreased myocardial oxygen demand (via decreased preload and afterload)

5. Increased cardiac output by 500-1000 cc/min

6. Increased diastolic cerebral and renal blood flow

Indications and Contraindications (Table 37.1)

The most frequent indication for an IABP in the CCU is cardiogenic shock complicating acute myocardial infarction. Patients with a surgically correctable mechanical defect (acute ventricular septal defect, papillary muscle rupture, or ventricular aneurysm) are most likely to benefit. An IABP may also be helpful in stabilizing patients with severe, reversible myocardial stunning following reperfusion with a thombolytic agent or coronary angioplasty. Patients with irreversible global left ventricular dysfunction are not likely to obtain long-term benefit from balloon counterpulsation

Table 37.1
Indications and Contraindications for the IABP

Indications

    Severe congestive heart failure or shock due to:
        Acute ventricular septal defect
        Severe mitral regurgitation
        Left ventricular aneurysm (proven or suspected)
        Right ventricular infarction
        Critical aortic stenosis
        Myocardial stunning following coronary reperfusion
    Unstable angina refractory to maximum medical therapy
    Critical left main coronary stenosis with unstable angina,
        hypotension, or pulmonary edema
    Stabilization of severe CHF while awaiting cardiac surgery,
        including heart transplantation
    Ischemic ventricular tachycardia or fibrillation refractory
        to anti-arrhythmic therapy
    PTCA complications with impending infarction
    Inability to wean from cardiopulmonary bypass
    Severe septic shock

Contraindications

    Aortic dissection
    Large aortic aneurysm
    Significant aortic regurgitation
    Severe peripheral vascular disease
    Severe bleeding diathesis

unless cardiac transplantation is an option.   Other indications for
the IABP are less common in the CCU.

    Significant aortic insufficiency is a contraindication to the IABP
because the augmented diastolic blood pressure increases the severity
of regurgitation.   Aortic dissection or aneurysm, severe peripheral
vascular disease, and known hemorrhagic diathesis are associated with
an increased risk of complications, and therefore represent relative
contraindications to IABP therapy.

Management

    An IABP should be inserted only by a physician skilled in the
techniques of intravascular catheterization.   Once in place, the
position of the balloon should be verified by chest x-ray (the tip
should be 1-3 cm distal to the left subclavian artery or just below
the aortic arch).   The timing of inflation and deflation should be
checked (Fig. 37.1), and if necessary the balloon inflation point
should be adjusted so that the diastolic pressure rise begins at the
dicrotic notch (Fig. 37.1D).   Deflation may also need to be adjusted

in order to maximize afterload reduction, which is estimated by the difference between the unassisted and assisted end diastolic pressures (usual range: 10-15 mm Hg; Fig. 37.1D).

While the balloon is in place, patients should be at bed rest with no more than 30° elevation of the head of the bed and minimal hip flexion on the side of the balloon. Patients should be closely monitored with frequent assessments of the vital signs, pressure waveforms, peripheral pulses, and urine output. Hemodynamic monitoring with a pulmonary artery catheter is indicated in most patients with an IABP. Daily laboratory studies should include a complete blood count and coagulation profile, electrolytes, blood area nitrogen, chest x-ray (to assess position of the tip), and in most cases, an electrocardiogram. Dressings should be changed daily and the insertion site should be closely inspected for signs of infection. Full heparinization is indicated, and appropriate bleeding precautions should be observed.

During normal operation, the IABP is set to assist every beat (1:1 assist mode). However, at heart rates in excess of 120/min, the balloon may function better with a 1:2 assist ratio (every other beat).

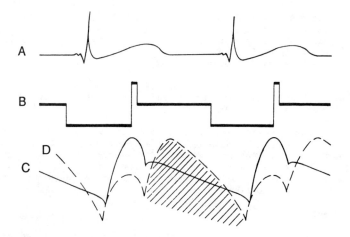

Figure 37.1   Balloon pump timing.   A. ECG trace.   B. Pump timing trace.   C. Unassisted arterial pressure trace.   D. Assisted arterial pressure trace.   Shaded area is diastolic augmentation.   Reproduced with permission from Bolooki H.   Clinical application of intra-aortic balloon pump.   Futura Publishing Co, Mount Kisco, New York, 1977:81.

Weaning

In the absence of complications, IABP support may be continued for periods of up to several weeks. However, the indications for continuation of the IABP should be reassessed daily. Once it is decided to terminate counterpulsation, support should be weaned over a period of 24-48 hours. The weaning protocol used at our institution is outlined in Table 37.2.

Table 37.2
Protocol for Weaning Off IABP Support

1. Weaning settings
   a. 1:2 assist mode for 8-12 hours
   b. 1:3 or 1:4 assist mode for 8-12 hours
2. Hemodynamic measurements q 15 min x 3 after each setting change
3. Arterial blood gases before and after each setting change
4. Discontinue weaning if:
   a. Hypertension or hypotension develops
   b. PAOP rises significantly
   c. Urine output declines
   d. Mental status changes occur
   e. Ischemic symptoms or ECG changes occur
   f. Ventricular ectopy increases significantly
5. Discontinue heparin 2-4 hours prior to balloon removal
6. Remove balloon if patient is stable for at least 8 hours on 1:3 or 1:4 assist
7. Hold pressure over arterial puncture site for 30-60 minutes, then "sandbag" for 6 hours over a pressure dressing
8. Evaluate distal pulses immediately prior to and after IABP removal, then every hour for 12-24 hours

Complications

Complication rates with the IABP are inversely related to the experience and skill of the operating physician and directly related to the severity of underlying vascular disease and the caliber of the vessel catheterized. In 5-20% of cases, successful percutaneous insertion of the balloon may not be possible. Leg ischemia, the most common complication, occurs in up to 25% of patients, and requires surgical intervention in 5-10%. Peripheral pulses should be checked at least hourly and the limb should never be allowed to remain pulseless for more than 2 hours. Leg ischemia may be exacerbated by vasopressors and diminished by inotropic agents and vasodilators.

Other major complications include aortic or iliac dissection or perforation (1-4%), major bleeding at the arteriotomy site (3-8%), and infection (1-3%). Balloon rupture, heralded by a gas leak or blood in the catheter, is uncommon and usually does not produce major sequelae (the CO_2 or helium is rapidly dispersed), but requires replacement of the balloon. Occasionally a patient will complain of abdominal pulsations; these can usually be minimized by using a smaller inflation volume.

FURTHER READING

1. Alcan KE, Stertzev SH, Wallsh E, Franzone AJ, Bruno MS, DePasquale NN. Comparison of wire-guided percutaneous insertion and conventional surgical insertion of intraaortic balloon pumps in 151 patients. Am J Med 1983;75:24-28.

2. Amsterdam EA, Awan NA, Lee G, et al. Intra-aortic balloon counterpulsation: Rationale, application, and results. Cardiovasc Clin 1981;11:79-96.

3. Bolooki H. Clinical application of intra-aortic balloon pump. Futura Publishing Co, Inc; Mount Kisco, New York, 1977.

4. Follard ED, Kemper AJ, Khuri SF, Josa M, Parisi AF. Intraaortic balloon counterpulsation as a temporary support measure in decompensated critical aortic stenosis. J Am Coll Cardiol 1985; 5:711-716.

5. Gottlieb SO, Brinker JA, Borkon AM, et al. Identification of patients at high risk for complications of intraaortic balloon counterpulsation: A multivariate risk factor analysis. Am J Cardiol 1984;53:1135-1139.

6. Kantrowitz A, Wasfie T, Freed PS, Rubenfire M, Wajszczuk W, Schork MA. Intraaortic balloon pumping 1967 through 1982: Analysis of complications in 733 patients. Am J Cardiol 1986;57:976-983.

7. McEnany MT, Kay HR, Buckley MJ, et al. Clinical experience with intraaortic balloon pump support in 728 patients. Circulation 1978;58(Supp I):I-124-132.

8. Scheidt S, Wilner G, Mueller H, et al. Intra-aortic balloon counterpulsation in cardiogenic shock. Report of a co-operative clinical trial. N Engl J Med 1973;288:979-984.

9. Willerson JT, Curry GC, Watson JT, et al. Intraaortic balloon counterpulsation in patients in cardiogenic shock, medically refractory left ventricular failure and/or recurrent ventricular tachycardia. Am J Med 1975;58:183-191.

10. Williams DO, Korr KS, Gewirtz H, Most AS. The effect of intraaortic balloon counterpulsation on regional myocardial blood flow and oxygen consumption in the presence of coronary artery stenosis in patients with unstable angina. Circulation 1982;66:593-597.

Chapter 38

Cardiovascular Drug Pharmacology

Jean T. Barbey, M.D.

In most clinical situations, medications are administered with the goal of achieving and maintaining a stable tissue concentration. Steady-state concentration will be directly proportional to the dose of drug administered and inversely proportional to its clearance. In emergency situations and for drugs with long elimination half-lives, the time necessary to reach steady-state (five half-lives) may be excessive. Under such circumstances, it may be desirable to administer a loading dose to promptly raise the concentration of drug to its projected steady-state value. The use of a loading dose does not, however, shorten the time required to achieve steady-state, since this is determined by the elimination half-life. Finally, disease states can alter pharmacokinetic parameters and thereby dictate dosage adjustments in individual patients. In this chapter, the pharmacology of cardiovascular drugs commonly used in the CCU will be reviewed.

I. Anti-arrhythmic Agents

Anti-arrhythmic drugs have a narrow margin between doses that suppress arrhythmias and those that cause adverse reactions. While it is evident that reversible precipitating factors should be sought and eliminated prior to considering drug therapy of arrhythmias, it is equally imperative that physicians using these drugs be familiar with their administration and potential toxicity and have a clearly defined therapeutic endpoint.

Classification of Anti-arrhythmic Drugs

As first suggested by Vaughn Williams, anti-arrhythmic drugs can be grouped according to their most prominent cellular electro-physiologic property.

Class I agents act primarily by blocking the rapid sodium channel. They are further subdivided on the basis of their rate of dissociation from the sodium channel and by their in vitro effects on refractoriness and repolarization. Quinidine, procainamide, and disopyramide dissociate from the sodium channel at a moderately slow rate and prolong refractoriness as well as repolarization, resulting in slight QRS widening and significant QT prolongation on the resting ECG. Lidocaine, mexiletine, and tocainide dissociate rapidly from the sodium channel and shorten repolarization to a greater extent than refractoriness, resulting in no change in QRS duration and a slight shortening of the QT interval. Flecainide and encainide dissociate from the sodium channel at a very slow rate and leave repolarization unchanged. Refractoriness is prolonged and conduction is markedly slowed, resulting in significant PR lengthening and QRS widening, but no additional prolongation of the QT interval.

Class II agents are the beta receptor blocking drugs, which act by inhibiting the effects of catecholamines.

Class III agents are those that act predominantly to prolong the action potential and its electrocardiographic correlate, the QT interval. Drugs from this class include amiodarone, bretylium, and N-acetylprocainamide.

Class IV agents are the calcium channel antagonists, which act by inhibiting intracellular calcium influx through calcium-specific channels.

Anti-arrhythmic drugs frequently possess properties of more than one class, and agents from a given class are not interchangeable. Thus, the above classification, although theoretically appealing, is of limited practical utility. Selected properties of specific anti-arrhythmic agents are reviewed below.

(a) Quinidine

Dosage, plasma concentrations: Loading with intravenous quinidine gluconate (0.5 mg/kg/min up to a maximum of 10 mg/kg) is rarely used outside the electrophysiology laboratory. The usual oral maintenance dose is 200-400 mg of quinidine sulfate every 6 hours. Therapeutic plasma concentration is 2-5 mcg/ml.

Disposition, elimination half-life: Quinidine undergoes extensive hepatic metabolism with generation of active metabolites. Elimination half-life is approximately 6 hours.

Adverse effects, drug interactions: The most frequent side effect of quinidine is diarrhea, which is usually noted early in the course of therapy and does not appear to be dose-related. Other non-cardiac adverse effects include nausea, vomiting, cinchonism, rash, and antibody-mediated thrombocytopenia. One to two percent of patients started on quinidine develop marked QT prolongation and torsade de pointes. Quinidine increases plasma digoxin concentration by displacing digoxin from tissue binding sites and by decreasing its renal clearance. Phenytoin, phenobarbital, and rifampin markedly enhance quinidine metabolism. The combination of quinidine with a lidocaine-like drug results in enhanced anti-arrhythmic efficacy.

(b) Procainamide and N-acetylprocainamide (NAPA) Procainamide has been in clinical use for over 30 years. Its major metabolite,

N-acetylprocainamide, is cardioactive but has different electro-physiologic, pharmacokinetic, and toxic properties.

Dosage, plasma concentrations: Intravenous loading with procainamide can be accomplished with a 25 mg/min infusion up to a maximum of 1.5 grams; this is usually followed by a 1-5 mg/min maintenance dose. Oral therapy is administered as the sustained release form in doses ranging from 500-1500 mg every 6 hours. Therapeutic plasma concentrations for procainamide are 4-10 mcg/ml. When NAPA is administered to patients with ventricular arrhythmias, it is effective at concentrations ranging between 4-19 mcg/ml, with adverse reactions occurring frequently at concentrations greater than 15 mcg/ml.

Disposition, elimination half-life: From 50-70% of procain-amide is eliminated unchanged in the urine, while 20-40% undergoes hepatic conversion to NAPA, which is also renally excreted. The elimination half-life of procainamide is approximately 4 hours; that of NAPA is about 8 hours. In patients with renal insufficiency, clearance is attenuated and dosage adjustment is often necessary to avoid toxicity.

Adverse effects, drug interactions: A frequent side effect encountered during procainamide therapy is the development of the lupus syndrome. This appears to be related to the cumulative dose of drug and is likely to occur more rapidly in the 50% of patients who are slow acetylators of procainamide. Other adverse reactions include nausea, rash, and, rarely, agranulocytosis. Procainamide can cause torsade de pointes and has negative inotropic properties which are most apparent after rapid intravenous administration. Procainamide clearance is decreased by amiodarone. Combining procainamide with lidocaine or one of its analogues results in enhanced anti-arrhythmic efficacy.

(c) Disopyramide

Dosage, plasma concentrations: Parenteral disopyramide is not available in this country. The usual oral dose is 150-450 mg of the extended-release preparation every 12 hours, with a therapeutic plasma concentration ranging from 2-5 mcg/ml.

Disposition, elimination half-life: Disopyramide is excreted unchanged by the kidney (50%) and is also metabolized by the liver (50%). The elimination half-life is approximately 6 hours.

Adverse effects, drug interactions: The most common side effects are anticholinergic and include dry mouth, urinary retention, and blurred vision. Disopyramide also has significant, concentration-dependent negative inotropic properties, and may cause torsade de pointes. Clearance of disopyramide is increased by concomitant phenytoin or rifampin administration. Combination with a lidocaine-like drug results in enhanced anti-arrhythmic efficacy.

(d) Lidocaine

Dosage, plasma concentrations: Several loading regimens have been used successfully. In one method, 100 mg is given over 2 minutes followed by 50 mg over 2 minutes at 10 minute intervals up to a maximum of 4 mg/kg, if necessary. The usual maintenance infusion rate is 1-5 mg/min. Lidocaine is not suitable for oral administration because of extensive first pass hepatic metabolism with generation of toxic metabolites. Therapeutic plasma concentration is 1-4 mcg/ml.

Disposition, elimination half-life: Lidocaine undergoes hepatic metabolism at a rate primarily dependent on liver blood flow. The elimination half-life is normally 1-2 hours, but may be prolonged in patients with liver disease or low cardiac output. In patients with CHF, the half-life may remain unchanged, since clearance and the volume of distribution may decline commensurately.

Adverse effects, drug interactions: The primary adverse effects of lidocaine are neurologic: paresthesias, nausea of central origin, slurred speech, somnolence, and convulsions. Cardiac toxicity (e.g. pro-arrhythmia or worsening of ventricular function) is rare. Lidocaine clearance is enhanced by liver enzyme inducers and decreased by cimetidine and propranolol. Combining lidocaine-like drugs with quinidine-like drugs results in enhanced anti-arrhythmic efficacy.

(e) Mexiletine

Dosage, plasma concentrations: The parenteral form of mexiletine is not currently available in this country. The usual oral maintenance dose is 150-400 mg every 8 hours. Therapeutic plasma concentration is 0.5-2.0 mcg/ml.

Disposition, elimination half-life: Mexiletine is cleared by the liver with an elimination half-life of 10-14 hours.

Adverse effects, drug interactions: Dose-related neurologic and gastrointestinal side effects frequently occur during treatment with mexiletine. They can be minimized by administering the drug with food. Hepatic enzyme inducers accelerate the clearance of mexiletine. Anti-arrhythmic efficacy is enhanced by combination with a quinidine-like drug.

(f) Tocainide

Dosage, plasma concentrations: Parenteral tocainide is not available in this country. The usual oral maintenance dose is 200-600 mg every 8 hours. Therapeutic plasma concentration is 3-9 mcg/ml.

Disposition, elimination half-life: Approximately 50% is excreted unchanged by the kidney; the remainder undergoes hepatic glucuronidation prior to excretion. Elimination half-life is 14-19 hours.

Adverse effects, drug interactions: The incidence of neurologic and gastrointestinal side effects is similar to mexiletine. In addition, a rash has been reported in 5-10% of patients, and agranulocytosis in 0.2% of patients receiving tocainide. No significant drug interactions have been reported other than an additive anti-arrhythmic effect when combined with a quinidine-like drug.

(g) Flecainide

Dosage, plasma concentrations: Parenteral flecainide is not currently available in this country. The usual oral maintenance dose ranges from 50 mg every 8 hours to 200 mg every 12 hours. Therapeutic plasma concentration is 0.2 to 1.0 mcg/ml.

Disposition, elimination half-life: Approximately 30% is excreted unchanged in the urine while the remainder is biotransformed in the liver before undergoing renal excretion. Elimination half-life can range from 12-24 hours and is prolonged in patients with heart failure. Dosage adjustments should be made no more frequently than every 3-5 days.

Adverse effects, drug interactions: Transient central nervous system side effects are not uncommon while the dose of flecainide is being adjusted. Other non-cardiac adverse effects are rare. Flecainide has significant negative inotropic properties, and provocation of serious ventricular arrhythmias may occur. While the incidence of pro-arrhythmia is probably no higher than with other anti-arrhythmic drugs in patients with preserved ventricular function, it approaches 20% in patients with severe ventricular dysfunction and a history of sustained ventricular tachycardia who are receiving doses in excess of 400 mg/day. Propranolol increases the plasma concentration of flecainide (and vice versa). Amiodarone decreases the clearance of flecainide and enhances its anti-arrhythmic efficacy.

(h) Encainide

Dosage, plasma concentrations: The parenteral form of encainide is not commercially available in this country. The usual oral maintenance dose is 25-60 mg every 8 hours. Therapeutic plasma concentrations in patients receiving encainide have not been fully defined. In extensive metabolizers (see below), ventricular arrhythmias are suppressed in the presence of $\geq$ 0.05 mcg/ml of O-desmethyl encainide (ODE) and $\geq$ 0.1 mcg/ml of 3-methoxy-ODE (3-MODE) in the absence of the parent compound. In poor metabolizers, arrhythmia suppression occurs at encainide plasma concentrations above 0.25 mcg/ml in the absence of ODE and 3-MODE. Plasma concentrations above which adverse effects are likely to occur have not been established.

Disposition, elimination half-life: In 92% of patients, encainide undergoes extensive first-pass hepatic metabolism with generation of the active metabolites O-desmethyl encainide and 3-methoxy-O-desmethyl encainide. In these "extensive metabolizers," the elimination half-life of encainide is 2-3 hours, while the half-life of ODE and 3-MODE is much longer (5-37 hours). Approximately 8% of patients are deficient in the enzyme needed to oxidize encainide. In these "poor metabolizers," encainide accumulates at high concentrations and has an elimination half-life of 8-22 hours. Thus, regardless of metabolizer type, the dosage should be increased no more frequently than every 3-5 days. Encainide, ODE, and 3-MODE are renally excreted so that the encainide dose should be decreased in the presence of renal insufficiency.

Adverse effects, drug interactions: The incidence of central nervous system symptoms and pro-arrhythmia during encainide therapy is similar to that described with flecainide. Encainide appears less likely than flecainide to exacerbate congestive heart failure. No significant drug interactions have been documented at this time.

(i) Bretylium

Dosage, plasma concentrations: Only the parenteral form of bretylium is available. It is usually administered as a loading infusion of 300-600 mg over 30 minutes, followed by a 1-4 mg/min drip. Plasma concentrations are not routinely available; the therapeutic range appears to be from 3-6 mcg/ml.

Disposition, elimination half-life: Over 85% is excreted unchanged in the urine. The average elimination half-life is 10 hours.

Adverse effects, drug interactions: The most commonly described adverse reactions include postural hypotension, nausea, vomiting, and bradyarrhythmias. Marked sensitivity to catecholamines is usual during bretylium administration.

(j) Amiodarone

Dosage, plasma concentrations: The parenteral form of amiodarone is not commercially available in this country. Because of amiodarone's extremely long half-life, a loading regimen is used to hasten the onset of its anti-arrhythmic effect. This usually consists of an initial high dose period, 800-1600 mg/day in divided doses for approximately 2 weeks, followed by an intermediate dose period (600-800 mg/day) lasting approximately 4 weeks. The usual maintenance dose is about 400 mg/day (range 100-600 mg/day). Therapeutic plasma concentration is 1.0-2.5 mcg/ml. Desethylamiodarone (DEA), the principal metabolite of amiodarone in man, also has anti-arrhythmic activity that contributes to the effect of amiodarone. At steady-state, DEA is usually present at concentrations comparable to the parent compound.

Disposition, elimination half-life: Surprisingly little is known about the excretion of amiodarone and DEA. Only negligible amounts can be recovered from the urine. Although significant concentrations have been demonstrated in bile, the extent of fecal elimination remains unknown. No disease state has been shown to alter the pharmacokinetics of amiodarone. The elimination half-life ranges from 27-52 days; that of DEA is even longer.

Adverse effects, drug interactions: The adverse effect of greatest concern is pneumonitis, which has been described in up to 10% of patients receiving long-term therapy. Although the syndrome is usually reversible if amiodarone is discontinued, fatalities have been reported in 10% of cases. Other side effects include sun sensitivity and skin discoloration, weakness, ataxia and neuropathy, nausea, constipation, elevation of liver enzymes (usually asymptomatic), hypothyroidism, and hyperthyroidism. Corneal deposits eventually develop in all patients but are rarely bothersome. Cardiovascular adverse reactions, including pro-arrhythmia, worsening heart failure, and conduction system disease, have been reported in 2-5% of patients. Multiple drug interactions have been described with amiodarone, resulting in increased drug effects and increased plasma concentrations. Dosage of the following agents should be decreased by 30-50% when administered with amiodarone: digoxin, flecainide, phenytoin, procainamide, quinidine, and warfarin. The potential for drug interactions may persist long after amiodarone has been stopped.

II.   Calcium Channel Blockers

Calcium channel antagonists are a heterogeneous group of compounds that share the property of blocking calcium selective ion channels in the membranes of a variety of excitable cells. The effects of calcium channel blockers on the cardiovascular system can be understood in terms of their ability to reduce both the chemical and electrical signals that are generated when calcium enters cells of the heart and vascular smooth muscle. The effects of each agent on different tissues varies, so that a given agent may be best suited for use in a specific clinical setting. Selected properties of currently available calcium antagonists are shown in Table 38.1.

III.   Beta Adrenergic Blocking Drugs

Beta adrenergic blocking drugs are effective in treating hypertension, angina, and arrhythmias. However, because individual agents differ in terms of pharmacokinetic and ancillary properties, they should not be considered interchangeable (Table 38.2).

In low doses, beta-1 selective agents produce little blockade of beta-2 vascular and bronchial smooth muscle receptors, a feature that may be advantageous in patients with asthma or peripheral vascular disease. At higher doses, beta-1 selectivity disappears. Nonselective beta blockers decrease the hypokalemia associated with epinephrine release and may theoretically offer better protection against lethal arrhythmias during periods of acute stress. Beta adrenergic blockers with intrinsic sympathomimetic activity (ISA) slightly activate the beta receptor in addition to preventing its access to catecholamines. Whether this property actually constitutes

Table 38.1
Characteristics of Calcium Channel Blockers

	Verapamil	Nifedipine	Diltiazem
Decreases calcium influx	+	+	+
Fast sodium channel blockade	+	0	+
Slowing of AV conduction	+	0	+
Negative inotropism in vivo	+/++	0/+	+
Negative chronotropism in vivo	+	0	+
Peripheral vasodilation	+	++	+
Coronary vasodilation	+	+	+
Pulmonary vasodilation	+	+	+
Absorption	90%	90%	90%
Bioavailability of oral dose	10-30%	50-60%	40-50%
Metabolism	Hepatic	Hepatic	Hepatic
Elimination half-life	3-7 hours	5-10 hours	4-6 hours
Usual oral dose (q 8 hrs)	40-120 mg	10-40 mg	30-120 mg
Usual intravenous dose	5-20 mg	N/A	N/A

0 = minimal, + = mild to moderate, ++ = marked

an advantage is debatable; it may lessen some of the adverse effects associated with therapy but also appears to lessen the cardio-protective effect in patients recovering from myocardial infarction. Lipid solubility is an important determinant of beta blocker metabolism. Whether it has an important effect on the development of central nervous system side effects is controversial. At plasma concentrations greater than those necessary to achieve beta receptor blockade, propranolol has additional electrophysiologic properties, referred to as membrane stabilizing activity, which may contribute to its anti-arrhythmic effect in some patients.

Although well absorbed, some beta adrenergic blockers undergo significant first-pass hepatic metabolism. As a result, only a fraction of the parent compound reaches the systemic circulation. This can produce significant interpatient variability in plasma drug concentrations, a nonlinear dose-response curve, and alterations in pharmacokinetics when other hepatically metabolized drugs are adminis-tered. The route of elimination has obvious clinical implications when selecting a drug for a patient with renal or hepatic impairment. As with other drugs, the elimination half-life determines the time necessary to achieve steady-state and the appropriate dosing interval. However, with beta adrenergic blocking agents the relationship between plasma concentration and therapeutic effect is variable, so that pharmacokinetic and pharmacodynamic half-lives do not necessarily coincide. Table 38.2 summarizes these properties in currently available beta blockers.

Table 38.2
Characteristics of Beta Adrenergic Blocking Drugs

	Beta-1 Selectivity	ISA	Lipid Solubility	MSA	First Pass Metabolism	Route of Elimination	T 1/2 (hrs)	Daily Oral Dose (mg)	Usual IV Dose
Acebutolol	+	+	0	+	+	H,R	3-4*	400-1200	N/A
Atenolol	++	0	0	0	0	R	6-9	25-200	N/A
Esmolol	++	0	?	0	N/A	H	0.15	N/A	50-400 mcg/kg/min
Labetalol	0	0	0	0	++	H	3-4	400-2400	200-300 mg
Metoprolol	++	0	+	0	++	H	3-4	50-400	5-15 mg
Nadolol	0	0	0	0	0	R	14-24	40-240	N/A
Pindolol	0	++	+	+	0	H,R	3-4	10-30	N/A
Propranolol	0	0	++	++	++	H	3-4	40-320	1-10 mg
Timolol	0	0	0	0	+	H,R	4-5	10-45	N/A

ISA = intrinsic sympathomimetic activity; MSA = membrane stabilizing activity; H = hepatic; R = renal;
0 = low; + = moderate; ++ = high. * 8-12 hours for active metabolites.

IV. Sympathomimetic Amines

   A. Catecholamines

      Epinephrine: Potent alpha and beta agonist. Raises blood pressure by increasing myocardial contractility, increasing heart rate, and constricting most vascular beds. Improves coronary blood flow. Relaxes bronchial smooth muscle. Indications: cardiac arrest, severe bronchospasm, hypersensitivity reactions. Dosage: 0.2-1 mg subcutaneously, 0.2-0.5 mg IV (slowly), may be repeated at 5-minute intervals.

      Norepinephrine (Levarterenol): Potent beta-1 agonist, somewhat less potent alpha agonist than epinephrine, not much effect on beta-2 receptors. Norepinephrine bitartrate (Levophed) is the water soluble crystalline monohydrate salt. Indication: hypotension. Dosage: titrate infusion to maintain adequate blood pressure, usual dose 2-4 mcg/min.

      Isoproterenol (Isuprel): Potent beta-1 and beta-2 agonist with almost no effect on alpha receptors. Indications: as a temporizing measure in severe bradyarrhythmias or torsade de pointes; used rarely in the treatment of cardiogenic shock or severe bronchospasm. Dosage: titrate infusion to achieve desired effect, usual dose 1-5 mcg/min.

      Dopamine (Intropin): The immediate metabolic precursor of norepinephrine and epinephrine. In low doses (< 4 mcg/kg/min), it increases renal and mesenteric blood flow by stimulating specific dopaminergic receptors. In moderate doses (4-10 mcg/kg/min), it acts primarily as a beta-1 agonist with persistence of enhanced renal blood flow. At higher doses (> 10 mcg/kg), alpha stimulation becomes the dominant effect, leading to vasoconstriction without further increases in cardiac output. Indications: hypotension and shock; also used to increase renal blood flow (low doses) and as an inotropic agent (moderate doses). Dosage: titrate infusion to achieve desired effect.

      Dobutamine (Dobutrex): Direct acting agent with selectivity for beta-1 receptors. More pronounced inotropic than chronotropic effect. No specific effect on renal vasculature. Indication: increase cardiac output in patients with hemodynamic decompensation due to depressed myocardial contractility. Dosage: titrate infusion to achieve maximal benefit, usual dose 2.5-20/mcg/kg/min.

   B. Non-Catecholamines

      Metaraminol (Aramine): Direct and indirect alpha and beta stimulant. Effects comparable to norepinephrine but less potent and longer acting. Indication: acute hypotension. Dosage: 0.25-5 mg IV or 0.25-1.0 mg/min as continuous infusion.

Phenylephrine (Neosynephrine): Powerful alpha-1 stimulant with little effect on beta receptors. Indications: acute hypotension, also a second line agent for terminating paroxysmal supraventricular tachycardia. Dosage: initially 0.2-0.5 mg IV, may repeat at 10 minute intervals and increase up to 1 mg; usual maintenance infusion rate: 40-60 mcg/min.

Methoxamine (Vasoxyl): Similar to phenylephrine but initial dose is 3-5 mg IV which may be repeated at 10-minute intervals and increased up to 10 mg.

V. Digitalis

Cardiac glycosides consist of an aglycone, which is responsible for the pharmacodynamic properties of the drug, and one or more sugars, which determine its pharmacokinetic properties. Digoxin is by far the most commonly prescribed glycoside in the United States, with digitoxin a distant second. Digitalis and related compounds increase the force of myocardial contraction and slow conduction through the AV node. At the molecular level, cardiac glycosides inhibit sodium-potassium ATPase, the membrane-bound enzyme associated with the sodium pump. This causes a transient increase in intracellular sodium which, in turn, enhances calcium influx by the sodium-calcium exchange mechanism. In addition, digitalis possesses parasympathomimetic properties. Table 38.3 summarizes the major characteristics of digoxin and digitoxin.

Several important interactions between digoxin and other drugs have been documented. Concomitant administration of cholestyramine, antacids, or bran can affect gastrointestinal absorption of digoxin and decrease its plasma concentration by up to 25%. Erythromycin and tetracycline have been reported to increase the bioavailability of digoxin in some patients by inhibiting the flora that converts digoxin to inactive reduction products in the bowel. Neomycin, sulfasalazine, and aminosalicylic acid decrease plasma digoxin concentrations, presumably by altering its aborption. Quinidine, amiodarone, and verapamil increase plasma digoxin concentration. All three drugs decrease the clearance of digoxin so that decreased maintenance doses should be used. Only quinidine appears to modify the volume of distribution, which requires the loading dose of digoxin to be decreased as well.

VI. Vasodilators

A. Nitrovasodilators: Several compounds containing nitrogen oxide have the ability to dilate blood vessels directly. Although their exact mechanism of action is not fully understood, it appears these agents react with specific sulfhydryl-containing receptors and stimulate production of cyclic-GMP in vascular smooth muscle. Recent evidence indicates that the coronary and anti-anginal effects of nitrates become attenuated in some patients during sustained therapy.

Table 38.3
Characteristics of Digoxin and Digitoxin

	Digoxin	Digitoxin
Oral Bioavailability	60–75%*	90–100%
Percent Protein Binding	20–40%	90%
Onset of Action after IV Dose	15–30 min	60–120 min
Peak Effect	2–5 hrs	6–12 hrs
Elimination Half-Life	36–48 hrs	4–6 days
Enterohepatic Circulation	Small	Large
Route of Excretion	Renal	Hepatic
Usual Daily Oral Dose	0.125–0.375 mg	0.05–0.2 mg
Rapid Load (over 24 hrs)	Oral: 1.0–1.5 mg IV: 0.75–1.25 mg	Oral: 0.8–1.2 mg IV: 0.8–1.2 mg
Therapeutic Plasma Level	0.5–2.0 ng/ml	10–25 ng/ml

*90–100% with Lanoxicaps

The causes for this "nitrate tolerance" are probably multiple, reflecting neurohumoral activation as well as sulfhydril group depletion. In such patients, maximal benefit from nitrate therapy may be achieved by a regimen incorporating a daily nitrate-free interval, rather than by one aimed at maintaining high plasma nitrate concentration throughout a 24-hour period.

Glyceryl trinitrate (Nitroglycerin) is well absorbed from the gastrointestinal tract, skin, and mucous membranes. Despite extensive first-pass hepatic metabolism, significant hemodynamic and anti-anginal effects can be achieved after oral administration of the drug. It has an extremely short half-life, which has led to the development of preparations designed to maintain therapeutic plasma concentrations over prolonged periods of time.

Isosorbide dinitrate is the most commonly prescribed oral nitrate for the prophylaxis of angina pectoris. Like glyceryl trinitrate, it undergoes extensive first-pass hepatic metabolism, but its elimination half-life is longer, and it has active metabolites which probably contribute to its effect.

Sodium nitroprusside (Nipride) is available for intravenous administration only. It is a potent, rapidly acting vasodilator with a balanced effect on arterioles and veins (Table 38.4), even at low concentrations. Infusions must be carefully titrated to avoid excessive hypotension; rebound hypertension may occur following abrupt discontinuation of nitroprusside. After prolonged administration, cyanide and thiocyanate may accumulate, particularly in patients with renal impairment. Early manifestations of thiocyanate toxicity include nausea, vomiting, mental status changes, and metabolic acidosis.

Indications for administration of intravenous nitrovasodilators include:

1. Anginal syndromes (glyceryl trinitrate)

2. Control of severe hypertension (sodium nitroprusside)

3. Afterload reduction in severe aortic or mitral insufficiency or peri-infarctional ventricular septal defect (sodium nitroprusside or nitroglycerin)

4. Congestive heart failure or low cardiac output states associated with a high "wedge" pressure (nitroglycerin or nitroprusside alone or in combination with an inotrope)

5. Acute aortic dissection (sodium nitroprusside in combination with a beta blocker)

Table 38.4
Site of Action of Commonly Used Vasodilators

	Venous Dilation	Arteriolar Dilation
Glyceryl trinitrate Isosorbide dinitrate	+++	+
Sodium nitroprusside	+++	+++
Hydralazine, Minoxidil, Diazoxide	0	+++
Phenoxybenzamine, Phentolamine, Tolazoline	++	++
Prazosin, Terazosin	+++	++
Captopril, Enalapril, Lisinopril	+	++

Dosage and Administration: Glyceryl trinitrate is available in many forms. Intravenous infusions usually begin at 5 mcg/min, and are titrated up by 5-10 mcg increments at 3-5 minute intervals until the desired effect is achieved. Sodium nitroprusside infusions begin at 0.5 mcg/kg/min and are also titrated up at 3-5 minute intervals to achieve the desired effect. Isosorbide dinitrate is not available in parenteral form in this country.

B. Direct Acting Vasodilators

Diazoxide (Hyperstat) is a nondiuretic benzothiadiazine capable of relaxing arteriolar smooth muscle. It is indicated in the setting of hypertensive emergencies not associated with aortic dissection or coarctation. It is administered at doses of 1-2 mg/kg over no more than 30 seconds and can be repeated at intervals of 5-15 minutes. Diazoxide may produce hyperglycemia and fluid retention.

Hydralazine (Apresoline) causes direct relaxation of arteriolar smooth muscle. It is used in the treatment of hypertension and in patients with congestive heart failure (in combination with nitrates). Usual oral doses are 25-100 mg BID-QID. Chronic administration of more than 300 mg/day has been associated with drug-induced lupus in some patients. A parenteral form of hydralazine is also available.

Minoxidil (Loniten) is a potent vasodilator with a mechanism of action similar to hydralazine. It is indicated in the treatment of severe hypertension in doses of 5-20 mg twice daily.

C. Alpha Adrenergic Blocking Agents

Phenoxybenzamine (Dibenzyline) is a long-acting irreversible alpha adrenergic blocker used to control the hypertension associated with pheochromocytoma. It does not affect beta receptors. The usual dose is 20-40 mg two or three times daily.

Phentolamine (Regitine) and Tolazoline (Priscoline) are shorter acting reversible alpha adrenergic blockers. Phentolamine is indicated for treatment of hypertension associated with pheochromocytoma, and in the local treatment of dermal necrosis caused by extravasation of norepinephrine. The usual dose is 5 mg IV (10 mg subcutaneously for dermal necrosis). Tolazoline is occasionally used in the treatment of persistent pulmonary hypertension in the newborn. Rarely it may be used in the cardiac catheterization laboratory to assess the reversibility of pulmonary hypertension.

Prazosin (Minipress) exerts its action by blocking post-synaptic alpha-1 receptors. It is used primarily in the treatment of hypertension. Although sometimes used for congestive heart failure, tachyphylaxis is a major problem. The starting dose is 1 mg at bedtime; the usual maintenance dose ranges from 6-30 mg daily in divided doses.

Terazosin (Hytrin) is a recently released alpha-1 blocker with properties similar to prazosin. It has a longer elimination half-life and may be taken once a day in most cases.

Labetalol (Normodyn, Trandate) combines competitive alpha-1 blockade with non-selective beta blockade. The ratio of alpha to beta blockade is approximately 1:3 during oral administration and 1:7 after IV administration. Labetalol is indicated in the treatment of hypertension. The intravenous dosage is 200-300 mg, and the usual oral maintenance dose is 100-400 mg twice a day.

D. Angiotensin Converting Enzyme Inhibitors

Captopril (Capoten), Enalapril (Vasotec), and Lisinopril (Prinivil, Zestril) are the first of a class of agents that inhibit angiotensin I converting enzyme. Additional mechanisms of action include a reduction in aldosterone secretion, inhibition of the degradation of vasodilatory bradykinins, and possibly specific renal arteriolar vasodilation. Converting enzyme inhibitors are mixed vasodilators effective in treating hypertension and congestive heart failure. Selected properties of currently available converting enzyme inhibitors are shown in Table 38.5.

Table 38.5
Comparison of Angiotensin Converting Enzyme Inhibitors

	Captopril	Enalapril	Lisinopril
Active principle	Captopril	Enalaprilat*	Lisinopril
Time to peak effect	60-90 min	4-6 hrs	6 hrs
Elimination half-life	3 hrs	11 hrs	12 hrs
Sulfhydryl group	Yes	No	No
Immune-mediated side effects	Yes	No	No
Clinical experience	Several years	Fewer years	Fewest years
Dosage	6.25-50 mg q 8 hrs	2.5-20 mg q 12-24 hrs	10-40 mg q 24 hrs

* Generated in the liver

E. Phosphodiesterase Inhibitors

Amrinone (Inocor) has both inotropic and vasodilating properties. Its hemodynamic effects are similar to those of dobutamine. The intravenous form has been approved for the management of patients with severe congestive heart failure. Treatment is usually initiated with a bolus of 0.75 mg/kg over 5 minutes (repeated if necessary), followed by an infusion of 5-10 mcg/kg/min. Amrinone has an elimination half-life of 3.5-6 hours and is excreted unchanged in the urine. Aggravation of arrhythmias and thrombocytopenia are the two principal adverse effects.

FURTHER READING

1. Abrams J. Tolerance to organic nitrates. Circulation 1986; 74:1181-1185.

2. Anderson JL, Pritchett LC, eds. International symposium on supraventricular arrhythmias: Focus on flecainide. Am J Cardiol 1988; 62:10D-67D.

3. Campbell RWF. Mexiletine. N Engl J Med 1987;316:29-34.

4. Colucci WS, Wright RF, Braunwald E. New positive inotropic agents in the treatment of congestive heart failure. N Engl J Med 1986; 314:290-299 & 349-358.

5. Duff HJ, Roden D, Primm RK, Oates JA, Woosley RL. Mexiletine in the treatment of resistant ventricular arrhythmias: Enhancement of efficacy and reduction of dose-related side effects by combination with quinidine. Circulation 1983;67:1124-1128.

6. Frishman WH. Clinical pharmacology of the beta-adrenoreceptor blocking drugs, 2nd ed. Appleton-Century-Crofts, Norwalk, CT, 1984.

7. Katzung BG. New concepts of antiarrhythmic drug action. In: Yu PN, Goodwin JF, eds. Progress in cardiology. Lea & Febiger, Philadelphia, 1987;15:5-18.

8. Mason JW. Amiodarone. N Engl J Med 1987;316:455-466.

9. Packer M, Frishman WH, eds. Calcium channel antagonists in cardiovascular disease. Appleton-Century-Crofts, Norwalk, CT, 1984.

10. Roden DM, Woosley RL. Flecainide. N Engl J Med 1986;315:36-41.

11. Roden DM, Woosley RL. Tocainide. N Engl J Med 1986;315:41-45.

12. Romankiewicz JA, Brogden RN, Heel RC, Speight TM, Avery GS. Captopril: An updated review of its pharmacologic properties and therapeutic efficacy in congestive heart failure.   Drugs 1983; 25:6-40.

13. Smith TW. Digitalis: Mechanism of action and clinical use.   N Engl J Med 1988;318:358-365.

14. Taylor P, Weiner N. Drugs acting at synaptic and neuroeffector junctional sites.   In: Gilman AG, Goodman LS, Rall TW, Murad F, eds. The pharmacologic basis of therapeutics, 7th ed.   MacMillan Publishing Co, New York, 1985:66-235.

15. Todd PA, Heel RC. Enalapril: A review of its pharmacodynamic and pharmacokinetic properties and therapeutic use in hypertension and congestive heart failure.   Drugs 1986;31:198-248.

16. Woosley RL, Wood AJ, Roden DM. Encainide.   N Engl J Med 1988; 318:1107-1115.

ABG	arterial blood gases
ACV	assist-control ventilation
AI	aortic insufficiency
AIVR	accelerated idioventricular rhythm
APC	atrial premature contraction
APSAC	anisoylated plasminogen-streptokinase activator complex
AV	atrioventricular or arterial-venous
BBB	bundle branch block
BP	blood pressure
BSA	body surface area
CCU	coronary care unit
CHF	congestive heart failure
COPD	chronic obstructive pulmonary disease
CK	creatine kinase
CPR	cardiopulmonary resuscitation
CXR	chest x-ray
DVT	deep vein thrombosis
ECG	electrocardiogram
ESR	erythrocyte sedimentation rate
ETT	endotracheal tube
HR	heart rate
IABP	intra-aortic balloon pump
ICU	intensive care unit
IM	intramuscular
IMV	intermittent mechanical ventilation
ISA	intrinsic sympathomimetic activity
IV	intravenous
LA	left atrium
LAFB	left anterior fascicular block
LBBB	left bundle branch block
LDH	lactic dehydrogenase
LPFB	left posterior fascicular block
LV	left ventricle
LVH	left ventricular hypertrophy
MAT	multifocal atrial tachycardia
MI	myocardial infarction
N/V	nausea, vomiting
PAOP	pulmonary artery occlusive pressure
PE	pulmonary embolus
PEEP	positive end-expiratory pressure
PMD	papillary muscle dysfunction
PSV	pressure-sensitive ventilation
PSVT	paroxysmal supraventricular tachycardia
PTCA	percutaneous transluminal coronary angioplasty

RA	right atrium
RAD	right axis deviation
RBBB	right bundle branch block
RV	right ventricle
TPA	tissue plasminogen activator
VF	ventricular fibrillation
VPC	ventricular premature contraction
VSD	ventricular septal defect
VT	ventricular tachycardia

APPENDIX B   Formulas

Hemodynamic Data

1. Cardiac output (CO) = Heart rate (HR) X Stroke volume (SV)

2. Cardiac index (CI) = Cardiac output/Body surface area (BSA)

3. Fick equation:

   (1) Cardiac output (CO) = (O_2 consumption)/(A-V O_2 content difference)

   (2) Oxygen consumption = O_2 content of inspired air - O_2 content of expired air

       = (ml O_2 consumed/liter expired air) X Minute ventilation

   Correcting for body surface area (BSA):

   (3) O_2 consumption index = (ml O_2 consumed/liter expired air) X (Minute ventilation)/BSA

       Normal range in basal state: 110-150 ml O_2/min/M^2

   (4) A-V O_2 difference = (arterial O_2 content) - (mixed venous O_2 content)

   (5) O_2 content (ml O_2/L) = 1.36 ml O_2/gm Hgb X Hgb (gm/dl) X O_2 saturation X 10 dl/L

   From (4) and (5),

   (6) A-V O_2 diff = 1.36 ml O_2/gm Hgb X Hgb (gm/dl) X 10 dl/L X (arterial - venous saturation)

   Combining (1), (3), and (6) in the basal state and correcting for body surface area:

   (7) Cardiac index (CI) = (O_2 consumption index)/A-V O_2 difference

       $\approx$ (125-130 ml/min/M^2)/(A-V O_2 difference)

       Normal range: 2.6-4.2 L/min/M^2

4. Systemic vascular resistance (SVR) = (MAP − RAP) X 80/(Cardiac output in L/min)

   where MAP = mean systemic arterial pressure, and RAP = mean right atrial pressure

   Normal range: 800–1500 dynes-sec/cm^5

5. Pulmonary vascular resistance (PVR) = (MPAP − PAOP) x 80/(Cardiac output in L/min)

   where MPAP = mean pulmonary artery (PA) pressure, and PAOP = mean PA occlusive pressure

   Normal range: 40–150 dynes-sec/cm^5

6. Mean arterial pressure (MAP) = [(SBP−DBP)/3] + DBP = (SBP + 2DBP)/3

   where SBP = systolic blood pressure, DBP = diastolic blood pressure

7. Stroke volume (SV) = EDV − ESV = (Cardiac output)/(Heart rate)

   where EDV = end diastolic volume, ESV = end systolic volume

Pulmonary Calculations

1. Alveolar oxygen concentration ($p_A O_2$)

   $p_A O_2 = F_I O_2$ X (barometric pressure − 47 mm Hg H2O pressure) − ($p_a CO_2$/R)

   where $F_I O_2$ = fraction O_2 in inspired air, R = respiratory gas exchange ratio (usu. 0.8)

2. Alveolar-arterial oxygen gradient (A−a gradient)

   A−a gradient = $p_A O_2$ − $p_a O_2$ (Normal < 20 mmHg)

   where $p_A O_2$ = alveolar oxygen concentration, $p_a O_2$ = arterial oxygen concentration

Pressures (mm Hg)

Systemic arterial	100–140/60–90
Mean arterial (MAP)	70–105
Right atrium	2–8
Right ventricle	15–30/2–8
Pulmonary artery (PA)	15–30/4–12
Mean pulmonary artery	8–18
PA occlusive ("wedge")	3–12
Left ventricle	100–140/3–12

Flows and Volumes

Cardiac output	Varies with body size
Cardiac index (L/min/M^2)	2.6–4.2
Stroke volume	Varies with body size
Stroke volume index (ml/M^2)	30–65

Resistances (dynes–sec/cm^5)

Systemic vascular resistance (SVR)	800–1500
Pulmonary vascular resistance (PVR)	40–150

Oxygen consumption index (basal)   110–150 ml/min/M^2

Arteriovenous O_2 content difference   30–50 ml/L

*Adapted from Grossman W. Cardiac catheterization and angiography.
Lea & Febiger, Philadelphia, 1986:545–546. Used with permission.

APPENDIX D   Dosages of Dopamine and Dobutamine*

Dopamine dosage in microdrops = [Wt(kg) X Dose (mcg/kg/min) X 60 (drops/cc)]/Concentration (mcg/cc)

Concentration of solution: 400 mg/250 cc = 1.6 mg/cc = 1600 mcg/cc

Weight | Dosage (mcg/kg/min)

lb	kg	2.5	5.0	7.5	10.0	15.0	20.0
88	40	4	8	11	15	22	30
99	45	4	8	13	17	25	34
110	50	5	9	14	19	28	38
121	55	5	10	15	21	31	41
132	60	6	11	17	22	34	45
143	65	6	12	18	24	37	49
154	70	7	13	20	26	39	52
165	75	7	14	21	28	42	56
176	80	8	15	22	30	45	60
187	85	8	16	24	32	48	64
198	90	8	17	25	34	51	68
209	95	9	18	27	36	53	71
220	100	9	19	28	38	56	75

Flow rate in drops/min, based on 60 drops = 1 cc

Dobutamine dosage in microdrops = [Wt (kg) X Dose (mcg/kg/min) X 60 (drops/cc)]/Concentration (mcg/cc)

Concentration of solution: 500 mg/500 cc = 1.0 mg/cc = 1000 mcg/cc

Weight		Dosage (mcg/kg/min)					
lb	kg	2.5	5.0	7.5	10.0	15.0	20.0
88	40	6	12	18	24	36	48
99	45	7	14	20	27	40	54
110	50	8	15	22	30	45	60
121	55	8	16	25	33	50	66
132	60	9	18	27	36	54	72
143	65	10	20	29	39	58	78
154	70	10	21	32	42	63	84
165	75	11	22	34	45	68	90
176	80	12	24	36	48	72	96
187	85	13	26	38	51	76	102
198	90	14	27	40	54	81	108
209	95	14	28	43	57	86	114
220	100	15	30	45	60	90	120

Flow rate in drops/min, based on 60 drops = 1 cc

*Adapted from Campbell JW, Frisse M. Manual of medical therapeutics, 24th edition. Little, Brown & Company, Boston, 1983:435. Used with permission.

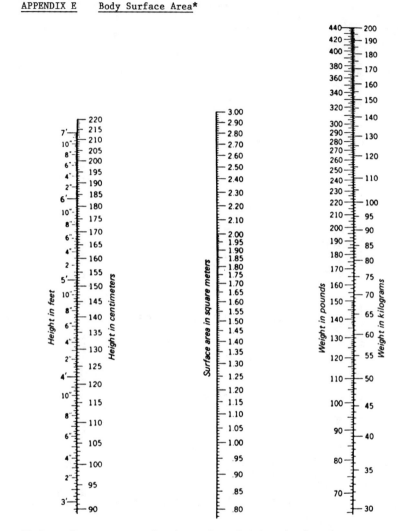

*Body surface area may also be estimated using the formula:

$$BSA\ (M^2) = 0.007184 \times Height\ (cm)^{0.725} \times Weight\ (kg)^{0.425}$$

$$\approx \sqrt{Ht(in) \times Wt(lb)/3131} \qquad \approx \sqrt{Ht(cm) \times Wt(kg)/3600}$$

From Mosteller RD. Simplified calculation of body surface area. N Engl J Med 1987;317:1098.

Index

Page numbers in *italics* denote figures; those followed by "t" denote tables.

A-a gradient, *See* Alveolar-arterial oxygen gradient
A-wave, 118
  giant (cannon), 120
Abbreviations, used in text, 251–252
Accelerated idioventricular rhythm, complicating acute myocardial infarction, 96
Acid-base
  disorders, 47, 53
    simple, 51t
  equilibrium, 51, 52, *See also* pH
  status, 47
Acidosis
  metabolic, 39, 52t
  respiratory, 52, 52t, 56
  treatment, 39
Activity, in elderly, 206
Acute myocardial infarction
  angioplasty for, acute, 92–93
  anterior, 139
  arrhythmias complicating, 95t, 95–97
  bypass surgery for, 92, 93
  cardiac rehabilitation after, 160–164
  cardiogenic shock in, intra-aortic balloon pump for, 228
  chest pain in, 8t, 12
  complications, by age, 204t
  conduction disturbances complicating, 95t, 97–99
  coronary care unit and, 1
  death from, causes, 137
  depression from, 199
  diagnosis, 64–67
  in elderly, *See* Elderly
  hemodynamic disturbances complicating, 109
    congestive heart failure, 109t, 111–114

hypoperfusion, 109–111
  management, guidelines for, 112–113
  shock, 114–115
  hemodynamic monitoring in, invasive, *See* Hemodynamic monitoring
  infarct size and location, prognostic indications, 147
  infarct size limitation, 67–68, 70–71, 75
    beta blockade for, 88–91
    calcium antagonists, 73–74
    general measures, 71–73
    metabolic agents for, 74–75
    nitroglycerin and other vasodilators, 73
    thrombolytic therapy for, *See* Thrombolytic therapy
  inferior, A-V dissociation in, 21
  mechanical complications, 135
    free wall rupture, 137–138
    left ventricular aneurysm and pseudoaneurysm, 138–139
    papillary muscle dysfunction and rupture, 136–137
    ventricular septal defect, 135–136
  non-Q wave, 64, 147
    chest pain in, management, 11–12
  non-transmural, *See* Acute myocardial infarction, non-Q wave
  occurrence, 70
  pacemaker for, temporary, 102, *See also* Pacemakers
    indications for, 102, 104–105
    for inferior myocardial infarction, 102, 104
    for right ventricular infarction, 132
  troubleshooting, 105–107
  pericardial disease in, 143–144

259

Acute myocardial infarction—*continued*
  pericarditis from, 173t
  prognosis, 147
    during hospital phase, 147–149
    during post-hospital phase, 149–150
    risk stratification, 150
  Q-wave, 147
  recurrent cardiac events, secondary
    prevention of, 154, 157
    invasive treatment strategies, 157
    pharmacologic treatment, 155–157
    risk factor modification, 154–155
  recurrent ischemia and infarction, 80,
    84, 142–143
  reinfarction, 80, 84
  right ventricular infarction, 130–133, *See
    also* Right ventricular infarction
  risk factors
    unstable angina and, 166
    variant angina and, 167
  "rule out MI," 4, 5
  silent infarcts, 64
  subendocardial, *See* Acute myocardial
    infarction, non-Q wave
  thromboembolic phenomena in, 142
  transmural, 143
    chest pain in, 10–11
  ventricular fibrillation following, late,
    31
Admission orders, coronary care unit, routine, 4–5
Adult respiratory distress syndrome, 43
Afterload, reduction, 137
Age
  acute myocardial infarction and
    complications incidence by, 204t
    prognosis, 148
  thrombolytic therapy and, 81
Age-related changes, in cardiovascular
  system, 202
Agitation, 55
Airway
  care, in mechanical ventilation, 62
  function, improvement, in mechanical
    ventilation, 60
  pressure, increased, 62
  upper, trauma to, 62
Alcohol, 180t, 25t, 27t, 225

Alkalosis, 72
  metabolic, 52, 52t
  respiratory, 52t, 56
Allen's test, 225
Allopurinol, 75
Alpha adrenergic blocking agents, *See also*
  specific agent
  pharmacology, 246–247
Alprazolam, 199
Alveolar-arterial oxygen gradient (A-a gra-
  dient), 48, 49
  formulas, 254
Alveolar gas exchange, 47–49, 54
Alveolar oxygen concentration, *See* PAO$_2$
Alveolar ventilation, 48
  abnormalities, 47
Aminoglycosides, 60
Aminophylline, 60, 90
  for pulmonary edema, 182
Aminosalicylic acid, 243
Amiodarone, 39
  pharmacology, 238–239, 243
Amrinone (Inocor), 24, 25t, 115
  for congestive heart failure, refractory
    chronic, 183
  disadvantages, 183
  pharmacology, 248
Analgesics, 143, *See also* specific agent
Anemia, 72
Aneurysms
  false, *See* Pseudoaneurysm
  left ventricular, 137–139
Angina, 8t, 143
  unstable, 165
    pathophysiology, 165
    prognosis, 166–167
    treatment, 165–166
    variant (Printzmetal's), 167–168
Angiography
  contrast, in aortic dissection, 195
  digital subtraction, 195
  nuclear, in right ventricular infarction,
    130
Angioplasty, 84, 147
  percutaneous transluminal coronary, 92,
    190–191
  for angina, variant, 168
Angiotensin converting enzyme inhibitors,

See also specific agent
for congestive heart failure, 181
pharmacology, 247–248
Anisoylated plasminogen-streptokinase
activator complex (APSAC), 81
effect on mortality and ventricular function, 78, 79t
efficacy, 81
Antecubital fossa, 216
Anti-anginal therapy, 13, *See also* specific
agent
Anti-arrhythmic agents, 22t, 27t, 37, 111,
180t, 233, *See also* specific agent
for atrial premature contractions, 25
classification, 233
excess, 41
pharmacology
amiodarone, 238–239
bretylium, 238
disopyramide, 235
encainide, 237–238
lidocaine, 236
mexiletine, 236
procainamide and N-acetylprocainamide, 234–235
quinidine, 234
tocainide, 236–237
post myocardial infarction, secondary
prevention with, 156
use with cardioversion, 211
for ventricular fibrillation, 31
for ventricular premature contractions,
28
for ventricular tachycardia, 97
non-sustained, 28–29
Anti-coagulation, 111, *See also* specific
agent
in atrial fibrillation or flutter, 26
in cardioversion for, 210
for left ventricular mural thrombi, 142
pericarditis and, 174
post-myocardial infarction, secondary
prevention with, 156–157
Antidepressants, tricyclic, 27t
Antidiuretic hormone, secretion, increased, 62
Anti-inflammatory agents, non-steroidal,
71t, 143, 180t

infarct size limitation by, 75
Anti-oxidants, 71t, 75, *See also* specific
agent
Anti-platelet agents, post-myocardial infarction, 157
Anxiety, in CCU patient, 198
Anxiolytic agents, 115, 198–199
Aorta
dissection of, 186, 193
acute, 195
chest pain from, 8t
chronic, 195
classification, 193
clinical presentation, 194
diagnosis, 194–195
management, 195
prognosis, 195–196
normal, 193
rupture of, 194
Aortic contour, in aortic dissection, 194
Aortic insufficiency
acute, in aortic dissection, 194
Aortic stenosis, congestive heart failure
from, 181
Aortic valve disease, shock and, 114
Apresoline, *See* Hydralazine
Aramine, *See* Metaraminol
Arrhythmias, 10, *See also* specific
arrhythmia
A-V dissociation, 19–22
bradyarrhythmias, *See*
Bradyarrhythmias
complicating acute myocardial infarction, 95t, 95–97
congestive heart failure from, 179t
in elderly, 203
following cardioversion, 210
pacemaker-induced, 107
reperfusion, 83
supraventricular, 24–27
tachycardias, *See* Tachycardias
treatment, 16–17, *See also* Anti-
arrhythmic agents
algorithm for, *35–38*
ventricular, 27–31
Arterial blood gases
in cardiac arrest, 34
in chest pain, 6

Arterial blood gases—*continued*
  interpretation, 47
    acid-base equilibrium, 51–53
    alveolar gas exchange, 47–50
    indications, 47
    oxygen tension and saturation, 50–51
Arterial carbon dioxide tension, 56
Arterial lines, 225
  care of, 226–227
  femoral and brachial, 226
  radial artery cannulation, technique,
    225–226
Arterial oxygen saturation, 72
Arterial oxygen tension, 48, 50
Arterial pressure, mean, formulas, 254
Arterial sheath, 190, 191
  French, 190
Arteriovenous O_2 content difference, 255
Aspiration, needle, 42–43
Aspirin
  for angina
    unstable, 166
    variant, 167
  for chest pain in acute myocardial in-
    farction, 12
  enteric coated, 4
  for pericardial disease
    for pericarditis, acute, 174
    post-myocardial infarction, 143, 144
  post-myocardial infarction, 157
  use with streptokinase, 78, 80
ASSET trial, 79, 81
Assist-controlled ventilation, 56–57
Asystole, 31
  cardiac arrest from, *37*, 38
Atherosclerosis, 194
  progression, inhibition of, 154
Atrial activity, in tachycardias, 15
Atrial contractions, 120
  premature, 25
Atrial fibrillation, 17t, 18, 26
  A-V dissociation and, 20, *21*
  cardioversion for, 209, 210–211
  conversion of multifocal atrial tachycar-
    dia to, 27
  in congestive heart failure, 181, 182
  in right ventricular infarction, 132
Atrial flutter, 15, 17t, 18, 26

cardioversion for, 209, 210
in congestive heart failure, 181
Atrial "kick," 182
Atrial sequential pacing, 222
Atrial tachyarrhythmias, 111
Atrial tachycardia, 17t
  multifocal, 16, 17t, 27
Atrioventricular (A-V) block, 83
  complicating acute myocardial infarc-
    tion, 97, 98t, 98
  first degree, 98
  second degree, 18
    differential features of, 19t, 19
    Mobitz I, 18, 20, 98
    Mobitz II, 18, 19, 31
    Wenckebach, 19, 98
Atrioventricular (A-V) dissociation, 16, 18,
    19, 120
  causes, 21, 22t
  diagnosis, 19–20
  incomplete, 20
  isorhythmic, 20, *21*
  mechanism, 20–21
Atrioventricular sequential pacing, 132,
    222, *223*
Atropine, 11, 39, 90, 132
  for bradycardia, 31, 32
Ausculation
  in cardiogenic shock, 114
  in chest pain, 10
  in hypoxemia, 44

Balloon pump, intra-aortic, 228
  beneficial hemodynamic effects, 228
  complications, 231–232
  deflation, 229–230
  indications and contraindications,
    228–229
  management, 229–*230*
  weaning from, 231, 231t
Balloon-tipped pacing wire, 221
Barbiturates, 43
Barotrauma, 62
Basilic vein, 217
  for central venous access, 212
Beckman metabolic cart, 125
Bed rest
  for angina, unstable, 166

for pericarditis, acute, 174
prolonged, complications of, 160
Behavior, type A, 155
Benzodiazepines, 67, 199, See also specific
  agent
Beta adrenergic blocking agents, 1, 22t, 26,
  37, 71t, 88, 111, 143, 180, See also specific agent
  acute myocardial infarction prognosis
  and, 147, 149
  adverse reactions to, management of,
  89, 90
  for angina
  unstable, 166
  variant, 167
  for aortic dissection, 195, 196
  for atrial premature contractions, 25
  for chest pain, 13
  in acute myocardial infarction, 11, 12
  combined with thrombolytic therapy,
  90–91
  for congestive heart failure, 182
  dosage and administration, 89
  effectiveness, in elderly, 205
  indications and contraindications, 88,
  89t
  pharmacology, 234, 238, 240, 241t
  post-myocardial infarction, secondary
  prevention with, 155–156
  for sinus tachycardia, 25
  for ventricular premature contractions,
  28
Bicarbonate, 41, See also Sodium
  bicarbonate
Bleeding
  from intra-aortic balloon pump, 231
  from thrombolytic therapy, 79, 83
Blood, pH, 51, 52
Blood gases, See also Arterial blood gases
  criteria, in mechanical ventilation, 54
Blood pressure
  post-myocardial infarction, normalizing
  of, 155
  systolic
  in aortic dissection, 195
  in pericardial tamponade, 175
Blood tests, in aortic dissection, 194
Body surface area, 258

correcting for, 253–254
Brachial arterial lines, 226
Brachial vein, for central venous catheterization, 216–217
Bradyarrhythmias, 18–19
  in acute myocardial infarction, management, 103
  pacemaker for, 104, 105
  management, 31–32
Bradycardia, 21, 83, 132
  cardiac arrest and, 37, 38, 43, 44
  drug-induced, 11
  beta-blockade, 89
  digitalis, 39
  etiologies, 18, 37
  sinus, See Sinus bradycardia
  treatment, 31
Brain, protection, in cardiac arrest, 43, 44t
Breathing, decreasing work of, 60
Bretylium, 31
  pharmacology, 238
Brevital, See Methohexital
Bronchodilators, 90
Bronchospasm, from beta blockers, 90
Bumetamide (Bumex), for congestive
  heart failure, 181
Bumex, See Bumetamide
Bundle branch block
  in acute myocardial infarction, 95t,
  97–98, 102
  left, 104
  right, 104

Calcification, pericardial, 177
Calcium, 69
  uses, 38
Calcium antagonists, 43, 71t, 111, 143, 188t,
  191, See also specific agent
  for acute myocardial infarction, for infarct size limitation, 73–74
  for angina, variant, 167
  for chest pain, 15
  for congestive heart failure, 182
  intoxication, 38
  pharmacology, 239, 240t
Cancer, pericarditis from, 173
Cannon waves, 120

Cannulation
  brachial artery, 226
  femoral artery, 226
  radial artery, 225–226
Captopril (Capoten), 186
  for congestive heart failure, 181
  for left ventricular aneurysm, 139
  pharmacology, 247, 247t
  site of action, 245t
Capture, pacemaker, failure of, 106
Carbon dioxide
  poisoning, 50
  production, increased, 61
  tension
    arterial, 56
    measurement, 47
Cardiac arrest, 34
  complications, 43–44
  management, 34, 39
    of asystole, 37, 38
    of bradycardia and electromechanical
      dissociation, 37–38
    of digitalis intoxication, 39–41
    of hyperkalemia, 41
    of pericardial tamponade, 41–42
    pericardiocentesis, 42, 42t
    post-arrest, 43–44
    of pulmonary embolus and tension
      pneumothorax, 42–43
    of ventricular fibrillation and ven-
      tricular tachycardia, 34, 35, 36, 37
  recurrent, prevention of, 44–45
Cardiac Arrhythmia Suppression Trial, 156
Cardiac catheterization, See Catheterization
Cardiac events, recurrent, in acute myo-
      cardial infarction, See Acute myo-
      cardial infarction, recurrent
      cardiac events
Cardiac examination, in congestive heart
      failure, 112
Cardiac failure, See Congestive heart
      failure
Cardiac index, formulas, 254
Cardiac life support, 31
Cardiac output
  determination, 124–126
  formulas, 253
  inspiratory fall in, 121

Cardiac pressure, waveforms, abnormal,
      etiologies of, 122t
Cardiac rupture, 12
Cardiac standstill, See Asystole
Cardiac tamponade, See Pericardial
      tamponade
Cardiogenic shock, 56
  in acute myocardial infarction
    clinical manifestations, 114
    intra-aortic balloon pump for, 228
  in right ventricular infarction, 132
Cardiomyopathy
  congestive heart failure from, 179t
  constrictive, 120, 177
  dilated, 211
Cardiopulmonary resuscitation, 31
  for cardiac arrest, 34
Cardiovascular causes, of chest pain, 7t
Cardiovascular complications, in hyper-
      tensive emergencies, 186
Cardiovascular system, age-related
      changes in, 202
Cardioversion, 16, 197, 209
  for atrial fibrillation and flutter, 26,
      210–211
  complications, 210
  indications and contraindications, 209
  technique, 209–210
  for ventricular tachycardia, sustained,
      29
Carotid sinus, massage, 15
Catecholamines, See also specific agent
  pharmacology, 242
Catheter(s)
  balloon-tipped, for percutaneous trans-
      luminal coronary angioplasty, 190
  central venous, care of, 218
  pulmonary artery, 124, 126–128, 212
    care of, 218
    for congestive heart failure, refrac-
      tory chronic, 183
    insertion of, 217–218
    positioning of, 215
    Swan-Ganz, 117
    in right ventricular infarction, 132
    tip, failure to wedge, 127
Catheterization
  for acute myocardial infarction, 84

in angina, unstable, 165
central venous, 212
  brachial vein, 216–217
  complications, 218–219t
  femoral vein, 215–216
  internal jugular vein, 212–214
  subclavian vein, 214–215
in pericardial effusion, 174–175
in pericardial tamponade, 176
in pericarditis, constrictive, 177
post-myocardial infarction, 157
pulmonary artery, 104, 112, 217–218
  complications, 218–219t
  in papillary muscle dysfunction or
    rupture, 136–137
  in right ventricular infarction, 131
  in ventricular septal defect, 136
Central venous system, access to, see
  Catheterization, central venous
Cephalic vein, 216–217
  for central venous access, 212
Chest pain, 5
  in acute myocardial infarction, 143
  anginal, 143, See also Angina
  in aortic dissection, 196
  causes
    common, 6, 7t
    selective, 6, 8t
  in congestive heart failure, 112
  ischemic, 88, 142
    management, 73
  management, 10–14
  in myocardial rupture, 138
  in percutaneous transluminal coronary
    angioplasty, 190
  pericardial, 172
  peri-infarctional, 10, 11
Chest x-ray
  in aortic dissection, 194, 196
  in chest pain, 6
Chlorothiazide, for congestive heart
    failure, 181
Cholesterol, lowering of, 154
CK-MB
  in acute myocardial infarction, 64–65
  elevations, false positive, 65, 66t
  peaking of, thrombolytic therapy and, 83
Circulatory dysfunction, 58

Clonidine, for hypertensive emergencies
    and urgencies, 186, 188t
Cocaine, 180t
Collagen vascular disorders, pericarditis
    from, 173t
Collateral flow, improvement, for infarct
    size limitation, 71t
Collateral vessels, in elderly, 202
Computed tomography, 177
  in aortic dissection, 195
  in pericardial effusion, 174
Conduction disturbances complicating
    acute myocardial infarction, 97–99
  management, 103
  pacemaker for, 104
Conduction system, disease, primary, su-
    praventricular arrhythmias from,
    25t
Congestive heart failure, 179
  in acute myocardial infarction, 111–114
    hemodynamic monitoring of, 117
    prognostic implications, 147
  from beta blockade, 89
  diagnosis and etiology, 179, 179t, 180,
    180t, 194
  in digitalis intoxication, 40
  in elderly, 203, 205
  intra-aortic balloon pump for, 228, 229t
  pulmonary edema, acute, 182
  refractory chronic, 183–184
  removal from ventilatory support, 60
  treatment, 112, 181–182
  in ventricular septal defect, 136
Converting enzyme inhibitors, 183, See
    also Angiotensin converting en-
    zyme inhibitors
  for congestive heart failure, 113
Coronary artery, cannulation, 190
Coronary artery bypass grafting (CABG)
  for acute myocardial infarction, 92, 93
  for angina, variant, 168
Coronary artery disease, See also Coro-
    nary heart disease
  surgical treatment for, 167
  variant angina with, 168
Coronary care unit
  admission
    for chest pain, 5

admission—*continued*
routine, 4–5
description, 1
Coronary heart disease, *See also* Coronary
artery disease
development, risk factors for, 154
Coronary occlusion, thrombotic, 78
Coronary ostia, 194
Corticosteroids, 43, 143, 180t, *See also*
Glucocorticoids
Coumadin
for atrial fibrillation, prior to cardioversion, 210–211
for left ventricular mural thrombi, 142
in percutaneous transluminal coronary
angioplasty, 191
Counterpulsation, intra-aortic balloon, 71t,
136, 184
in angina, unstable, 166
for cardiogenic shock, 115
for myocardial infarction, 75
right ventricular infarction, 132
in papillary muscle dysfunction and
rupture, 137
Creatine kinase (CK)
in acute myocardial infarction, 64–65,
67
early peaking of, thrombolytic therapy
and, 83
elevations, false positive, 65, 66t
"Crosstalk," 223

Deep vein thrombosis, 142
Default, in A-V dissociation, 20, 22t
Defibrillation, 29, 31
defined, 209
Demerol, *See* Meperidine
Demoralization, sense of, 199
Denial, 198
Depression, in CCU patient, 199
Diaphoresis, 55
Diastolic function, in congestive heart
failure, 182
Diastolic pressures, equalization of, in
right ventricular infarction, 131
Diazepam (Valium), 199, 209
Diazoxide (Hyperstat)
for hypertensive emergencies and

urgencies, 188t
pharmacology, 245t, 246
Dibenzyline, *See* Phenoxybenzamine
Diet, post-myocardial infarction, 154
Digibin, *See* Fab fragments, digoxin-
specific
Digitalis, digitalis glycosides, 22t, 26, 27t,
37, *See also* Digoxin
for atrial fibrillation or flutter, 26
effectiveness, in elderly, 205
for junctional tachycardia, 26
pharmacology, 243, 244t
supraventricular arrhythmias from, 24,
25t
toxicity, *21*
paroxysmal supraventricular tachycardia from, 26
treatment, 39–41
Digitoxin, pharmacology, 244t
Digoxin, 113, *See also* Digitalis
for congestive heart failure, 181
pharmacology, 243, 244t
serum levels, 39
Digoxin-specific fab fragments, 39–41
Dilaudid, *See* Hydromorphone
Diltiazem, 22t, 26, 37, 143
for acute myocardial infarction
for chest pain in, 12
for infarct size limitation, 74
pharmacology, 240t
post-myocardial infarction, secondary
prevention with, 156
Disopyramide, 25
pharmacology, 233, 235
Diuretics, 67, 136, 137, *See also* specific
agent
for congestive heart failure, 112, 181, 182
for hyperkalemia, 41
for hypertensive emergencies and
urgencies, 186
Dobutamine (Dobutrex)
for cardiogenic shock, 115
for congestive heart failure, refractory
chronic, 183
dosage, 256, 257
effectiveness, in elderly, 205
Dobutrex, *See* Dobutamine
Docusate sodium, 4

Dopamine (Intropin)
for cardiac arrest, 43
for cardiogenic shock, 115
for congestive heart failure, refractory chronic, 183
dosage, 256
effectiveness, in elderly, 205
pharmacology, 242
Doppler color flow techniques, in ventricular septal defect, 136
Douglas bag, 125
Dressler's post-myocardial infarction syndrome, 144
Drugs, See also specific agent; specific type
A-V dissociation from, 22t
bradycardia from, 37
cardiovascular, pharmacology, 233
anti-arrhythmic drugs, 233–239
beta-adrenergic blocking agents, 239, 240, 241t
calcium channel blockers, 239, 240t
digitalis, 243, 244t
sympathomimetic amines, 242–243
vasodilators, 243–248
congestive heart failure from, 180
for myocardial infarction, for infarct size limitation, 71t
pericarditis induced by, 173t
supraventricular arrhythmias from, 25t
ventricular arrhythmias from, 27t
Dyspnea, 67
in acute myocardial infarction, 203

Echocardiogram
in aortic dissection, 195
in left ventricular mural thrombi, 142
in papillary muscle dysfunction and rupture, 137
in pericardial effusion, 174
in pericardial tamponade, 175
in right ventricular infarction, 130
Ectopy, ventricular, 28, 150
Edema, pulmonary, 136, 182
Ejection fraction
effect of thrombolytic therapy on, 78
related to left ventricular infarction prognosis, 149, 149

Elderly, acute myocardial infarction in, 202
clinical presentations, 203–204
ethical issues, 206
management, 204–206
pathology in, 202
prognosis, 206
Electric shock, transthoracic direct current, 209, See also Cardioversion
Electrocardiogram
in acute myocardial infarction, 64
in chest pain, 6, 10
related to prognosis, 147, 148
in hyperkalemia, 41
in pericardial tamponade, 175
in pericarditis
acute, 172, 173–174
constrictive, 177
in right ventricular infarction, 130
Electrode, pacing, flow-directed, 222
Electrode paddles, for cardioversion, 209–210
Electromechanical dissociation
cardiac arrest from, 37, 38, 38
from pericardial tamponade, 41
Electrophysiologic testing
in ventricular fibrillation, 97
in ventricular tachycardia, 97
Embolectomy, 42
Embolic events, following cardioversion, 210
Embolization
arterial lines and, 227
Embolus, pulmonary, See Pulmonary embolus
Enalapril (Vasotec)
for congestive heart failure, 181
pharmacology, 247, 247t
site of action, 245t
Encainide, 25, 156
pharmacology, 234, 237–238
End-diastolic pressures
equalization of, 121
pulmonary artery, 123
Endocardial pacing, transvenous, 221
Endocarditis, from pacemakers, 223–224
Endotracheal tube, complications, 61
Enoximone, 184

Environment, CCU, 198
Enzymatic method, for acute myocardial
    infarction diagnosis, 64–65
Enzymes, serum levels, in myocardial in-
    farction, in elderly, 203
Epinephrine
    pharmacology, 242
    for stridor, 62
Ergonovine, 167
Erythromycin, 243
Escape beats, ventricular, 31
Escape rhythm
    in A-V dissociation, 20
    junctional, 102
        narrow QRS, 102
    ventricular, accelerated, 28
Esmolol, for aortic dissection, 195
Esophageal lead, 16
Ethical issues, related to elderly, 206
Examination
    cardiac, See Cardiac examination
    physical, See Physical examination
Exercise, See also Rehabilitation
    post-myocardial infarction, 155
    range of motion, 160
Exercise testing, in pericarditis, acute, 172
External transthoracic pacing, 220

Fab fragments, digoxin-specific, 39–41
"Failure to wedge," 127
Fascicular block, left anterior, 104
Femoral arterial lines, 226
Femoral vein, 212
    for central venous catheterization, 215–
        216
Fever
    in acute myocardial infarction, 68
    oxygen demand and, 72
Fick equation, 253
Fick method, for cardiac output measure-
    ment, 124, 126, 136
F_IO_2, 48
    in mechanical ventilation, 55, 58
Firing, pacemaker, failure of, 106–107
Flecainide, 25, 156
    pharmacology, 234
Flows, normal values, 255
Fluid

accumulation, in pericardial space, 174
administration, excess, congestive heart
    failure from, 111
    in sinus tachycardia, 25
Fluoroscopy, 176
Formulas, 253–254
    for body surface calculation, 258
Free wall, rupture, in acute myocardial in-
    farction, 137–138
Friction rub, pericardial, 143, 172
Furosemide
    in cardiac arrest, 43
    for congestive heart failure, 112, 181
    for pulmonary edema, 182

Gas exchange
    alveolar, 47–50, 54
    in mechanical ventilation, 56
Gastrointestinal causes, of chest pain, 7t,
        8t
Geriatric patient, See Elderly
GISSI trial, 79, 80, 82
Glucocorticoids, 71t, See also
        Corticosteroids
    infarct size limitation by, 74–75
Glucose, 41, 71t
    availability, increasing of, 75
Glutamate oxalocetic transaminase
    (GOT), in acute myocardial infarc-
    tion, 67
Glyceryl trinitrate, See Nitroglycerin
Glycosides, cardiac, 243
Goldberger's sign, 139

Haloperidol, 199
"Heart attack," 5
Heart block, 15, 132
    A-V dissociation and, 20, 21, 22t
    from beta blockers, 90
    complete, 18, 31, 104
Heart failure, See Congestive heart failure
Heart rates, intra-aortic balloon pump
        and, 230
Hematoma
    dissecting, propagation of, 195
    enlarging, 191
Hemodynamic alterations, 62
Hemodynamic compromise, 28, 29

from beta blockers, 90
Hemodynamic consequences, of ventricular septal defect, 135
Hemodynamic data
in acute myocardial infarction, interpretation
cardiac output determination, 124–126
hemodynamic calculations, 126–127
normal physiology and waveforms, 118–120
oximetry, 124
pathology and abnormal waveforms, 120
formulas, 253–254
Hemodynamic deterioration, in papillary muscle dysfunction and rupture, 137
Hemodynamic disturbances, complicating acute myocardial infarction, See Acute myocardial infarction
Hemodynamic instability, persistent, in cardiac arrest, 43
Hemodynamic monitoring, See also Arterial lines
intra-aortic balloon pump and, 230
invasive, 117, in acute myocardial infarction, See also Hemodynamic data
indications, 117
troubleshooting, 126–128
Hemodynamic values, normal, 255
resting, 121t
Hemodynamics, in right ventricular infarction, 130, 131
Hemoglobin, serum levels, 72
Hemothorax, 214, 215
Henderson-Hasselbach equation, 51
Heparin, 4, 143
for angina, unstable, 166
intra-aortic balloon pump and, 230
for left ventricular mural thrombi, 142
in myocardial infarction, 12
in percutaneous transluminal coronary angioplasty, 191
post-myocardial infarction, secondary prevention with, 156
Hepatomegaly, 177
History, for chest pain, 6

Hospital discharge, in acute myocardial infarction, 160
Hospital phase, of acute myocardial infarction, prognosis during, 147–149
Hyaluronidase, 71t
infarct size limitation by, 74
Hydralazine (Apresoline), 114, 173t, 183
for congestive heart failure, 181
for hypertensive emergencies and urgencies, 186, 188t
pharmacology, 245t, 246
Hydrogen ion, concentration, 51
Hydromorphone (Dilaudid), 11
Hypercholesterolemia, treatment of, 154
Hyperkalemia, 38
cardiac arrest from, 41
Hyperstat, See Diazoxide
Hypertension
in aortic dissection, 194
in cardiac arrest, 43
life-threatening complications of, 187, See also Hypertensive emergencies and urgencies
oxygen demand and, 72
post-myocardial infarction, treatment, 155
pulmonary arterial, 123
Hypertensive emergencies and urgencies, 186, 187, 187t
management, 186, 187–188t
Hyperventilation, 39, 48
chest pain from, 8t
Hypocalcemia, 38
Hyponatremia, 62
Hypoperfusion in acute myocardial infarction, 109t, 109–111
hemodynamic monitoring of, 117
Hypotension
in aortic dissection, 194
from beta blockade, 89
in cardiac arrest, 43
defined, 109
oxygen demand and, 72
in right ventricular infarction, 130, 132
from thrombolytic therapy, 79
Hypothermia, 43
Hypoventilation, 48
etiologies, 49t

Hypoxemia, 199
  in cardiac arrest, 43, 44
  from V/Q mismatching, 50
Hytrin, *See* Terazosin

Idioventricular rhythm, accelerated, 28, 95
Incisura, *118*, 119
Indomethacin, for pericarditis, acute, 174
Infections, from pacemakers, 223
Infectious disease, pericarditis induced by, 173t
Inocor, *See* Amrinone
Inotropic agents, 60, 67, 89, 90, 136 *See also* specific agent
  for acute myocardial infarction, for infarct size limitation, 71t
  for cardiogenic shock, 115
  for congestive heart failure, 113, 114, 182
    refractory chronic, 183
Inspiratory pressure, in mechanical ventilation, 57
Insulin, 41, 71t, 75
Intensive care nursing facility, *See* Coronary care unit
Intensive care unit, mobile, 1
Interference, in A-V dissociation, 20, 22t
Intermittent mandatory ventilation, 57
Internal jugular vein, for central venous catheterization, 212–214
Intima, aortic, tear, 195
Intra-aortic, balloon pump, *See* Balloon pump, intra-aortic
Intrapericardial pressure, rise in, 175
Intrathoracic pressure
  increased, 62
  negative, 120
  positive, 60
Intrinsic sympathomimetic activity, beta blockers with, 239, 240
Intropin, *See* Dopamine
Intubation, prolonged, 61
Inverse ratio ventilation, 50
Ischemic heart disease, 166
  acute, 2, 28, 190
    metoprolol for, intravenous, 90t
  in acute myocardial infarction, recurrent, 142–143

arterial lines and, 227
beta blocker effects on, 88
chest pain from, management, 12–13
congestive heart failure from, 179t
differentiated from pericarditis, acute, 172, 173–174
silent, 166
symptomology, 10
tissue response to, alteration of, 71t
ISIS-2 trial, 79, 81
Isoniazid, 173t
Isoproterenol (Isuprel), 29, 31, 90
  pharmacology, 242
Isosorbide dinitrate, pharmacology, 244, 245t
Isuprel, *See* Isoproterenol
Italian streptokinase trial, 204

Jugular veins, for central venous access, 212–214
Jugular venous distension, 130
Jugular venous waveform, 175
Junctional escape beats, 20
Junctional rhythm, accelerated, *21*
Junctional tachycardia, 15, 17t, 26
  paroxysmal, 26

Kayexelate, 41
Killip classification, of congestive heart failure, 111, 112t, 112
Kussmaul's sign, 121, 130
  in pericarditis, constrictive, 177

Labetolol (Normodyn, Trandate), 195
  for hypertensive emergencies and urgencies, 188t
  pharmacology, 247
Lactic dehydrogenase (LDH), in acute myocardial infarction, 64, 65, *67*
  ratios, reversed, 66t
Left anterior fascicular block, in acute myocardial infarction, 104
Left atrial pressure, 123
  waveforms, 119
Left bundle branch block, 104
Left ventricle
  aneurysms and pseudoaneurysms, in

acute myocardial infarction, 138–139

dysfunction, 60

intra-aortic balloon pump for, 228, 229

function, acute myocardial infarction prognosis and, 149

thrombi, mural, 142

Left ventricular assist device, 184

Left ventricular filling, in right ventricular infarction, 130, 131

Left ventricular pressure, waveforms, 119

Leg, ischemia, from intra-aortic balloon pump, 231

Levarterenol, See Norepinephrine

Levodopa, for congestive heart failure, refractory chronic, 184

Lidocaine, 28, 29, 31, 39, 199

adverse effects, 96

contraindications, 96

pharmacology, 96, 233, 236

prophylactic, 5

in elderly, 205

ventricular fibrillation and, 95, 95t

for ventricular tachyarrhythmias, 44

Life support

advanced, 34

basic, 34

Lipid, 61

solubility, 240, 241t

Lisinopril (Prinivil, Zestril)

pharmacology, 247, 247t

site of action, 245t

Loniten, See Minoxidil

Lung

disease, diffusion, 59

function, abnormal, 48

stiff, 56

Magnesium, 60

Magnesium sulfate, for torsade de pointes, 29

Magnetic resonance imaging, 177, 195

in pericardial effusion, 174

Mannitol, in cardiac arrest, 43

Marfan's syndrome, 196

Mean arterial pressure, formula, 254

Mechanical complications, of acute myocardial infarction, See Acute myocardial infarction, mechanical complications

Median vein, 216

Medical therapy, for angina, unstable, 166

Membrane stabilizing activity, 240

Meperidine (Demerol), 11

Metabolic acidosis, 52t

treatment, 39

Metabolic agents, See also specific agent

for myocardial infarction, for infarct size limitation, 74–75

Metabolic alkalosis, 52, 52t

Metaraminol (Aramine), pharmacology, 242

Methohexital (Brevital), 209

Methoxamine (Vasoxyl), pharmacology, 243

3-Methoxy-ODE (3-MODE), 237

Methyldopa, for hypertensive emergencies and urgencies, 186, 188t

Metolazone, for congestive heart failure, 181

Metoprolol, 89, 195

adverse reactions to, 90

for angina, unstable, 166

for chest pain in acute myocardial infarction, 11

intravenous, protocol, in acute ischemia, 90t

post-myocardial infarction, secondary prevention with, 155t

Mexiletine, pharmacology, 233, 236

Midolazam (Versed), 209

Minipress, See Prazosin

Minoxidil (Loniten)

for hypertensive emergencies and urgencies, 186, 188t

pharmacology, 245t

Mitral regurgitation, in papillary muscle dysfunction and rupture, 136, 137

Mitral valve prolapse, chest pain from, 8t

Mobile intensive care unit, 1

Mobitz I A-V block, 18, 20, 98

Mobitz II A-V block, 18, 19, 31

Moricizine, 156

Morphine, morphine sulfate, 112
    for acute myocardial infarction, 67
    for chest pain in, 10–11, 12
    for pulmonary edema, 182
Mortality
    in acute myocardial infarction, 204t, 204
    effect of thrombolytic therapy on, 78,
        79t
Mural thrombi, left ventricular, 142
Murmur
    holosystolic, 135
    systolic, 135, 136
Musculoskeletal causes, of chest pain, 7t,
    8t
Myocardial cell, necrosis, 64
Myocardial function, residual, 70
Myocardial infarction, See Acute myocar-
    dial infarction
Myocardial ischemia, See Ischemic heart
    disease
Myocardial rupture, 42
Myocardial salvage, by beta blockers, 88
Myocardium, damage to, 70

N-acetylprocainamide, pharmacology, 235
Naloxone (Narcan), 11
Narcan, See Nalaxone
Narcotics, 115, See also specific agent for
    chest pain, in acute myocardial in-
    farction, 11
Nasal intubation, in mechanical ventila-
    tion, 55
Neck vein, examination, in pericardial
    tamponade, 175
Necrosis, myocardial cell, 64
Needle aspiration, in tension pneu-
    mothorax, 42–43
Neosynephrine, See Phenylephrine
Neurologic deficit, in aortic dissection, 194
Neurologic findings, in elderly, 203
Neurologic sequelae, in cardiac arrest, 43
Niacin (Nicotinic acid), 154
Nicotinic acid (niacin), 154
Nifedipine
    for acute myocardial infarction
        for congestive heart failure in, 113
        for infarct size limitation, 74, 74t

for angina, unstable, 166
for hypertensive emergencies and
    urgencies, 186, 188t
pharmacology, 240t
Nipride, See Sodium nitroprusside
Nitrates, 114, 143, See also specific agent
    for angina
        unstable, 166
        variant, 167
    for chest pain, 12, 13
        in acute myocardial infarction, 12
    for congestive heart failure, 181
    post-myocardial infarction, secondary
        prevention with, 156
    tolerance to, 181, 244
Nitroglycerin, (glyceryl trinitrate), 112, 114,
    132, 191
    for acute myocardial infarction
        for chest pain in, 11
        for congestive heart failure in, 113
        for infarct size limitation, 71t, 73
    for angina, unstable, 166
    for chest pain, ischemic, 12
    for congestive heart failure, 181, 186, 223
        refractory chronic, 183
    for hypertensive emergencies and
        urgencies, 186, 188t
    pharmacology, 244, 245t
    for pulmonary edema, 182
Nitroprusside, sodium nitroprusside
    (Nipride), 114, 132, 136, 186
    for acute myocardial infarction, for in-
        farct size limitation, 73
    for aortic dissection, 195
    for congestive heart failure, 181, 186
        refractory chronic, 183
    for hypertension in cardiac arrest, 43
    for hypertensive emergencies and
        urgencies, 187, 188t
    pharmacology, 245, 245t
Nitrovasodilators, See also specific agent
    pharmacology, 243, 244–246
Norepinephrine (Levarterenol)
    for cardiogenic shock, 115
    pharmacology, 242
Normodyn, See Labetolol
Nosocomial pneumonia, 61
Nuclear imaging, See Angiography, nu-

clear, Magnetic resonance imaging;
specific agent

O-desmethyl encainide, 237
Obtundation, 55
Oliguria, 16
  in cardiac arrest, 43
Otitis media, 55
"Overwedging," 127
Oxazepam, 199
Oximetry, 124
Oxygen
  consumption
    formulas, 253
    measurement, 125
  demand
    myocardial, beta blocker effects on,
      88
    reduction, infarct size limitation by,
      71t
  supply, improvement, for infarct size
    limitation, 71t, 72
Oxygen administration
  for acute myocardial infarction, 67
  for pulmonary edema, 182
Oxygen consumption index, 255
Oxygen gradient, alveolar-arterial, 48, 49,
  254
Oxygen saturation, 50–51, 136
  arterial, 72
  mixed venous, 50
Oxygen "step-up," 114, 136
Oxygen tension, 50–51
  arterial, 48, 50
Oxygenation, 54
  abnormalities, 47
  assessment, 47, 48
  mechanical ventilation and, 58
Oxyhemoglobin dissociation curve, 50–51
  of normal blood, 72, 72

P-waves, 15
Pacemaker, 31, 90
  for A-V dissociation, 21
  function, normal, 105
  permanent, for A-V block, 98–99
  temporary, 39, 220
    for acute myocardial infarction, See

Acute myocardial infarction
  for bradycardia, 44
  complications, 223–224
  function, testing of, 222–223
  insertion, techniques, 221–223
  methods of therapy, 220–221
Pacemaker box, temporary, 222, 223
Pacing
  in torsade de pointes, 29
  overdrive, 105
  temporary, 89
Pacing wire, temporary, 190, 221
$PaCO_2$, 254
Paddles, for cardioversion, 209–210
Pain, chest, See Chest, pain
Pancuronium bromide (Pavulon), 43,
  for respiratory distress, 56
PaO_2, 48, 50
  in mechanical ventilation, 58
PAO_2
  formulas, 254
  mechanical ventilation and, 54
Papillary muscle, dysfunction and rupture, in acute myocardial infarction, 136–137
Parenteral agents, for hypertensive
  emergencies and urgencies, 186
Paroxysmal supraventricular tachycardia,
  15, 17, 24, 26
Pavulon, See Pancuronium bromide
pCO_2, alterations, 48
  arterial, 48
Percutaneous transluminal coronary angioplasty (PTCA), See Angioplasty,
  percutaneous transluminal
  coronary
Percutaneous transthoracic pacing, 221
Pericardial constriction, 120
Pericardial disease, 172
  in acute myocardial infarction, 143-144
  hemodynamic findings in, 121
  pericardial effusion, See Pericardial
    effusion
  pericardial tamponade, See Pericardial
    tamponade
  pericarditis, See Pericarditis
Pericardial effusion, 174, 175
  in acute myocardial infarction, 143–144

Pericardial effusion—*continued*
  diagnostic evaluation, 174–175
Pericardial friction rub, 143
  in pericarditis, acute, 172
Pericardial space, obliteration of, 176
Pericardial tamponade, 175–176
  in acute myocardial infarction, 111
  cardiac arrest from, 41–42
  clinical evaluation, 175–176
  hemodynamic findings in 120, 121
  treatment, 176
    pericardiocentesis, emergency bedside, 176
Pericardiocentesis, 176
  for cardiac arrest, 42, 42t
  emergency bedside, technique, 176
Pericardioscopy, flexible fiberoptic, 175
Pericardiotomy, 176
Pericarditis, 12, 174
  acute, 172
    clinical manifestations, 172, 173–174
    etiology of, 173t
    management, 174
    chest pain from, 8t
  constrictive, 176
    clinical presentation, 176–177
    treatment, 177
  post-myocardial infarction, 143, 144
  viral, 176
pH, 48, 50, 56, *See also* Acid-base, equilibrium
  blood, 51, 52
Phenoxybenzamine (Dibenzyline)
  pharmacology, 246
  site of action, 245t
Phentolamine (Regitine)
  for hypertensive emergencies and urgencies, 186, 188t
  pharmacology, 246
  site of action, 245t
Phenylephrine (Neosynephrine), pharmacology, 243
Phenytoin, 29, 39, 173t, 224
Phlebitis, 224
Phlebotomy, for pulmonary edema, 182
Phosphodiesterase inhibitors, *See* Amrinone; specific agent

Phosphorus, 60
Physical activity, *See also* Exercise; Rehabilitation
  post myocardial infarction, 160
Physical examination
  in aortic dissection, 194
  in chest pain, 6
Plaque, atherosclerotic, ruptured, 165
Plasminogen activator, *See* Tissue plasminogen activator
Platelet activation, in angina, unstable, 165
Pneumonia, nosocomial, 61
Pneumothorax, 62
  risk of, 213, 214
  tension, 42–43
pO_2, in mechanical ventilation, 58
Positive-end expiratory pressure (PEEP), 50, 58, 119
  "intrinsic" or "auto PEEP", 58
Potassium, 60, 71t, 75
  levels
    in bradycardia, 39
    in digitalis intoxication, 39, 40
    in ventricular tachycardia, 97
Prazosin (Minipress), 183
  pharmacology, 246
  site of action, 245t
Prednisone, for pericarditis, acute, 174
Premature contractions, ventricular, *See* Ventricular premature contractions
Pressure(s)
  normal values, 255
  waveforms, abnormalities in, 120, 122t
Pressure support ventilation, 57–58
Prinivil, *See* Lisinopril
Printzmetal's angina, 167–168
Priscoline, *See* Tolazoline
Procainamide, 25, 31, 97, 173t
  pharmacology, 233, 234, 235
Propranolol, 29, 39, 195
  for chest pain in acute myocardial infarction, 11
  post-myocardial infarction, secondary prevention with, 155t
Pseudoaneurysms, left ventricular, 139
Psychiatric consultation, 199
Psychogenic causes, of chest pain, 7t

Psychosis, in CCU patient, 199
Psychosocial aspects of coronary care, 198–200
Psychosocial factors
acute myocardial infarction outcome and 155
in elderly, 206
Pulmonary artery
catheterization, See Catheterization, pulmonary artery
end-diastolic pressure, 123
occlusive ("wedge") pressure (PAOP), 58, 111, 119, 123, 217
in cardiogenic shock, 114
continuous tracing, 127
interpretation of, 123–124
obtaining of, failure in, 127
waveform, *118*, 119
pressure rise in, 119
Pulmonary artery catheter, See Catheters, pulmonary artery
Pulmonary calculations, formulas, 254
Pulmonary causes, of chest pain, 7t
Pulmonary congestion, in acute myocardial infarction, 109t, 110–111
Pulmonary disorders
acute, 180
supraventricular arrhythmias from, 25t
Pulmonary edema, 136
in congestive heart failure, 182
Pulmonary embolus, emboli, 142
cardiac arrest from, management, 42–43
chest pain from, 8t
Pulmonary vascular resistance, formulas, 254
Pulsus alternans, 10
Pulsus paradoxus, 111, 175
Pyrophosphate, See Technetium pyrophosphate

QRS complex, 15
in A-V dissociation, 20
impulse synchronization with, 209
QRS junctional escape rhythm, narrow, 102

Quinidine, quinidine sulfate, 15, 26, 39, 211
pharmacology, 233, 234, 243

R-on-T phenomenon, 95, 96, 107
Radial artery, cannulation, technique of, 225–226
Radicals, oxygen-free, 75
Range of motion exercises, 160
Reassurance, providing of, 198
Regitine, See Phentolamine
Rehabilitation, See also Exercise
cardiac, after acute myocardial infarction, 160–164
Renal failure, acute, in cardiac arrest, 43
Reocclusion, thrombotic, 12
Reperfusion arrhythmias, 83
Resins, exchange, in hyperkalemia, 41
Resistance, normal values, 255
Respiratory acidosis, 52, 52t, 56
Respiratory alkalosis, 52t, 56
Respiratory compromise, 11
Respiratory distress, mechanical ventilation and, 55, 56
Respiratory failure, mechanical ventilation for, 54, 55–56
Respiratory muscle, fatigue, 60–61
Respiratory system, function, 47
Resuscitation bag, 55
Right atrial pressure
elevation, 120
fall in, 118
in right ventricular infarction, 132
waveform, normal resting, 118
Right bundle branch block, 104
Right ventricle
filling, 121
free wall, blood flow to, 130
perforation, from pacemaker insertion, 224
pressure
systolic, elevated, 123
waveforms, 118, 119
Right ventricular infarction, 111
clinical course and prognosis, 132–133
diagnosis, 130, 131t
hemodynamics, 130, 131–132
treatment, 132

"Rule out MI," 4, 5, 127
Rupture
    aortic, 194
    cardiac, 12
    free wall, 137–138
    myocardial, 42
    papillary muscle, 136

S_4 gallop, 130
Saline, for right ventricular infarction, 132
Scavengers, free-radical, 43
Sedatives, 4
Sensing, pacemaker, failure of, 105–106
Sequential pacing, 222, 223
Shock
    in acute myocardial infarction, 114–115
    in aortic dissection, 194
    cardiogenic, See Cardiogenic shock
Shunt, shunting, right-to-left, 49, 50, 132
Silent ischemia, 166
    acute myocardial infarction, 64
Sinus bradycardia, 18
    in acute myocardial infarction, pace-
        maker for, 102
Sinus rhythm, 211
Sinus tachycardia, 15, 17t, 24, 25
    treatment, 25
Sinusitis, 55
Skeletal muscle, paralysis, 56
Sleeping pills, 4
Smoking, cessation, post-myocardial in-
        farction, 154–155
Sodium bicarbonate, in cardiac arrest, 39
Sodium nitroprusside (Nipride), See
        Nitroprusside
Spasm, in angina, variant, 167
Spironolactone, for congestive heart
        failure, 181
"Square root sign," 120, 177
Stenosis, aortic, 181
Sternocleidomastoid muscle, 212, 213
Steriods, See Corticosteroids
Stool softeners, 4, See also specific agent
Streptokinase, 78
    age and, 81
    choosing of, 81
    clinical course and complications, 79–
        81

combined with PTCA, 92
complications, 83
effect on mortality and ventricular func-
        tion, 78, 79t
efficacy, 82
use
    in elderly, 204, 205
    protocols for, 84t
Stridor, 62
Stroke volume, formula, 254
Subclavian artery, 215
Subclavian vein
    for central venous access, 212
    for central venous catheterization, 214–
        215
Sudden cardiac death
    from ventricular fibrillation, late, 31
Superior vena cava, for central venous ac-
        cess, 212
Superoxide dismutase, 75
Supraventricular arrhythmias
    atrial fibrillation and atrial flutter, 26
    atrial premature contractions, 25
    etiologies, 24, 24t
    junctional tachycardia, 26
    multifocal atrial tachycardia, 27
    paroxysmal supraventricular tachycar-
        dia, 15, 17t, 24, 26
Supraventricular tachycardia, 16
    distinguishing features, 17t
    paroxysmal, 15, 17t, 24, 26
Surgery
    for angina, unstable, 167
    coronary bypass, 92, 93, 168
    for free wall rupture, 138
    for left ventricular aneurysm, 139
    for papillary muscle dysfunction and
        rupture, 137
    for ventricular septal defect, 136
Swan-Ganz pulmonary artery catheter, 117
Sympathomimetic activity, intrinsic, 239,
        240
Sympathomimetic amines, 24, 25t, 26, 27t,
        See also specific agent
    digitalis intoxification and, 40
    pharmacology
        catecholamines, 242
        non-catecholamines, 242–243

Systemic arterial pressure waveforms, 119
Systemic vascular resistance, formulas, 254
Systolic murmur, 135
  in papillary muscle dysfunction, 136
Systolic pressure, right ventricular, 122

"T" tube trial, 60, 61
Tachyarrhythmias, See Tachycardias; specific type of arrhythmia
Tachycardias, 15, See also specific type of tachycardia
  atrial, See Atrial tachycardia
  differential diagnosis of, 16t
  narrow QRS 16
    distinguished from wide, 15
  ventricular, See Ventricular tachycardia
  wide QRS, 15-16, 16t
    differential diagnosis, 18t
    treatment, 18
Tachypnea, mechanical ventilation for, 57
Tamponade, See Pericardial tamponade
Technetium-99m pyrophosphate, in acute myocardial infarction, 65
  in right ventricular infarction, 130
Tension pneumothorax, cardiac arrest from, management, 42-43
Terazosin (Hytrin)
  pharmacology, 247
  site of action, 245t
Tetracycline, 243
Thallium scintigraphy, in acute myocardial infarction, 65
Theophylline derivatives, 24, 25t, 27t
  in junctional tachycardia, 26
Thermodilution method, cardiac output determination by, 124-126, 136
Thrombi, non-occlusive, 165
Thromboembolic complications, from pacemakers, 224
Thromboembolic events, post-myocardial infarction, 156
Thromboembolic phenomena, in acute myocardial infarction, 142
Thrombolysis in myocardial infarction (TIMI) trial, 90-91
Thrombolytic therapy, 1, 12, 30, 42, 78, 111, 143, See also specific agent

acute myocardial infarction prognosis and, 147, 149
agents
  choice of, 81-82
  use of, protocol for, 82-84
  for angina, unstable, 166
  for chest pain, ischemic, 12
  clinical course and complications, 79-80
  clinical trials, 78
  combined with beta blockade, 90-91
  contraindications to, 83t
  effect on mortality and ventricular function, 78
  in elderly, 204, 205
  indications for, 82t
  patient selection for, 80-81
  PTCA timing after, 92
Thrombosis, deep vein, 142
Thump pacing, 220
Timolol, 155t
Tissue plasminogen activator (TPA), 78
  age and, 81
  clinical course and complications, 79-81
  effect on mortality and ventricular function, 78, 79t
  PTCA following, 92
  recombinant, 81
  use
    in elderly, 204-205
    protocols for, 84t
Tocainide, pharmacology, 233, 236-237
Tolazoline (Priscoline)
  pharmacology, 246
  site of action, 245t
Torsade de pointes, 29, 29t
  in acute myocardial infarction, pacing for, 105
  causes, 30t
Tracheomalacia, 62
Trandate, See Labetolol
Tranquilizers, 27t
Transaminase, levels, in acute myocardial infarction, 65
Transthoracic pacing
  external, 220
  percutaneous, 221

Transvenous endocardial pacing, 221
Trauma, pericarditis induced by, 173t
Trendelenburg position, 115
Triazolam, 4
Tricuspid regurgitation, 130
Trimethaphan, 195
    for hypertensive emergencies and
        urgencies, 186, 188t

Unstable angina, *See* Angina, unstable
Urokinase, 81
    efficacy, 82
Usurption, in A-V dissociation, 20

V-lead, 222
V/Q, *See* Ventilation/perfusion
V-wave, 118, 120
    in papillary muscle dysfunction or rup-
        ture, 136–137
Vagal stimulation, 15
Valium, *See* Diazepam
Valsalva maneuver, 15
Valvular heart disease
    congestive heart failure from, 111, 179t
    supraventricular arrhythmias from, 25t
Variant angina, *See* Angina, variant
Vascular resistance
    pulmonary, 254
    systemic, 254
Vasodilators, 60, 90, 136, *See also* specific
        agent
    for acute myocardial infarction, for in-
        farct size limitation, 71t, 73
    adverse effects, 182
    for congestive heart failure, 113, 181, 182
        refractory chronic, 183, 184
    pharmacology
        of alpha adrenergic blocking agents,
            246–247
        of angiotensin converting enzyme in-
            hibitors, 247, 247t
        of direct acting vasodilators, 246
        of nitrovasodilators, 243, 244–246
        of phosphodiesterase inhibitors, 248
    site of action, 245t
    for ventricular septal defect, 136
Vasotec, *See* Enalapril
Vasoxyl, *See* Methoxamine

Ventilation
    alveolar, 48
    abnormalities, 47
    inverse ratio, 50
    mechanical, 54
        assist-controlled, 56–57
        in cardiogenic shock, 115
        complications, 61–62
        controlled, 56
        discontinuation of, 59–61
        initiation of, 54–56
        intermittent mandatory, 57
        maintenance of, 56-59
        mode of, 56–57
        oxygenation and, 58
        pressure support, 57–58
    manual, 55
Ventilation/perfusion (V/Q), 58
    mismatch, 49, 50
Ventilator
    dependency on, 58
    malfunction, 62
    settings, 55
Ventilatory dead space, increase in, 49
Ventilatory drive, inadequate, 61
Ventricular arrhythmias, *See also* specific
        arrhythmia
    accelerated idioventricular rhythm, 28
    acute myocardial infarction prognosis
        and, 150
    in elderly, 205
    etiology, 27, 27t
    fibrillation, *See* Ventricular fibrillation
    pacemaker-induced, 107
    premature contractions, 28
    tachycardia, *See* Ventricular tachycardia
    torsade de pointes, 29, 30t
Ventricular contractions, premature, 28
Ventricular ectopy, 28
    acute myocardial infarction prognosis
        and, 150
Ventricular escape beats, 31
Ventricular escape rhythm, accelerated, 28
Ventricular fibrillation, 29, 30–31
    cardiac arrest from, 34, *35*, 37
    complicating acute myocardial infarc-
        tion, 95t, 95–96, 97
    in elderly, 205

management, 31
from pericardial tamponade, 41
primary, 29, 30, 31, 95t, 97
secondary, 31
complications, 95t, 97
Ventricular filling, in congestive heart
failure, 182
Ventricular function
assessment, in cardiogenic shock, 114
effect of thrombolytic therapy on, 78,
79t
following PTCA, 92
Ventricular premature contractions, complicating acute myocardial infarction, 95t, 95–96
Ventricular septal defect, 111, 123
in acute myocardial infarction, 135–136
Ventricular tachyarrhythmias, 111
Ventricular tachycardia, 16, 44
cardiac arrest from, 34, *35*, *36*, 37
management, 39
cardioversion for, 209
complicating acute myocardial infarction, 95t, 96–97
non-sustained, 28–29
paroxysmal, 96
sustained, 29
torsade de pointes, 29, *30*, 30t
Verapamil, 22t, 26, 37, 39
for acute myocardial infarction
for chest pain in, 11
for infarct size limitation, 74
for angina, unstable, 166

for aortic dissection, 195
pharmacology, 240t, 243
for tachycardia
multifocal atrial, 27
wide QRS, 18
Versed, *See* Midolazam
Vitamin E, 75
Vocal cord, damage to, 62
Volume(s), normal values, 175
Volume expansion, for pericardial tamponade, 176
Volume loading, in right ventricular infarction, 132

Waveforms
in acute myocardial infarction
abnormal, 120–124
interpretation of, 118–120
jugular venous, 175
over-damped, 127
"Wedge pressure," *See* Pulmonary artery,
occlusive pressure
Wenckebach A-V block, 19, 98

X-descent, 118
in pericarditis, constrictive, 177
X-ray, chest, *See* Chest, x-ray
Xylocaine, 60, 225

Y-descent, 118, 120, 130
in pericarditis, constrictive, 177

Zestril, *See* Lisinopril